Small Animal Nutrition

Editor

DOTTIE LAFLAMME

VETERINARY CLINICS
OF NORTH AMERICA:
SMALL ANIMAL PRACTICE

www.vetsmall.theclinics.com

May 2021 • Volume 51 • Number 3

ELSEVIER
1600 John F. Kennedy Boulevard • Suite 1800 • Philadelphia, Pennsylvania, 19103-2899
http://www.vetsmall.theclinics.com

VETERINARY CLINICS OF NORTH AMERICA: SMALL ANIMAL PRACTICE Volume 51, Number 3 May 2021 ISSN 0195-5616, ISBN-13: 978-0-323-77867-1

Editor: Stacy Eastman
Developmental Editor: Axell Purificacion

Veterinary Clinics of North America: Small Animal Practice (ISSN 0195-5616) is published bimonthly by Elsevier Inc., 360 Park Avenue South, New York, NY 10010-1710. Months of issue are January, March, May, July, September, and November. Business and Editorial Offices: 1600 John F. Kennedy Blvd., Ste. 1800, Philadelphia, PA 19103-2899. Customer Service Office: 3251 Riverport Lane, Maryland Heights, MO 63043. Periodicals postage paid at New York, NY and additional mailing offices. Subscription prices are $358.00 per year (domestic individuals), $933.00 per year (domestic institutions), $100.00 per year (domestic students/residents), $451.00 per year (Canadian individuals), $998.00 per year (Canadian institutions), $488.00 per year (international individuals), $998.00 per year (international institutions), $100.00 per year (Canadian students/residents), and $220.00 per year (international students/residents). To receive student/resident rate, orders must be accompained by name of affiliated institution, date of term, and the *signature* of program/residency coordinator on institution letterhead. Orders will be billed at individual rate until proof of status is received. Foreign air speed delivery is included in all *Clinics* subscription prices. All prices are subject to change without notice. **POSTMASTER:** Send address changes to *Veterinary Clinics of North America: Small Animal Practice*, Elsevier Health Sciences Division, Subscription Customer Service, 3251 Riverport Lane, Maryland Heights, MO 63043. Customer Service (orders, claims, online, change of address): Elsevier Periodicals Customer Service, Elsevier Health Sciences Division Subscription **Customer Service 3251 Riverport Lane Maryland Heights, MO 63043. Tel: 1-800-654-2452 (U.S. and Canada); 314-447-8871 (outside U.S. and Canada). Fax: 314-447-8029. E-mail: journalscustomerservice-usa@elsevier.com (for print support); journalsonlinesupport-usa@elsevier.com (for online support).**

Reprints. For copies of 100 or more of articles in this publication, please contact the Commercial Reprints Department, Elsevier Inc., 360 Park Avenue South, New York, NY 10010-1710. Tel.: 212-633-3874; Fax: 212-633-3820; E-mail: reprints@elsevier.com.

Veterinary Clinics of North America: Small Animal Practice is also published in Japanese by Inter Zoo Publishing Co., Ltd., Aoyama Crystal-Bldg 5F, 3-5-12 Kitaaoyama, Minato-ku, Tokyo 107-0061, Japan.

Veterinary Clinics of North America: Small Animal Practice is covered in *Current Contents/Agriculture, Biology and Environmental Sciences, Science Citation Index, ASCA, MEDLINE/PubMed (Index Medicus), Excerpta Medica, and BIOSIS.*

Contributors

EDITOR

DOTTIE LAFLAMME, DVM, PhD, DACVN
Diplomate, American College of Veterinary Nutrition; Floyd, Virginia, USA

AUTHORS

SARAH K. ABOOD, DVM, PhD
Consultant, Sit, Stay, Speak Nutrition, LLC, Dimondale, Michigan, USA

HEATHER L. ACUFF, MS
Department of Grain Science & Industry, Kansas State University, Manhattan, Kansas, USA

GREG ALDRICH, PhD
Department of Grain Science & Industry, Kansas State University, Manhattan, Kansas, USA

LINDSEY E. BULLEN, DVM
Diplomate, American College of Veterinary Nutrition; Clinician, Clinical Nutrition Service, Veterinary Specialty Hospital of the Carolinas, Cary, North Carolina, USA; Adjunct Professor, College of Veterinary Medicine, Lincoln Memorial University, Harrogate, Tennessee, USA; Private Veterinary Nutrition Consultant, Apex, North Carolina, USA

JULIE A. CHURCHILL, DVM, PhD
Diplomate, American College of Veterinary Nutrition; Veterinary Clinical Science Department, University of Minnesota College of Veterinary Medicine, St Paul, Minnesota, USA

RONALD JAN CORBEE, DVM, PhD
Diplomate, European College of Veterinary and Comparative Nutrition; Assistant Professor, Department of Clinical Sciences, Faculty of Veterinary Medicine, Utrecht University, Utrecht, the Netherlands

AMANDA N. DAINTON, MS
Department of Grain Science & Industry, Kansas State University, Manhattan, Kansas, USA

JANAK DHAKAL, DVM, PhD
Department of Grain Science & Industry, Kansas State University, Manhattan, Kansas, USA

LAURA EIRMANN, DVM
Diplomate, American College of Veterinary Nutrition; Oradell Animal Hospital, Oradell, New Jersey, USA; Nestle Purina PetCare, St Louis, Missouri, USA; Oradell Animal Hospital, Paramus, New Jersey, USA

SAMUEL KIPROTICH, MS
Department of Grain Science & Industry, Kansas State University, Manhattan, Kansas, USA

GARY M. LANDSBERG, DVM, MRCVS
Diplomate, American College of Veterinary Behaviorists; Diplomate, European College of Animal Welfare and Behavior Medicine; Consultant in Veterinary Behavior, Richmond Hill, Ontario, Canada

CATHERINE E. LENOX, DVM
Diplomate, American College of Veterinary Nutrition; Regulatory Veterinary Manager, Royal Canin USA, St Charles, Missouri, USA

VALERIE J. PARKER, DVM
Diplomate, American College of Veterinary Internal Medicine; Diplomate, American College of Veterinary Nutrition; Associate Professor, Clinical, Veterinary Clinical Sciences, The Ohio State University, Columbus, Ohio, USA

RACHEL PILLA, DVM, PhD
Gastrointestinal Laboratory, Department of Small Animal Clinical Sciences, Texas A&M University, Texas A&M College of Veterinary Medicine & Biomedical Sciences, College Station, Texas, USA

DONNA M. RADITIC, DVM, CVA
Diplomate, American College of Veterinary Nutrition; Nutrition and Integrative Medicine Consultants, Athens, Georgia, USA

KORINN E. SAKER, MS, DVM, PhD
Diplomate, American College of Veterinary Nutrition; Associate Professor, Department of Molecular and Biomedical Sciences, NC State University College of Veterinary Medicine, Raleigh, North Carolina, USA

SHERRY LYNN SANDERSON, BS, DVM, PhD
Diplomate, American College of Veterinary Internal Medicine; Diplomate, American College of Veterinary Nutrition; Department of Veterinary Biosciences and Diagnostic Imaging, The University of Georgia College of Veterinary Medicine, Athens, Georgia, USA

MEGAN SHEPHERD, DVM, PhD
Diplomate, American College of Veterinary Nutrition; Clinical Assistant Professor, Nutrition, Department of Large Animal Clinical Sciences, Virginia-Maryland College of Veterinary Medicine, Blacksburg, Virginia, USA

JONATHAN STOCKMAN, DVM
Diplomate, American College of Veterinary Nutrition; Assistant Professor, Department of Clinical Veterinary Sciences, LIU College of Veterinary Medicine, Long Island University, Brookville, New York, USA; Affiliate Faculty, Colorado State University, Department of Clinical Sciences, Fort Collins, Colorado, USA

JAN S. SUCHODOLSKI, Dr Vet Med, PhD, AGAF
Diplomate, American College of Veterinary Microbiology; Gastrointestinal Laboratory, Department of Small Animal Clinical Sciences, Texas A&M University, Texas A&M College of Veterinary Medicine & Biomedical Sciences, College Station, Texas, USA

VALARIE V. TYNES, DVM
Diplomate, American College of Veterinary Behaviorists; Diplomate, American College of Animal Welfare; Ceva Animal Health, Lenexa, Kansas, USA

SHOSHANA VERTON-SHAW, RVT, VTS-Nutrition
Veterinary Nutrition Technician, Ontario Veterinary College, University of Guelph, Guelph, Ontario, Canada

CECILIA VILLAVERDE, BVSc, PhD
Diplomate, American College of Veterinary Nutrition; Diplomate, European College of Veterinary and Comparative Nutrition; Consultant and Co-founder, www.expertpetnutrition.com, Fermoy, Cork, Ireland

Contents

VETERINARY CLINICS OF NORTH AMERICA: SMALL ANIMAL PRACTICE

FORTHCOMING ISSUES

July 2021
Working Dogs: An Update for Veterinarians
Maureen McMichael and Melissa Singletary, *Editors*

September 2021
Effective Communication in Veterinary Medicine
Christopher A. Adin and Kelly D. Farnsworth, *Editors*

November 2021
Diagnostic Imaging: Point-of-Care Ultrasound
Gregory R. Lisciandro and Jennifer M. Gambino, *Editors*

RECENT ISSUES

March 2021
Forelimb Lameness
Kevin Benjamino and Kenneth A. Bruecker, *Editors*

January 2021
Advances in Gastroenterology
Frédéric P. Gaschen, *Editor*

November 2020
Emergency and Critical Care of Small Animals
Elisa M. Mazzaferro, *Editor*

SERIES OF RELATED INTEREST

Veterinary Clinics of North America: Exotic Animal Practice
https://www.vetexotic.theclinics.com/

Preface
Small Animal Nutrition

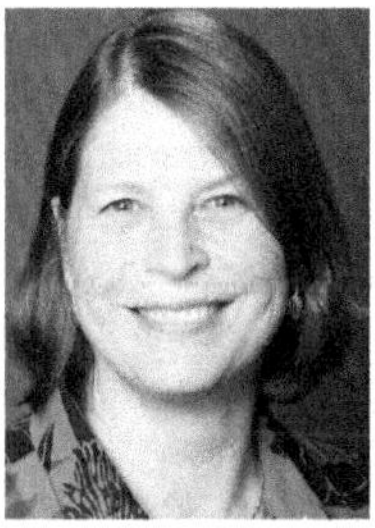

Dottie Laflamme, DVM, PhD, DACVN
Editor

Nutrition plays a critical role in maintaining the health of pets or managing those with various health problems. The importance of veterinarians and the veterinary health care team in assessing the nutritional needs of their patients and in guiding the pet owners' decisions about feeding their pets cannot be overstated. As of now, veterinarians remain the most important source of information about pet care and nutrition for pet owners, but this role is being overtaken by "Dr Google" and other social media and Internet sources. In order to address their clients' questions and provide appropriate recommendations for them, veterinarians need to be confident in their own nutrition knowledge and ability to communicate about nutritional issues. This issue of *Veterinary Clinic of North America: Small Animal Practice* on Small Animal Nutrition was designed to help veterinarians expand their knowledge and skills in key nutrition topics. It covers a spectrum of topics, from commercial pet foods for healthy pets to nutritional management of common nutrient-sensitive diseases. Although most articles focus on dogs and cats, one article is dedicated to other small animals commonly seen by veterinarians, including gerbils, rabbits, and ferrets.

The first article in this issue deals with communication: how to efficiently and effectively talk about nutrition with your clients. A common issue raised by those in primary veterinary practice is the lack of time to pursue nutrition conversations with their clients. Members of the veterinary health care team will find tips and tools in this article to help make the most of the available time, relative to nutritional conversations.

Two articles on commercial pet food provide very different viewpoints. Although commercial pet foods have been around for well over a century, nutritionally balanced diets have only been generally available in the United States since the 1950s. With the widespread use of these diets, the prevalence of conditions related to nutritional deficiencies has been all but eliminated and nearly forgotten. In the modern era, nutritional deficiencies are novel and often justify written case reports or, if due to errors in commercial diets, product recalls. Nevertheless, as concerns about processed foods for

Vet Clin Small Anim 51 (2021) xiii–xiv
https://doi.org/10.1016/j.cvsm.2021.02.001

human consumption increase, concerns related to commercial pet foods have emerged. Sometimes these concerns are driven by marketing, sometimes by pet owners' personal preferences and opinions on healthy foods, and sometimes by social media. Readers are encouraged to review both articles on commercial pet foods for different, evidence-based perspectives that will be of value while addressing your clients' questions.

An emerging area of importance, due in part to climate change and the ever-increasing human population, is the need for sustainable pet foods. Small animal veterinarians have a central role as an information and guidance resource for clients on diet selection, feeding management, and proper pet waste disposal practices relative to sustainability and impact of pets and pet foods on climate change. If you believe that mankind has any role in climate change, you will want to be informed about the potential role of the veterinary health care team in educating clients and contributing toward a sustainable future.

Two areas of active research in both human and veterinary medicine deal with the microbiome, and with the emerging roles of macrominerals and vitamin D in various health conditions. The gut microbiome, reflecting all of the microorganisms within the gut, plays an important role not only in gut health but also in systemic health as well. The macrominerals, calcium and phosphorus, have received considerable attention in recent years. The excellent review on this subject highlights the role different dietary phosphorus sources may play in renal health, as well as the role of both minerals in urolithiasis. Research with vitamin D, long recognized for its role in calcium metabolism and skeletal health, now indicates that vitamin D may have roles in immune function, enteropathies, and neoplasia. Although it is currently too early to make clinical recommendations relative to these new benefits, veterinarians should be watchful as this research continues.

The balance of this issue provides up-to-date information about the role of nutrition in managing patients with various health issues, or with aging. An interesting message that is fairly consistent across these articles is that nutrition must be tailored to the individual patient, so it is necessary to complete both physical and nutritional evaluations on patients in order to provide the best dietary options.

I would like to thank the contributing authors for volunteering their time and expertise, especially during this particularly trying year of pandemic, wildfires, hurricanes, and social unrest. I hope that all members of veterinary health care teams find this issue to be relevant and helpful.

Dottie Laflamme, DVM, PhD, DACVN
Floyd, VA, USA

E-mail address:
JunqueDr@yahoo.com

Talking About Dog and Cat Nutrition with Clients

Sarah K. Abood, DVM, PhD[a,*], Shoshana Verton-Shaw, RVT, VTS-Nutrition[b]

KEYWORDS

- Communication strategies • Readiness to change • Motivational interviewing
- Nutrition assessment

KEY POINTS

- Pet owners want their veterinarian to provide diet or feeding management recommendations.
- Understand why client resistance to recommendations occurs and how to recognize "change talk".
- Inquire about a client's readiness to change in order to evaluate the likelihood of adherence to recommendations.
- Use a team approach for each nutritional assessment to improve efficiency in delivering effective recommendations for patients.
- Invest in communication training, and coaching in motivational interviewing, to enable clients to overcome their own resistance to changing behaviors.

INTRODUCTION

In order to make successful dietary recommendations, recommendations about nutrition, food choices, and feeding management that clients are willing to accept and execute in the home setting, veterinary health care teams (VHCT) must develop, practice, and refine their communication skills on a regular basis. Effective communication skills are important because most pet owners want their veterinarian to provide diet or feeding management recommendations. Many VHCT, including the veterinarians, licensed technicians or nurses, practice managers and receptionists, assistants, and animal care attendants, pay close attention to their own listening skills, empathic statements, written and verbal instructions, and accurate documentation in medical records. However, despite the time and energy devoted to improving communication skills, we are not always successful at getting clients to consistently follow our dietary or feeding management recommendations.

[a] 8817 Bridge Highway, Dimondale, Michigan, MI 48821, USA; [b] Department of Clinical Sciences, Ontario Veterinary College, University of Guelph, 50 Stone Road East, Guelph, Ontario N1G 2W1, Canada
* Corresponding author.
E-mail address: sabood@uoguelph.ca

Vet Clin Small Anim 51 (2021) 517–528
https://doi.org/10.1016/j.cvsm.2021.01.008 vetsmall.theclinics.com

Why, when, and how do we fail? *Why don't clients follow our recommendations* and do all that we say? Busy VHCT will legitimately point to the lack of adequate time available in scheduled appointments to address client questions, or bring up what might be perceived as a "touchy" subject (eg, weight gain, use of supplements like CBD oil, or unbalanced homemade or raw diets). As a strategy for implementing written communications, many practices have found unique and creative ways to deliver nutrition messages that fit into their clinic culture (**Box 1**). Clients often use language that might give the impression they are resistant to following dietary recommendations; however,

Box 1
Examples of incorporating nutrition messages into a clinic culture

Displays

1. Mount and display body condition, muscle condition, and fecal score charts in every examination room to facilitate nutrition discussions.
2. Brochures and pamphlets can be on display in the reception area or examination rooms; pdf documents of the same nutrition handouts should be available on your clinic Web site.
3. Professionally printed or homemade flyers with fun facts about the nutritional needs of dogs and cats could be mounted in examination rooms, at the weight scale, or in a reception area. Flyers and posters designed to engage pet owners can provide an easy format for sharing nutritional truths and demonstrating the expertise of the veterinary health care team.

Client Information

4. Use of social media "nutrition sound bites" via the clinic account on Facebook, Twitter, or LinkedIn.
5. Three-minute nutrition videos made to educate and entertain wherever monitors are mounted or on the clinic Web site.
6. Incorporating nutrition information into puppy and kitten packets is a great way to educate owners about nutrient needs, use of training treats, and transitioning from growth food to adult food. Most new owners want to know what their family veterinarian recommends, so a separate handout outlining the clinic's "top picks" (5–8 brands) of food and the criteria that were used would be ideal.
7. Most pet parents like seeing their pet's photo, so creating posters of patients with before and after pictures could be hung in waiting areas or examination rooms.
8. Appointment reminders could include nutrition messages and mentions of the need for clients to bring digital pictures of food products, treats, and supplements fed to the pet.
9. Blog posts at the clinic Web site could be designed to address nutritional topics several times each year.

Staff Training

10. Client care staff should remind owners to have pets fasted (or come hungry) for their appointment so the veterinary health care team can use treats to improve the pet experience.
11. Hold a clinic "lunch and learn" 2 or 3 times a year to focus on the importance of body condition scoring and make sure everyone on the health care team is consistently scoring and recording the same way.
12. Ensure that the client service or "intake team" asks diet history questions at every patient visit; this approach trains clients to know that some nutrition/diet questions are coming and sets the stage for more thorough answers than "the white bag with a colorful logo." Reminder calls or e-mails should encourage clients to take digital pictures of all food products, treats, and supplements currently being fed.
13. All pets scheduled for a spay or neuter should receive a "complimentary" nutrition consult. The offer could be good for 1 month post–spay/neuter and would allow the health care team to realign the patient's feeding plan and account for calorie reduction. The cost of this service should be included in the cost of the surgical procedure and would bring the client/patient back at a separate time to talk about prevention of weight gain.

they may simply be trying to engage their family veterinarian in a conversation about an issue they have questions about. For example, comments about distrust for pet food companies or wanting more control over what their pet eats could stem from the desire to explore homemade diets and the supplements necessary to balance a recipe. By ignoring or downplaying what might sound at first like a negative comment, we could be missing an opportunity to discover our client's concern or future intention about the recommendation or recommendations we have made.

At several points in the life of each pet, there is the potential for an owner to show some resistance to recommendations made by the VHCT. A few examples include deciding on the choice of puppy or kitten food, when to spay or neuter, how often to vaccinate, when/what to select for an adult food, how/when to manage weight gain, and how/when to transition to a senior pet food. Resistance can stem from several areas,[1,2] such as a client misunderstanding the need for a recommendation; the recommendation made by the veterinarian might be unclear; a lack of trust on the part of the client; either the client or the veterinarian feeling overwhelmed or stressed; lack of competence or self-efficacy on the part of the client; lack of control (or not being included in the decision); fear of new problems developing at home or for the pet; and a lack of rewards or benefits connected to whatever change is required. The Health Belief Model has been shown to be a promising research tool to identify factors associated with pet owners' likelihood of adhering to nutrition or dietary management recommendations.[3,4]

A popular trend in the pet food industry has been the expansion of raw diets. Despite the evidence suggesting that feeding raw meat–based diets is a behavior linked to increased risks of zoonotic infections,[5–9] many clients strongly believe that "feeding raw" can offer better health benefits for their pet. Another emerging niche market is plant-based diets, which have potential risks for 1 or more nutrient deficiencies.[10] Marketing messages about these trends are aimed at supporting pet owners' belief systems on several levels; the result often being that VHCT feel as if they are "arguing on behalf of science" and losing the battle.

Perhaps what is most commonly experienced by VHCT across North America are clients expressing comments about information they learned from a pet store employee, or advice heard from their groomer, or a YouTube video made by a popular pet expert with no formal training in either animal nutrition or veterinary medicine. As the Internet has expanded (and social media has exploded), and pet owners' attitudes have changed, general practitioners, licensed veterinary technicians, as well as board-certified veterinary nutritionists have realized that anyone can claim to be a nutrition expert, and many clients are willing or able to be persuaded by a wide variety of individuals offering products or information on pet nutrition.

DISCUSSIONS ABOUT NUTRITION

Nutrition is recognized as the fifth vital assessment and should be incorporated into every veterinary evaluation at each pet visit.[11] A recent study surveyed 100 dog and cat owners referred to a veterinary teaching hospital in Belgium and used the World Small Animal Veterinary Association (WSAVA) nutritional risk checklist (**Fig. 1**) to identify potential risk factors.[12] Results suggested there were several risk factors present in the referred patients, including unconventional diets, abnormal body condition scores, and abnormal muscle condition scores, which had not been diagnosed by the referring veterinarian. An additional finding was that fewer than 20% (15/85) of dog owners and 47% (7/15) of cat owners reported receiving a dietary recommendation from their family veterinarian.[12] The researchers concluded that greater use of the

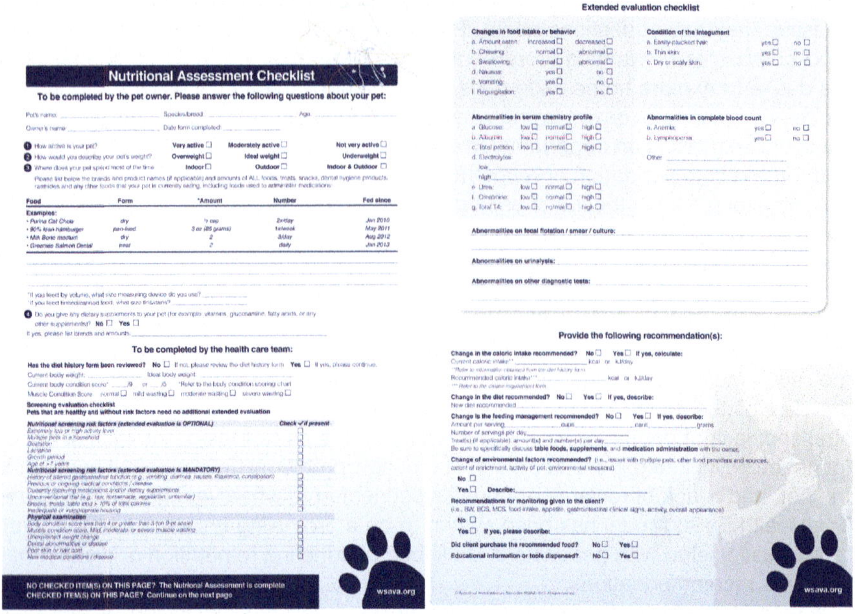

Fig. 1. WSAVA nutritional risk checklist. Global Nutrition Committee Toolkit material provided courtesy of the World Small Animal Veterinary Association.

WSAVA guidelines by general practitioners could improve the nutritional management of more companion animals.

A systematic method for collecting nutrition information is the iterative process commonly referred to as the "Circle of Nutrition," promoted for more than 25 years by the American College of Veterinary Nutrition (**Fig. 2**).[13] Details on using communication skills and the iterative process in each nutritional assessment have been previously reported.[11,14] The technique of asking open-ended questions is routinely taught in many veterinary schools around the world, but not all open questions elicit the same types of information (**Box 2**). Many of us are inclined to revert to the use of direct, closed questions, citing the fear of long-winded clients. Coe and colleagues[15] found that the combination of open and closed questions allowed a conversation to be refocused when necessary and overall took less time while gathering more information. These researchers examined the amount and type of information collected in a general practice setting when clients were asked 1 of 2 open questions followed by specific, closed questions. Clients were randomly assigned to 1 of 2 groups and asked, "What are you feeding?" or "Tell me everything that your pet eats from the time s/he gets up in the morning until s/he goes to bed." Framing a question like "Tell me everything you're feeding…" might be perceived as requiring significantly more time for a client to answer; however, the researchers discovered that this question resulted in a greater number of foods and treats being recorded than when clients were simply asked, "What are you feeding?"

Although the purpose of asking open-ended questions is to elicit diet history details regarding what and how much is being fed, there is also an opportunity to discern the client's attitude toward recommendations the VHCT might make. Before concluding that a client sounds "difficult" or "resistant" to recommendations, the VHCT should explore the pet owner's "readiness to change." Using basic communication skills to

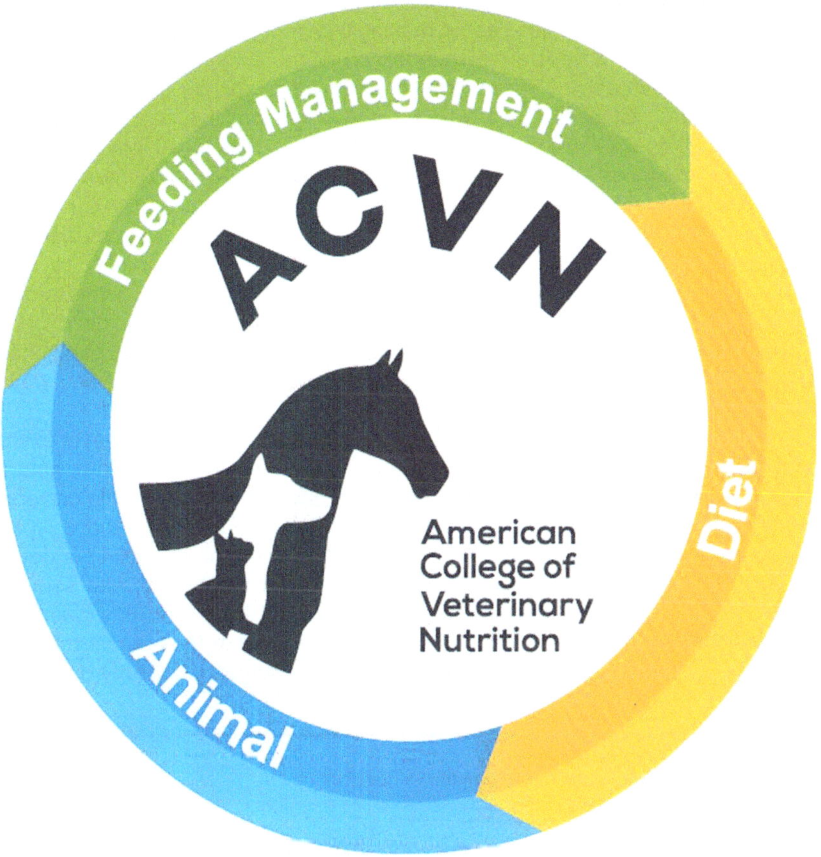

Fig. 2. American College of Veterinary Nutrition's "Circle of Nutrition." (Reprinted with permission from the American College of Veterinary Nutrition.)

Box 2
Application in action: open versus closed questions

Busy health care teams may wonder how open-ended questions can be effective as an information-gathering technique when time is so limited in short appointments. To illustrate this point, try this brief game of "20 questions" at a future staff meeting. Print an image (from a zoo or amusement park) from your computer and keep it hidden from all but 1 person on the team who acts as the "client." Others on the team are allowed to ask closed-ended questions, which require only "yes" or "no" responses. A second volunteer acts as the "vet" and must draw the image based solely on answers provided to the questions asked. A third volunteer serves as the timekeeper. The group is given 5 minutes with no more than 20 questions allowed to try and guess the accuracy of the image. The exercise can then be repeated using a different image, and this time the group can ask 1 or 2 open-ended questions. The timekeeper is instructed to note how long it takes for the group to guess the accuracy of the second image. Most teams find it interesting that the level of detail shared can be significant in less than a minute or 2 when people are invited to respond to an open-ended question.

identify the client's "stage of change" has been described for small animal practice.[16] When clients have been thinking about making a change, we can appreciate whether they are prepared to accept a new suggestion or recommendation by listening for what's called "change talk." These types of pet owners typically express themselves using statements, such as "I want to..." or "I might be able to..." or "We really should..." or "This week we started..." Expressions such as these indicate an openness to considering or implementing a new recommendation for either diet, treats, feeding management, and/or exercise. Change talk signals a person's motivation about (or toward) making changes to improve their pet's health. Examples of this relative to overweight pets are given in **Box 3**. This approach is not specific to obesity management and can be used with clients considering different approaches to dietary modifications for their dog or cat. Many of these pet parents require little direction from the VHCT but could benefit from periodic support, whereas other pet parents need more (or request specific) guidance in addition to positive affirmations and ways to build their confidence.

Opposite of those who are prepared to consider changing their pet's diet or exercise are those who are not yet ready; they are either uninterested or resistant to a recommendation that requires them to alter their own behavior in some way. We can appreciate this position by listening for what is called "sustain talk" with these types of statements: "This seems too hard right now" or "I don't think the timing is good..." or "I don't think I'll be able to get my spouse to do that." There is also something referred to as "resistance talk" from clients who verbalize their unwillingness to make a change in the present moment; an example of what the authors might hear in their clinical nutrition service sounds like this: "The surgeons said my dog needed

Box 3
Stages of change: are clients ready to address obesity?

Clients who are ready to make a change tend to exhibit 1 or more of the following:
1. Able to identify on the body condition score (BCS) chart that their pet is *not* at its ideal body condition
2. Have attempted to make 1 or more changes on their own, often without success
3. May specifically ask for help in addressing a weight or health issue
4. Understand 1 or more health risks associated with pets not in ideal body condition

Clients who may be ready for some degree of change tend to exhibit 1 or more of the following:
1. May or may not accurately identify on the BCS chart that their pet is not at ideal body condition
2. Perception of "ideal" for their pet dog tends to be closer to a 6 (rather than 4–5) on a 9-point scale
3. Able to equally perceive that a score of 1 or 9 on a 9-point scale is unhealthy
4. May express something in the history suggesting they will not be able to fully commit to a change (work schedule, job demands, lifestyle change, loss or addition of a family member, illness, and so forth)
5. Understand 1 or more health risks associated with obesity

Clients who are not ready to make changes tend to exhibit 1 or more of the following:
1. Unable to perceive on a BCS chart that their pet is not at an ideal body condition
2. Find images of ideal body weight (on a BCS chart) to be unhealthy
3. Use positive descriptors of an obese pet as "well-loved" or "spoiled" or "pleasantly plump" or even "he's just big boned"
4. May admire some of the symptoms of strained health with comments like: "We're glad she doesn't jump on the table anymore" or "He's far more calm" or "She no longer pulls on walks"

to lose 20 lbs before they would do the surgery, but I would rather see my dog happy than wasting away." Clients may not always voice opposition or resistance in the examination room; however, observant practitioners and technicians can watch for cues and clues from the client's body language. Pet owners who are not yet ready to change may assume a "closed" or defensive posture, with arms and legs crossed in front of them. They may not maintain direct eye content, may avoid smiling, and may focus their attention on their pet. Clients who are receptive to considering a change will often mimic the body language of the person talking to them. They may lean forward, move closer, and have their arms at their sides or on their pet as they directly face the practitioner or technician. They are more likely to maintain eye contact, and to show focused attention on a handout or product offered in the appointment. Their facial expressions tend to convey interest, and they often ask questions about the information provided.

When clients sound or appear ambivalent about accepting a new diet or feeding management recommendation, members of the VHCT often feel they must somehow instill motivation through education. In 1 form or another, we attempt to outline or discuss risks of continuing undesired behaviors and emphasize health benefits for the pet by changing to a different food or a different feeding method or more exercise/activity. This commonly used approach to attempt to change client behavior fails to consistently result in successful or sustained change. Despite decades of nutrition research and controlled clinical trials examining the role of diet modification (with or without exercise modification), there is no single best practice that works for every overweight or obese dog or cat. The fact that obesity remains a prevalent medical condition among many companion animals[17,18] suggests we have not yet found the appropriate solution to effect lasting change.

MOTIVATIONAL INTERVIEWING

As a method for helping clients uncover their own reasons to change, the principles and skills of motivational interviewing (MI) may be the paradigm shift that the veterinary profession needs. Used for decades in numerous human health fields, MI is a communication method that is based on collaboration. Much like learning to play a musical instrument, MI requires training, feedback, and regular practice to specifically select and reinforce a client's own arguments and motivations for changing their behavior.[19,20] A client-centered approach is the fundamental underpinning of MI, which means the clinician must avoid directive or paternalistic language; he/she must think and act less like an orchestral conductor and more like a personal coach. The key communication skill lies in the clinician using reflective listening to strategically respond to "change talk" and then guiding the person toward resolving their ambivalence, and strengthening their motivation, to change.

MI has been extensively examined over 3 decades in human health care settings, addiction clinics, specialty clinics, and general practice settings. It is described as an evidence-based methodology that supports autonomy in order to help individuals explore and resolve their own ambivalence to behavioral change.[19,20] A meta-analysis evaluated almost 50 human studies conducted between 1983 and 2011 and the calculated odds ratio suggested a 55% increased chance of MI producing a positive outcome when compared with other interventions.[21] It was concluded that the MI approach can be used to boost self-efficacy of clients in their ability to make health-related behavioral changes across a wide spectrum of conditions.

MI has only recently been investigated in veterinary medicine. Bard and colleagues[22] reported on simulated (role-play) communication interactions between a trained actor and a small group of UK cattle veterinarians. The style and type of veterinary advice were largely directive and revealed deficits in empathy and collaboration. The researchers proposed that a paradigm shift was needed across the profession in order to counteract current communication strategies that tend to be paternalistic in nature or that focus on "find the problem and fix it." Communication training in MI was suggested as a method requiring more of a collaborative partnership between client and clinician.

In work that is ongoing, Sutherland and colleagues[23] introduced a "readiness ruler" in an assessment survey that clients of overweight or obese pets volunteered to take at a well-pet visit. The readiness ruler was adapted for use in veterinary medicine and based on the transtheoretical model of change behavior,[24] it is used with individuals to evaluate on a 1 to 10 scale how ready they feel about making a change in their personal behavior. Sutherland proposed that by identifying a client's self-rating of their own stage of change, members of the VHCT will be better positioned to apply appropriate MI communication techniques to support each pet owner. Three questions can be used to explore where an individual is, in terms of importance, confidence, and readiness[25]:

Example 1: "On a scale from 1 to 10, where 1 is not important at all, 5 is somewhat important, and 10 is very important, how important is it for you to make this change for your pet's health?"

Example 2: "On the same scale from 1 to 10, how are confident are you that you can begin to work on changes in the next few weeks or months?"

Example 3: "How ready are you at this point to start some of these changes in your home (or with your family and your pet)?"

By reviewing past successes with clients and offering different strategies, skills, and resources at various points in time, general practitioners and their teams can collaborate, as pet owners take incremental steps in the direction of goals that they have established for their pet's health.

MAKING NUTRITIONAL RECOMMENDATIONS

As a critical communication strategy, VHCT should set up their work environment (eg, clinic culture) to be supportive of nutrition conversations; in this context, it is important to develop a nutrition toolkit with ample resources for training members of the team and for educating clients (**Box 4**).

When clients are not receptive to suggestions or recommendations that might require a change in terms of choice of diet or feeding management, the VHCT should acknowledge this position and note in the medical record that a suggestion or recommendation was made but the pet owner decided to wait. Documenting the outcome of the recommendation is valuable so that future appointments can include inquires about whether the prior recommendation should be revisited, and whether the client has reached a different "stage of change."[16]

For those clients who are receptive to change and/or willing to consider recommendations from the VHCT, a specific recommendation should be verbally articulated and clearly written to avoid any confusion on the part of the client. Research studies[1,26] and reports[18,27] indicate that many pet owners want their veterinarian to provide diet or feeding management recommendations and that they would like to know about all of the options. However, many veterinarians do not provide succinct advice or diet recommendations by the conclusion of every appointment. Practitioners are sometimes uncomfortable or hesitant to make specific brand recommendations when there

Box 4
Building a resource toolkit to support nutrition conversations

1. An iterative model like the "Circle of Nutrition" is helpful to frame nutritional assessments and build diet recommendations
2. WSAVA diet history form (electronic and paper versions)
3. WSAVA body condition score and muscle condition score charts
4. Fecal score chart: https://www.purinainstitute.com/science-of-nutrition/exploring-molecular-nutrition/metagenomics
5. Calculator and weight tape
6. Monitoring diary or spreadsheet to record daily food intake, energy/attitude, bowel movements, activity/exercise, itch scale, vomiting, or seizures
7. Gram scale and how-to-use instructions are ideal, but measuring cups are also appropriate to demonstrate accuracy in measuring daily food portions
8. Handouts with recommended Web sites to explore (homemade diets, supplements, and so forth)
9. Handouts for targeted nutrition-related topics, such as puppy/kitten feeding, reading pet food labels, options for picky eaters, using treats for training, or feeding tube FAQs
10. Resource handouts featuring topics like food puzzles, automatic feeders, local/regional rehabilitation services, local/regional dog parks, or dog-walking services

is no single "best diet," or they are worried clients may perceive that the VHCT is pushing a product sold at the clinic. Coe and colleagues[1] found that more than 90% of veterinarian-initiated dietary proposals included explanations for nutritional changes that referred to the patients' current (or future) health problems. They also found that veterinarians were more likely to suggest a change associated with dental disease than obesity.[26] Delivering advice remains an interesting area requiring more research to fully understand all the aspects of how and when members of a VHCT frame dietary proposals, and to learn how clients receive those recommendations.

A straightforward approach to framing nutrition recommendations is to focus on features, advantages, and benefits. Adapted from common business marketing methods, 1 or more members of the VHCT can prepare talking points for veterinary therapeutic products in the clinic, as well as over-the-counter brands recommended by doctors in the practice. Both product packaging and company Web sites typically list the main features of a diet in easy-to-understand language. While listening and gathering information during collection of the diet history, key points to be discussed can reflect what was conveyed as important to the client about feeding their pet. A few questions are used to frame the features or advantages of the diet and benefits to the pet owner; 3 examples are outlined in **Table 1**.

Similar to writing drug prescriptions, an analogous approach can be used for writing short- and long-term feeding plans for companion animals seen in either general practice or in specialty practice settings. The features of a medical prescription are the same features of a solid nutrition recommendation and include a specific product, dose (feeding amount), duration (feeding method), the doctor making the prescription, the name, address, and phone number of the clinic, and when and how to follow up. If a change in body weight, body condition, or fecal score is an anticipated outcome, the client should have a clear follow-up plan in place to ensure adequate monitoring of the pet. A practice's management software can be used to print a label to stick directly on

Table 1
Describing diets by features and benefits

Example 1: Restricted calorie diet featuring additional fiber		
Feature—How is it different? *This diet has been enhanced with fiber at higher levels than many over-the-counter adult foods.*	Advantage—How will it work? *The additional fiber creates a feeling of fullness while your pet eats fewer calories.*	Benefit—How will it help me? *When your pet feels full and eats less calories, they will be less likely to beg and you can enjoy your own meal in peace.*
Example 2: Large-breed growth diet		
Feature–How is it different? *This diet contains an appropriate amount of calcium and phosphorus for growing large-breed puppies.*	Advantage—How will it work? *By feeding a diet designed for large-breed puppies, you're providing the best nutritional building blocks and helping to decrease any risk for problems with bones and joints.*	Benefit—How will it help me? *You'll have an active and healthy companion, and the satisfaction of knowing that you've provided a complete and balanced diet for your large-breed puppy.*
Example 3: Veterinary therapeutic diet to aid in the treatment of urolithiasis		
Feature–How is it different? *This diet has an increased level of sodium (salt).*	Advantage—How will it work? *The increased salt content will motivate your pet to drink more water and this will help to dilute the urine. Diluting the urine helps reduce the risk of future stone formation.*	Benefit—How will it help me? *You should be able to experience less stress and expense for additional treatments.*

the bag, case, or measuring device. In the absence of this type of protocol, clients are more likely to miss the value of returning with their pet to the veterinary clinic for a recheck or to return and get more food.

SUMMARY

VHCT should practice nutritional assessments on every pet at every patient visit. Using consistent, regular, and unified nutrition (and health) messages from everyone on the team should be an overarching goal in every veterinary practice. To be successful, the clinic culture must support nutrition conversations, and the practice management team must invest in on-going communication training for everyone who has contact with clients. The traditional mindset of "find the problem and fix it" should be adjusted to one that is more client-centered and collaborative. Training in MI could offer an alternative mindset for the profession to improve success in changing owners' behaviors for the benefit of their pet health.

CLINICS CARE POINTS

Pearl #1: Basic communication skills of open-ended questions, reflective listening, and expressing empathy are required for veterinary health care teams to be effective in building rapport and maintaining trust with clients.

Pearl #2: The principles and skills of motivational interviewing may be the transformation that the veterinary profession needs.

Pearl #3: As part of a team approach, all doctors and staff should communicate consistent nutrition messages.

Pitfall #1: We have not been successful as a profession in combating pet obesity; obesity rates in dogs and cats have increased over the past 10 years.

Pitfall #2: Despite most pet owners reporting that their veterinary team remains a trusted source of nutrition information, the perception of many clients is that they have not received an unsolicited recommendation from their veterinarian.

Pitfall #3: By ignoring or downplaying what might sound at first like negative comments from clients, we could be missing an opportunity to discover their concerns or future intentions about a recommendation that was made.

DISCLOSURE

Dr S.K. Abood has her own consulting business: Sit, Stay, Speak Nutrition, and also does contract work with Veterinary Nutritional Consultations, Inc. S. Verton-Shaw is the Nestle Purina Veterinary Technician at the Ontario Veterinary College and does consulting, training, and teaching for the pet food industry.

REFERENCES

1. Coe JB, Adams CL, Bonnett BN. A focus group study of veterinarians' and pet owners' perceptions of veterinarian-client communication in companion animal practice. J Am Vet Med Assoc 2008;233:1072–80.
2. Phillips AM, Coe JB, Rock MJ, et al. Feline obesity in veterinary medicine: insights from a thematic analysis of communication in practice. Front Vet Sci 2017;4:117.
3. Painter MR, Tapp T, Painter JE. Use of the health belief model to identify factors associated with owner adherence to elimination diet trial recommendations in dogs. J Am Vet Med Assoc 2019;255:446–53.
4. Kamleh M. Perceptions and attitudes towards human and companion animal nutrition, nutrition education and nutrition guidance received from healthcare professionals. University of Guelph, Ontario (Canada), PhD thesis; 2019.
5. Weese J, Rousseau J, Arroyo L. Bacteriological evaluation of commercial canine and feline raw diets. Can Vet J 2005;46:513–6.
6. Lefebvre SL, Reid-Smith R, Borelin P, et al. Evaluation of the risks of shedding Salmonellae and other potential pathogens by therapy dogs fed raw diets in Ontario and Alberta. Zoonoses Public Health 2008;55:470–80.
7. Nemser SM, Doran T, Grabenstein M, et al. Investigation of Listeria, Salmonella, and toxigenic Escherichia coli in various pet foods. Foodborne Pathog Dis 2014; 11:706–9.
8. Fauth E, Freeman LM, Cornejo L, et al. Salmonella bacteriuria in a cat fed a Salmonella-contaminated diet. J Am Vet Med Assoc 2015;247:525–30.
9. van Bree FPJ, Bokken GCAM, Mineur R, et al. Zoonotic bacteria and parasites found in raw meat-based diets for cats and dogs. Vet Rec 2018;182:1–7.
10. Dodd SD, Dewey C, Kohsa, et al. Plant-based pet food. Proceedings of Global Animal Nutrition Summit, University of Guelph, Ontario (Canada), August 12–14, 2020.
11. WSAVA Nutritional Assessment Guidelines Task Force, Freeman L, Becvarova I, et al. 2011 WSAVA nutritional guidelines. J Small Anim Pract 2011;52:385–96.

12. Vandendriessche VL, Hesta M, Picaveet P. First detailed nutritional survey in a referral companion animal population. J Anim Physiol Anim Nutr 2017; 101(S1):4–14.
13. Buffington CA, LaFlamme DP. A survey of veterinarians' knowledge and attitudes about nutrition. J Am Vet Med Assoc 1996;208:674–5.
14. Abood SK. Effectively communicating with your clients. Top Companion Anim Med 2008;23:143–7.
15. Coe JB, O'Connor RE, MacMartin C, et al. Effects of three diet history questions on the amount of information gained from a sample of pet owners in Ontario. Can J Am Vet Med Assoc 2020;256:469–78.
16. Churchill JC. Increase the success of weight loss programs by creating an environment for change. Compend Contin Educ Vet 2010;32:E1–4.
17. Bomberg E, Birch L, Endenburg N, et al. The financial costs, behaviour and psychology of obesity: a one health analysis. J Comp Pathol 2017;156:310–25.
18. Association for Pet Obesity Prevention. Pet owner and veterinary professionals pet food survey results. 2018. Available at: PetObesityPrevention.org. Accessed August 2, 2020.
19. Miller WR, Rollnick S. Motivational interviewing: helping people change. 3rd edition. New York: Guilford Press; 2013.
20. Miller WR, Rollnick S. Ten things that motivational interviewing is not. Behav Cogn Psychother 2009;37:129–40.
21. Lundahl B, Moleni T, Burke BL, et al. Motivational interviewing in medical care settings: a systematic review and meta-analysis of randomized controlled trials. Patient Educ Couns 2013;93:157–68.
22. Bard AM, Main DCJ, Haase AM, et al. The future of veterinary communication: partnership or persuasion? A qualitative investigation of veterinary communication in the pursuit of client behaviour change. PLoS One 2017;12(3):e0171380.
23. Sutherland KAK, Coe JB, Parr JM, et al. Assessing pet owners' readiness for behaviour change relating to companion animal obesity. Proceedings of Global Animal Nutrition Summit, University of Guelph, August 12–14, 2020.
24. Prochaska JO, Redding CA, Evers KE. The transtheoretical model and stages of change. In: Glanz K, Rimer BK, Viswanath K, editors. Health behavior and health education. 4th edition. San Francisco: Jossey-Bass; 2008. p. 105.
25. Center for Evidence-Based Practices at Case Western Reserve University. Readiness ruler. Cleveland (OH): Center for Evidence-Based Practices, Case Western Reserve University; 2010. Available at: www.centerforepb.case.edu.
26. MacMartin C, Wheat HC, Coe JB, et al. Conversation analysis of veterinarians' proposals for long-term dietary change in companion animal practice in Ontario, Canada. JVME 2018;45:514–33.
27. American Animal Hospital Association. The path to high-quality care: practice tips for improving compliance. Lakewood (CO): American Animal Hospital Association; 2003.

Pros and Cons of Commercial Pet Foods (Including Grain/Grain Free) for Dogs and Cats

Sherry Lynn Sanderson, BS, DVM, PhD

KEYWORDS

- Commercial pet food • Misinformation • Regulation • Processed foods
- Grain-inclusive diets • Grain-free diets

KEY POINTS

- A lot of misinformation exists about commercial pet food, leading to pet owners feeling overwhelmed and confused about the best diet to feed their pets.
- Not all commercial pet food companies invest the same amount of resources into ensuring the quality of their diets.
- Many foods that both pets and people consume are processed; however the type and extent of processing does not always correlated with the nutritional value of the product.
- Commercial pet food is regulated at both state and federal levels, and many of the same standards apply to both the human food industry and the commercial pet food industry.
- Grains are a rich source of essential nutrients in diets of pets and people. Concerns about grains in pet food was based on marketing rather than science.

INTRODUCTION

The origins of commercial pet food date back to the mid-1800s, when James Spratt, an American living in the United Kingdom, developed large, hard biscuits and sold them to dog owners.[1,2] The biscuits were made from vegetables, beef blood, wheat, and beetroot. In the 1870s, James Spratt returned to the United States and sold his product to wealthy American dog owners. Later, in 1922, the Chappel Brothers of Rockford, Illinois, introduced Ken-L-Ration, the first canned food available to pet owners in the United States. However, during World War II, when metal and meat were rationed in the United States, canned pet food was not available. As a result, the production of pet food shifted to dry foods consisting of oven-baked, dry food broken into smaller, irregular pieces. The technology of making dry pet food changed in the 1950s when Ralston Purina developed a method of making dry pet food using an extrusion process. This method allowed dry pet food to consist of lighter, larger, uniform kibbles, and eventually this method replaced the older method of making dry pet

Department of Veterinary Biosciences and Diagnostic Imaging, The University of Georgia College of Veterinary Medicine, 501 DW Brooks Drive, Athens, GA 30602, USA
E-mail address: sherrys@uga.edu

Vet Clin Small Anim 51 (2021) 529–550
https://doi.org/10.1016/j.cvsm.2021.01.009
vetsmall.theclinics.com
0195-5616/21/

food. During the 1960s and 1970s, pet food companies around the world adopted canning and extrusion technologies to meet increased demand for pet nutrition and convenience. The landscape of the commercial pet food industry continues to change. Not only is the number of new pet food companies increasing but the numbers of new technologies used in making products and packaging are increasing. The commercial pet food industry now consists of a diverse range of diets available to the consumer, such as wet (canned, pouches, rolls) and dry food (extruded and baked), as well as fresh and frozen cooked and raw diets.

SOURCES OF PET NUTRITION INFORMATION FOR PET OWNERS

Challenges Pet Owners Experience When Choosing a Diet

The increasing number of pet food companies and variety of commercial pet foods available to consumers makes it increasingly difficult for pet owners to understand the differences between pet food companies and the products they produce. Surveys confirm that dog owners report feeling overwhelmed with the choices of dog food available.[3,4] In addition, availability of nutrition information and misinformation from the Internet, pet retail stores, veterinarians, and through pet food company marketing adds to this confusion. To illustrate the overwhelming amount of information readily available to pet owners, a Google search was performed using the phrase, "How safe is commercial pet food?" The search yielded about 608,000,000 results.[5] The first 10 results consisted of a variety of sources with often contrasting and conflicting information. For example, 1 site provides information published by a governmental agency (United States Food and Drug Administration [FDA]) involved with overseeing aspects of commercial pet food. Another site is from a trade magazine on pet food safety. However, more than half of the first 10 sites contain opinion-based information and misinformation that seems intent on evoking fear in pet owners regarding commercial pet food. One site discusses by-products but incorrectly lists multiple things contained in animal by-products used to make pet food, such as hooves, hair, and feathers. The Association of American Feed Control Officials (AAFCO), an organization that defines ingredients allowed in pet food, specifically excludes these in their definitions of meat by-products and poultry by-products.[6] However, most pet owners do not know that some of the information provided by the Web site is false. Another site, run by a human dentist, provides consumers with information about the operations of a rendering plant without mentioning that there are different types of rendering plants in the United States, or that most pet food manufactures in the United States do not obtain any ingredients from rendering plants of the type described on this Web site. Yet another site warns consumers how commercial pet foods are making pets sick. The site provides consumers with a long list of harmful ingredients that should not be in pet food, such as grains and meat meal, but it lacks any credible references to support these claims. It is easy to see why pet owners are so confused about what to feed their dogs and cats, and why some think negatively about commercial pet foods.

In addition to false or conflicting information about commercial pet food and pet nutrition available on the Internet and in other places, there are many other factors playing a role in determining the diet pet owners choose to feed their pets. One of these factors is the growing trend in humanization of pets.[7] A recent study evaluating the determinants of food purchasing decisions of both dog and cat owners showed that pet owners ranked health and nutrition as their top priority, followed by quality, ingredients, freshness, and taste.[8] The least important characteristics were that the product was on sale, followed by color, packaging, and being gluten free.

Pet Owners Want and Value Nutritional Advice from Veterinarians

One of the surveys showing that pet owners feel overwhelmed by the number of pet food choices available also asked pet owners, "Would you like your veterinarian to recommend a routine/maintenance diet for your pet?"[4] Most pet owners (68%) answered "Yes" to that question. Despite this, only 38% of pet owners reported their veterinarians had made a recommendation about a maintenance diet during the previous year. An additional 22% reported that they received recommendations from their veterinarian, but had to ask for it, although the rest reported they had received no dietary advice from their veterinarians. Similarly, other data show veterinarians are the primary source of pet nutrition information, as well as being viewed as the most important source of nutrition information for pet owners (**Table 1**).[8]

COMMERCIAL PET FOOD INDUSTRY CONTINUES TO GROW

Why Are There so Many Commercial Pet Food Companies?

The 2019 to 2020 American Pet Product Association (APPA) National Pet Owners Survey showed that 63.4 million US households own a dog and 42.7 million own a cat.[9] As of 2017, there were 89.7 million dogs[10] and 94.2 million cats[11] in the United States. The APPA survey showed Americans spent more than $95 billion on their pets in 2019,[9] versus $48.35 billion in 2010[12] (**Table 2**).

Consumers spend more on pet food and treats than on any other area of the pet industry, including veterinary care. This trend has been a consistent and growing for more than a decade so it is easy to see why making and selling pet food has become such an attractive industry for so many people. Lawyers, veterinarians without any advanced training in small animal nutrition, people with marketing degrees, and lay people are just a few examples of people making and marketing their own brands of pet food. This trend is in contrast with major pet food companies that employ a team of qualified experts, such as boarded veterinary nutritionists, PhD nutritionists, food safety specialists, toxicologists, microbiologists, and engineers, just to name a few.

Marketing Claims

As more and more companies enter into the pet food market, many use marketing as a way to distinguish their diets from their competitors' diets. However, many of the

Table 1
Survey results from 2181 pet owners regarding pet nutrition information sources[8]

Information Source	Primary Source of Pet Dietary or Nutrition Information (%)	Perceived Importance of Dietary Recommendations[a]
Veterinarian	40.65	3.82
Veterinary staff	2.91	3.12
Internet	24.57	2.62
Breeder/trainer	4.03	2.20
Books/magazine	5.67	2.17
Friends/family	3.32	2.12
Pet store staff	1.94	1.80

[a] Using a 5-point Likert scale (1, not important at all; 2, slightly important; 3, moderately important; 4, very important; and 5, extremely important).

Table 2
American Pet Products Association breakdown of consumer spending on pets in the United States

Total Consumer Spending on Pets in the United States in 2010[12] and 2109[9]	2010 ($ Billions)	2019 ($ Billions)
Pet Food and Treats	18.76	36.9
Vet Care and Product Sales	13.01	29.3
Supplies, Live Animals and Over-the-counter Medicine	13.07	19.2
Other Services[a]	3.51	10.3
Total Spending on Pets	48.35	95.7

[a] Includes boarding, grooming, insurance, training, pet sitting and walking, and all services outside of veterinary care.

marketing claims made about certain types of commercial pet food lack research to support these claims. For example, through marketing, some companies vilified certain ingredients used in pet foods, such as grains and by-products, while making claims that diets without these ingredients were healthier for dogs and cats.[13] This marketing resulted in some pet owners believing that the best diets to feed their pets were grain-free diets. It is ironic that recommendations to avoid pet food containing grains is occurring at the same time that experts in human nutrition are promoting greater consumption of whole grains in our own diets because of the health benefits associated with such diets.[14]

FEEDING COMMERCIAL PET FOOD

Most Pet Owners in the United States Feed Commercial Cooked Pet Food

Most dog and cat owners (>90%) in the United States feed their pets commercial cooked pet food.[4,9,15] In contrast, raw diets (both commercial and home prepared) and homemade pet foods were never fed to more than 73% of dogs and 88% of cats: among veterinary professionals participating in this survey, 85.9% did not consider raw meat–based diets to be healthier than commercial pet foods.[4]

The percentage of pet owners feeding cooked commercial pet food has remained high, and pets are living longer than they used to.[16] Although numerous factors may be involved, advances in companion animal nutrition and veterinary care play a role in the increasing lifespan of dogs and cats.[17,18]

Commercial Pet Food Industry and Human Food Industry in the United States Are Both Highly Regulated

Regulation of commercial pet food occurs at both the state and federal levels, and many of the same regulations that apply to the human food industry apply to the commercial pet food industry. For example, the FDA is a federal agency that regulates both industries.[19] The US Federal Food, Drug, and Cosmetic (FD&C) Act states that the FDA is responsible for making sure food for both people and animals is safe to eat, properly manufactured, contains no harmful substances, and is truthfully labeled. Congress further strengthened the food safety system in the United States in 2011 and amended the FD&C by passing the FDA Food Safety Modernization Act (FSMA). This act overhauled regulations regarding food production both for human and animal foods, and it gave the FDA more authority to oversee and enforce food supply chains. It also shifted the focus of the FDA from responding to contamination of the food supply to preventing contamination.

The FSMA requires animal food production facilities to register with the FDA and create and implement a food safety plan that includes both hazard analysis and steps to reduce or eliminate any potential food safety hazards identified. It also requires that these facilities comply with good manufacturing practices, including baseline standards for manufacturing, processing, packing, and holding commercial pet food to ensure it is safe for animals to eat. As a result, many of the same standards that apply to the human food industry also apply to the commercial pet food industry.

The AAFCO is a nongovernmental organization, comprising the State Feed Control Officials from each of the 50 states and Puerto Rico, plus Canada, which provides standards for the pet food industry. AAFCO establishes model animal feed regulations and ingredient definitions.[20] AAFCO is not a regulatory body: regulatory adoption and enforcement are done at the state level. The FDA is also a voting member of AAFCO, and it plays a role in many of AAFCO's standardization activities, including safety reviews of ingredients defined by AAFCO. Pet food industry representatives may attend AAFCO meetings, but they have no voting authority.

Concerns About Commercial Pet Foods

Misinformation published on the Internet[21] and on social media undermines consumer confidence in commercial pet foods. See **Box 1** for details regarding some common concerns about commercial pet food. This misinformation is one reason some pet owners believe they need to make their own pets' food at home. Although feeding a homemade diet may be appealing to some pet owners and something they enjoy doing, there is no evidence to support that home-prepared diets are healthier or safer to feed than good-quality complete and balanced commercial pet food. Nonetheless, if pet owners want to feed a homemade diet, they should have a board-certified veterinary nutritionist[24] formulate a diet for them. A study evaluating nutrient composition of 200 home-prepared maintenance diets for dogs obtained from veterinary textbooks, pet care books, and Web sites showed that 95% of recipes had at least 1 essential nutrient at concentrations that did not meet National Research Council (NRC) or AAFCO guidelines.[29] Multiple nutrient deficiencies were found in 83.5% of recipes, 9 recipes surpassed the safer upper limit for vitamin D, and 6 recipes surpassed the safe upper limit for the fatty acids eicosapentaenoic acid (EPA) and docosahexaenoic acid (DHA). This study reinforces the importance of working with a board-certified veterinary nutritionist[24] to formulate homemade diets.

Commercial pet food companies that employ a team of qualified experts invest significant financial resources overseeing all aspects of development and production of their pet foods and ensuring they are adhering to FSMA food safety requirements. Members of this team also conduct in-house research evaluating things such as digestibility and bioavailability of nutrients in their diets. Although in-house research is not always published, it is important for pet food companies to evaluate how diets perform when fed to animals before selling diets to pet owners. Some of these larger companies have fed these diets to their own colonies of dogs and cats for years to determine how they perform when fed to dogs and cats long term. These companies also conduct clinical research with specialists to support their claims and advance nutrition knowledge, and publish these results in peer-reviewed journals.

Occasional health problems have been associated with feeding both commercial pet foods as well as homemade diets. However, considering the millions of pets fed commercial diets each year,[4,15] the risks of nutrient deficiencies or excesses associated with these foods, especially those produced by companies that employ a team of

Box 1
Examples of perceived cons of commercial pet foods

1. Commercial pet food is the equivalent to eating fast food or junk food.[22]
   Claim: commercial pet food is heavily processed fast food, just like burgers, fries, tacos, potato chips, cake, and candy.
   Response: the type and extent of processing does not necessarily correlate with the nutritional content of food. Most commercial pet foods provide compete and balanced nutrition, unlike fast food, candy, cake, and ice cream.
2. Veterinarians receive little training on nutrition, and what they are taught is paid for by commercial pet food companies. That is why veterinarians recommend commercial pet foods.[22,23]
   Claim: veterinarians, like medical doctors, learn little about nutrition in school, and what they do learn about nutrition is paid for by pet food companies. The reason veterinarians recommend commercial pet food is because the commercial pet food companies have paid for their nutrition education.
   Response: 19 of 32 accredited veterinary colleges in the United States and Canada have at least 1 board-certified veterinary nutritionist[24] on faculty. These veterinarians have advanced training in veterinary nutrition and have passed a rigorous certification examination to become diplomats in the American College of Veterinary Nutrition (ACVN). They are experts in their field of veterinary medicine. ACVN diplomats teach nutrition to veterinary students at many accredited veterinary colleges. For veterinary colleges that do not have a board-certified veterinary nutritionist on faculty, some may have a board-certified veterinary nutritionist associated with a nonprofit organization teach students about nutrition, whereas others have other faculty teach nutrition. In addition, many veterinary conferences offer lectures devoted to nutrition, so, even after graduation, veterinarians continue to learn about nutrition.
   At the author's veterinary college, nutrition is a core course in the curriculum. In addition, there is a 3-week clinical nutrition rotation that students can take to learn even more about small animal nutrition.
3. Veterinarian get kickbacks and huge profit margins when they sell commercial pet food.[25,26]
   Claim: veterinarians are in the pockets of the big pet food companies, and, when they sell these diets to their clients, they get kickbacks and receive huge profit margins from doing so.
   Response: most veterinarians do sell some pet foods, including therapeutic diets, in their clinics for the convenience of the pet owners, for the welfare of the pet, or to help manage certain medical conditions. They do make some profit from these sales. However, they generally have the same markup fee that online retailers do, and this would happen whether they sold you a commercial diet, heartworm prevention, or a medication. Veterinarians are just like anyone else that owns a business: this is how they make a living. Veterinarians should not be expected to give their services away or sell products at cost, just as auto mechanics would not be expected to fix cars for free and sell parts at cost. Veterinarians love animals but they also need to make money to live on, just like anyone else.
4. Commercial pet food contains 4 D (dead, dying, diseased, disabled) meat, roadkill, and euthanized dogs and cats.[22,27]
   Claim: 4 D meat, roadkill, euthanized dogs and cats, and spoiled supermarket food is just some of the things that can legally be used in pet food.
   Response: many of the same regulations that apply to the human food industry also apply to the pet food industry, including that the food produced is safe to eat, properly manufactured, contains no harmful substances, and is truthfully labeled.[19] In addition, AAFCO[20] defines what ingredients can be legally used in pet food, and any food that contains pentobarbital is considered adulterated and illegal to sell.
   There are also 2 types of rendering plants: independent rendering plants and integrated rendering plants. Integrated rendering plants only receive animal products from the US Department of Agriculture (USDA)–inspected meat or poultry plants they are affiliated with, and these are the types of rendering plants that reputable pet food companies

purchase their ingredients from. Because 4 D meat, roadkill, euthanized dogs and cats, and spoiled supermarket food would not be associated with a USDA-inspected plant processing animal protein for human consumption, these types of materials would also not be found in by-product meals used in pet food.[28]

5. Commercial pet foods are loaded with cheap fillers.[22,28]
   Claim: things, such as corn and soy, are used as cheap fillers in commercial pet food. Fillers in commercial pet food are there for the benefit of the manufacturers, not for the animals that are fed these diets. The focus should be on ingredients.
   Response: a filler is an ingredient that adds bulk to the diet but provides no nutritional value or benefit to the animal. Ingredients such as corn or soy do not meet the definition of a filler (see text). Dietary fiber is also not a filler. Dietary fiber feeds the beneficial bacteria in the gastrointestinal (GI) tract, which in turn produce short-chain fatty acids that feed the intestinal cells lining the large intestines. Seventy percent of the immune system lies within the GI tracts, and having a robust population of beneficial bacteria in the GI tract not only affects the health of the gut but also has beneficial effects systemically. Fiber also affects stool quality.
   Animals require nutrients, not ingredients. Focusing on the nutrients that diets provide so that dogs and cats receive all the nutrients they require in a complete and balanced diet should be what is important to pet owners.

experts, are low. In contrast, there are numerous examples of health problems related to feeding an improperly balanced homemade diet to pets.[29–37]

The FDA reports recalls and withdrawals of both pet food and treats[38] as well as recalls of human food and beverages.[39] **Table 3** illustrates the total number of commercial pet foods or treats recalled during a 12-month time frame. Recalls of all pet food and treats averaged less than 3 per month, and recalls for commercial cooked pet foods and treats averaged less than 1 per month. Most recalls were not associated with any illnesses in dogs or cats; however, 1 canned dog food and 1 canned cat food were associated with illnesses, as were 3 brands of treats. One brand of pig-ear treats contaminated with *Salmonella* was associated with illnesses in both dogs and people.

Contrast the number of pet food and treat recalls during a 12-month period with the number of recalls of human food and beverages during that same time.[39] There were

Table 3
United States Food and Drug Administration commercial pet food and treat recalls from July 17, 2019 to July 17, 2020[38]

Type of Food Recalled	No. of Recalls	Reasons for Recalls
Raw or freeze-dried diets or treats	16	(15) Potential contamination or proven contamination with pathogens (*Salmonella*, *Listeria monocytogenes*, Shiga toxin-producing *Escherichia coli* 0128, *Clostridium botulinum*); (1) incorrect compliance guidelines
Pig-ear pet treats	7	Potential contamination or proven contamination with *Salmonella*
Cooked dog or cat diets	7	Increased levels of choline chloride, thyroid hormone, vitamin D; products not meeting company's quality and safety standards; low levels of thiamine (vitamin B1)
Cooked dog treats	2	Increased levels of thyroid hormone
Bully sticks	1	Potential contamination with *Salmonella*
Total	33	—

more than 800 human food and beverage recalls during this same time, and many of the recalls were for potential contamination with pathogens. Examples of the types of human foods recalled included fresh fruits and vegetables, eggs and cheese, and many other foods. These foods are the same foods pet owners often purchase to make homemade diets for their pets. The US Department of Agriculture (USDA) also reports recalls of meat and poultry products.[40–42] Meat and poultry products meant for human consumption can contain pathogens, undeclared allergens, foreign material, or be produced without the benefit of inspection. The FDA classifies commercial pet food contaminated with *Salmonella* to be adulterated, and therefore unfit for sale,[43] but it is not illegal to sell raw chicken to consumers that is contaminated with *Salmonella*, including strains resistant to multiple antibiotics, and other pathogens.[44,45] As a result, purchasing foods meant for human consumption to use in homemade diets for pets does not guarantee that it is safer than purchasing cooked commercial pet food products. In addition, there is no evidence that pets fed homemade diets are healthier or live longer than pets fed good-quality commercial complete and balanced diets.

Current Classification Systems of Processed Foods Does Not Equate to Nutrient Quality

There is no shortage of false information available on the Internet about the dangers of feeding processed commercial pet food.[46,47] These sites often present their false information in a tabloid fashion, with the intent of convincing pet owners that feeding their dogs and cats commercial pet foods "are wreaking havoc on our pets' lives."[46] They go on to make claims, such as "processed diets have created generations of sick pets"[47] and "prepared pet foods help provide patients for vets."[46] They further state that feeding commercial complete and balanced diets does not promote long-term health, but feeding a biologically appropriate raw diet does. These sites make these types of claims without any scientific studies or credible references to support them, and, at most, just provide testimonials from pet owners to support their claims. As a result, some pet owners refuse to feed commercial pet food because of negative perceptions that they have about processed foods and the belief that all processed foods are inherently unhealthy or biologically inappropriate.

The USDA defines processed food as any raw agricultural commodity that has been subject to washing, cleaning, milling, cutting, chopping, heating, pasteurization, blanching, cooking, canning, freezing, drying, dehydrating, mixing, packaging, or other procedures that alter the food from its natural state.[48–50] If the strict USDA definition of processed food is used, any food not eaten raw and unwashed is processed to some extent. The term processed has such a broad definition that it is almost meaningless when discussing food.

Processed foods may also include the addition of other nutrients to food products, such as vitamins, minerals, salt, sugars, and fat. The Institute of Food Technologists includes additional processing terms to this definition, such as storing, filtering, fermenting, extracting, concentrating, microwaving, and packaging.

The type and extent of processing does not necessarily correlate with the nutritional content of the food, and processing can improve the nutritional value of food. Some food processing techniques, such as enrichment and fortification, can add essential nutrients to foods that may be otherwise limited and enhance the nutritional value of that food. Some examples include the fortification of milk with vitamin D; fortification of wheat flour with folic acid or salt with iodine; ready-to-drink beverages fortified with protein, vitamins, or electrolytes; as well as vitamins and minerals added to commercial pet foods to provide complete and balanced nutrition. In contrast, adding a lot of salt or refined sugar to foods are examples where a processed food may be less healthy for a person to consume, but that is not the type of processing that applies to most commercial pet foods.

Numerous systems exist that distinguish human foods or drinks based on different levels of processing. These systems use terms such as minimally processed, moderately processed, moderately processed for flavor, moderately processed grain, highly processed, food processed for preservation, processed culinary ingredients, ultraprocessed, highly processed ingredients, highly processed stand-alone, ready-to-eat processed, prepared foods/meals.[49,51] However, these classification systems seem arbitrary and often contradict one another when defining this terminology. They also fail to acknowledge the benefit of different degrees of processing on the nutritional value of a food or its effect on food safety. Conclusions about the association between the degree of food processing and nutritional quality are inconsistent.[52,53]

Human foods classified as highly processed or ultraprocessed products are often characterized by foods that are energy dense; high in simple sugars, unhealthy fats, and salt; and low in dietary fiber. Examples of these types of foods include cookies, sweets and deserts, sugar-sweetened drinks, white bread, French fries and chips, and hot dogs. Humans consuming large quantities of these types of food may be at risk for adverse effects on their health. However, these characteristics are not typical of commercial pet food, and therefore classifying pet food using terminology used to describe ultraprocessed human foods and beverages is misleading.

Most dry commercial pet foods are produced by extrusion cooking. There is a lot of misinformation about this method of producing dry pet food. **Box 2** provides an overview of the steps involved with extrusion cooking, as well as the beneficial effects and the less desirable effects of this method of cooking.

Cooking food is an example of food processing that can increase or decrease the availability of nutrients. For example, some vegetables show greater antioxidant, carotenoids, and polyphenol availability when consumed cooked compared with when consumed raw, whereas others show the reverse.[59–61] Moist cooking enhances the digestibility of grains. **Box 3** lists the impact cooking has on dietary protein.

NOT ALL COMMERCIAL PET FOOD COMPANIES ARE THE SAME

Pet foods have been classified as either conventional or unconventional.[70] Commercial dry and canned diets are considered conventional diets, whereas homemade diets, whether fed raw or cooked, are considered unconventional diets. The line between conventional and unconventional diets has become less distinct as the variety of commercially available diets has expanded to include raw diets and diets that resemble homemade diets but are produced on a large commercial scale. Even conventional diets can no longer be thought of as monolithic diets because the number of pet food companies has expanded and the qualifications of the people behind companies has changed. As a result, the old adage that people should feed their pets any commercial diet because they are all very similar no longer holds true.

Anyone can make and sell commercial pet food, but not all companies or their products are of equivalent quality. For example, inappropriate processing can negatively affect the bioavailability of nutrients. It is often challenging and confusing for pet owners and veterinary professionals to evaluate commercial pet foods when there is so much information, including misinformation, about pet foods available on the Internet, at pet stores, and other places.

The World Small Animal Veterinary Association (WSAVA) is a global community of more than 200,000 veterinarians from around the world whose goal is “to advance

Box 2
Processing steps used in manufacturing dry kibble[1,54–58]

Step 1. Procure ingredients in various forms that meet specifications and safety standards.
- Whole, pellets, granules, powders, liquids

Step 2. Convert ingredients into appropriate particle size or consistency.
- Whole grains and pelleted ingredients: grinding
- Frozen blocks of raw meat: frozen block breaking, grinding, and mixing with water to create a meat slurry

Step 3. Dry ingredients weighed and added to standard mixer for blending.
- Dry blended ingredients are dropped into a hopper (holding container) and conveyed to either a final grinding step or to overhead bins above the preconditioner and extruder.

Step 4. Preconditioning stage.
- Water and steam are added to dry blended ingredients.
- Heat is applied to begin the cooking process of starches (gelatinization).
- Liquid additions, such as fat and meat slurries, if included in the diet, are added toward the middle to end of preconditioning stage.
- Temperature of ingredients at end of preconditioning is approximately 80°C (176°F).

Step 5. Once ingredients have completed the preconditioning phase, they are transferred to the extruder.
- The extruder consists of a single screw or twin screws within a barrel.
- Extrusion cooking is a thermomechanical process that uses a combination of moisture, pressure, temperature, flow rate, residence time, and mechanical shear energy exerted by the rotating screws.
  - Adjustments of these properties contributes to the overall nutritional value of the product.
  - Extrusion cooking is referred to as a high temperature short time method.
    - The residence time (time ingredients spend in extruder) can vary from 10 to 270 seconds.
    - The temperature within the extruder can vary from 80°C to 200°C (176°F–392°F).
    - Although the name states high temperatures, the temperatures used during extrusion cooking are consistent with oven temperatures people use to cook their own foods. However, by leveraging pressure to facilitate cooking during extrusion, the cooking time is much shorter than the standard cooking times people use for cooking their own foods.
- Examples of human and pet food products that use extrusion cooking include pasta, baby foods, texturized vegetable protein, ready-to-eat breakfast cereals, snack foods, dried soups, dry beverage mixes, dry pet food, and pet treats.

Step 6. A die plate is located at the end of the extrusion barrel that contains 1 or more openings.
- The materials exiting the die resemble a rope as it leaves the extruder.
- Pressure generated within the extrusion barrel forces the material through the openings in the die plate and a knife cuts the material as it exits the die plate. The speed at which the die plate rotates determines how long each piece is.
- Die inserts fitted onto the outside of the die plate determine the final shape of the food. Depending on the food, these shapes can vary from circles, stars, bones, and fish to flat ribbon shapes used for some pet treats and pastas.

Step 7. Once the food exists the extruder, it is conveyed to the dryer to achieve the desired moisture content of the food.
- The drying chamber consists of a conveyer belt (dryer deck) that the food rests on as it goes through the drying process.
- The depth of the product on the conveyer belt, zone temperatures, retention times, and humidity all influence the drying of the food.
- Different zones within the dryer use different temperatures to optimize the drying process as the food passes through it.
  - The first zone warms the food to 80°C to 100°C (176°F–212°F).
  - The food then moves to the primary drying zone with temperatures of 120°C to 150°C (248°F–302°F).

- The last zone is the cooling zone.
- The residence time within the dryer including a cooling zone varies from 20 to 30 minutes.

Step 8. The food then goes through the enrobing step, which adds liquid and dry coatings to the food.

- Fat is often added during this step because it disrupts starch gelatinization to prevent expansion of the product.
- Flavor enhancers are also added during this step.

Step 9. The last step is packaging, which protects the food from infestation, reduces oxidation of fat, and increases the shelf life of the product.

Beneficial effects of extrusion cooking include:

- Improved digestibility of starch and protein.
- Improved bioavailability of bioactive compounds by forming complexes with protein.
- Destruction of antinutritional factors that can inhibit protein digestibility, such as protease inhibitors, trypsin inhibitors, hemagglutinins (lectins), tannins, and phytates.
- Starch cooking (gelatinization) to enhance digestibility.
- Inactivation of lipoxygenases and peroxidases, which cause lipid deterioration during storage.
- Sterilization (destruction of pathogens, such as *Salmonella*).
- Retains natural colors and flavors of foods.

Some nutrient loss occurs during extrusion cooking.

- Vitamin loss.
  - The stability of vitamins during extrusion is variable and depends on the chemical structure and composition of the vitamin, as well as the conditions used during extrusion.
  - B vitamins, vitamin A, and vitamin E are negatively affected by extrusion cooking.
  - Although some loss of vitamins occurs during the extrusion process, these losses are compensated for upstream by adjusting the amount added to the food before extrusion.
- Amino acid loss.
  - Lysine, arginine, tryptophan, cysteine, and histidine are the most common amino acids affected by extrusion. These losses during extrusion must also be accounted for when formulating diets.
- Reduction in protein availability through Maillard reactions.
  - Maillard reactions occur between reducing sugars and amino acids in proteins.
  - Maillard reaction products (MRPs) occur during heating but also when food is placed at room temperature. MRPs also form endogenously in the body.
  - Maillard reactions occur during extrusion cooking of pet food but also in many foods people consume, including roasted or grilled meats, coffee, baked goods with darkened crust, toast, fried onions, malt whiskey and beer, dried and condensed milk, toasted marshmallows, roasted peanuts, and chocolate.
  - Parameters that promote Maillard reactions are temperature, moisture content, thermal duration, and pH value.
  - Mild extrusion conditions, defined as high moisture content, low residence time, and low temperatures, improve nutrition quality of food.
  - More extreme extrusion conditions, defined as high extrusion temperatures (≥200°C [392°F]), low moisture content (<15%), and improper formulation (presence of highly reactive sugars) can impair nutritional quality of food.
    - Extrusion temperature and duration (residence time) also seem to be important parameters determining the degree of Maillard reactions, with increases in both variables increasing the reaction rate.
    - Extrusion cooking of commercial dry pet food generally occurs at temperatures less than 200°C (<392°F), which is lower than temperatures used for extreme extrusion conditions.

the health and welfare of companion animals worldwide through an educated, committed and collaborative global community of veterinary peers."[71] WSAVA established the WSAVA Global Nutrition Committee, which has created guidelines comprising 8 criteria for selecting diets made by reputable companies (**Box 4**).[72]

Box 3
Benefits associated with cooking dietary protein

1. Cooking improves digestibility of protein.
   - Cooking can improve protein digestibility through protein denaturation, but it can also destroy some heat-sensitive amino acids.[62]
     - The impact of cooking depends, in great part, on the method of cooking and parameters such as moisture, temperature, and other variables.
       - For example, a study done in humans showed that digestibility of chicken eggs was increased by 45% to 78% when eggs were consumed microwaved versus raw.[63]
       - Another study in Burmese pythons evaluated the impact of cooking and grinding of beef sirloin on the cost of digestion.[64] Cooking reduced the energy cost of digestion by 12.7%, and grinding reduced the energy cost of digestion by 12.4%. The effects of both cooking and grinding are additive.
       - A study comparing apparent total tract macronutrient digestibility in cats fed extruded, raw beef-based and cooked beef-based diets showed that the raw and cooked beef-based diets were more digestible than the extruded diet. However, all diets used were highly digestible so the variation in digestibility among diets would be unlikely to affect the long-term health of the cats.[65] Commercial extruded diets vary considerably in their digestibility so comparison with one extruded diet, such as the diet used in this study, may not be representative of all dry pet foods.
2. Cooking has the potential to affect protein digestibility or losses.
   - Depending on the methods and temperatures used, cooking can either increase or decrease protein digestibility and nutritional value.
     - Cooking of foods (meats and grains) was a major factor in human evolution, including advances in brain function caused by better nutrition.[66]
   - Most commercial pet food companies are aware of the impact of cooking on protein digestibility or losses and can compensate to ensure the final product fed to the pet has adequate levels of protein and essential amino acids.
3. Cooking destroys antinutritional factors found in some foods.
   - Examples of antinutritional factors destroyed by cooking include thiaminases found in raw fish, which destroy thiamine; trypsin inhibitors found in raw soybeans, which interfere with protein digestion; and avidin found in raw eggs, which destroys biotin.
4. Cooking food is also important from a food safety standpoint.
   - The US Department of Health and Human Services and the FDA list food safety standards, including recommended cooking temperatures for meat, poultry, and seafood.[67,68]
   - It is also important to keep in mind that dogs can shed *Salmonella* in their feces for 1 to 7 days after consuming 1 *Salmonella*-contaminated meal. Most dogs fed raw meats are asymptomatic for salmonellosis but pose a potential zoonotic risk.[69]

Recommending diets made by companies that meet WSAVA Guidelines is one way to distinguish reputable and high-quality pet food companies from the rest.

Grain-Inclusive and Grain-Free Diets

Grains, such as corn, wheat, and rice, provide a rich source of nutrients in diets for humans, dogs, and cats. For example, corn is an excellent source of linoleic acid, an essential fatty acid required in the diets of all mammals. Corn also provides protein, essential amino acids, antioxidants, vitamins, minerals, fiber, and energy. Grains have been part of complete and balanced commercial pet foods for decades, and dietary guidelines for humans strongly recommend including more whole grains in the diet as a key element of healthy eating patterns.[73] Properly processed grains are highly digestible in both dogs and cats.[74,75]

Some pet owners have expressed concern that glutens in grains may be a source of allergies in dogs. Glutens are the protein component of grains, and it is the gliadin, a

Box 4
Examples of criteria that the World Small Animal Veterinary Association recommends for selecting pet foods[72]

- Does the company employ a full-time qualified nutritionist, such as a PhD in animal nutrition or someone board certified by the American College of Veterinary Nutrition (AVN) or European College of Veterinary Comparative Nutrition (ECVCN)?
  - Some companies employ a team of experts, including full-time nutritionists, food scientists, microbiologists, food safety scientists, and toxicologists.
- What are the credentials of the people that formulate the diets for the company?
- What AAFCO protocol does the company use to substantiate that their diets are complete and balanced? Do they use AAFCO feedings trials or the formulation method? If the formulation method is used, do their diets meet AAFCO nutrient profiles by formulation or do they have the finished product analyzed for nutrient content?
- Does the company produce their diets in their own manufacturing plants or do they subcontract production of their foods to a third-party manufacturer?
  - Owning their manufacturing plants allows oversight of all aspects of diet production
- What quality-control measures does the company use to ensure consistency and quality of ingredients and end products?
- Will the company provide the average content of important nutrients in their diet? Are they able to provide the average or typical analysis for their diets, rather than just the guaranteed analysis, which only lists minimums and maximums of nutrients and not exact amounts?
  - They should also be able to provide individual nutrients on an energy basis, rather than just an as-fed or dry-matter basis

•What kind of research does the company conduct? If they are developing a new or novel diet, have they conducted research to validate their claims and to ensure that the diet is safe to feed on a long-term basis? Do they do internal feeding trials on their diets, and do they conduct research that is published in peer-reviewed journals?

specific protein within the gluten from wheat, rye, and barley, that people with celiac disease have reactions to.[76] Gluten found in corn and rice does not contain this gliadin. As a result, people with celiac disease generally do not have a reaction to gluten from corn or rice. Gluten sensitivity in dogs is rare. A heritable form of gluten-sensitive enteropathy that is similar to celiac disease in people can occur in specific lines of Irish setters.[77,78] Some border terriers with epileptoid cramping syndrome responded well to what the investigators described as a gluten-free diet.[79] However, the diet fed to the dogs that showed improvement was not a grain-free or gluten-free diet because it contained rice. Thus, it seems that these dogs tolerate rice gluten, just like people with celiac disease do.

Concerns about the use of grains in commercial pet food began occurring about 10 to 15 years ago, and this concern seems to have been driven largely by marketing[13,80,81] and not science. Through marketing and the Internet, pet owners were told to focus on ingredients in pet food as a way to determine its quality. They were also told that grains in pet foods are fillers; grains rejected for use in human foods ended up in pet food, cause allergies and other health problems, and are harmful to have in pet food. Despite educational materials and articles written by board-certified veterinary nutritionists discussing the myths and misperceptions of grains in pet food,[82,83] demand for grain-free diets steadily increased. Alternative ingredients, such as legumes and potatoes, seem to have replaced grains in many over-the-counter grain-free diets. Long-term safety studies with these newer ingredients do not seem to have been done. Now some grain-free diets have been associated with dogs developing secondary dilated cardiomyopathy (DCM).[84–89] The FDA initiated an investigation into the problem, and it is an ongoing investigation (**Box 5**).

Studies validating the association between dogs consuming grain-free diets and DCM have been published since the FDA announced its investigation in 2018.[87,88] A Facebook group entitled Diet-Associated Dilated Cardiomyopathy (DCM) in Dogs, whose membership includes veterinary professionals, such as boarded veterinary cardiologists, nutritionists, internists, as well as pet owners, is continuing to collect information on the diets consumed by dogs developing DCM (the author is a consultant for this group). This group also has long-term follow-up on many of the cases of DCM reported to them. Just as the most recent report from the FDA shows, the DCM in many dogs with DCM is improving dramatically or even reversing completely after changing diets and receiving appropriate therapy, which is consistent with these dogs having secondary (nutritional) DCM. The author continues to receive consults about dogs diagnosed with DCM while consuming these grain-free diets, so the problem continues.

To date, no specific nutritional cause and effect has been found for the association between grain-free diets and DCM, but a significant association has been confirmed. Other observations include multiple unrelated dogs from the same household fed the same grain-free diet developing DCM. Echocardiogram clinics screening dogs for DCM show that some asymptomatic dogs have occult DCM, and, as a result, it is difficult to know the true extent of the problem at this time. In addition, the author and others involved with this group find that veterinarians are not consistently reporting these cases to the FDA or having their clients report these cases, so the problem is likely underreported. Veterinarians should advise pet owners about the risks for DCM associated with grain-free diets and should consider recommending a different diet for those already feeding grain-free diets.

Diet-associated DCM associated with grain-free diets is an example of problems that can occur when marketing, not science, drives sales of a certain types of commercial pet food. Therapeutic grain-free diets for dogs have been around for almost 2 decades and have not been associated with DCM. These therapeutic diets are made by pet food companies that meet (and exceed) WSAVA guidelines. They also established their diets as complete and balanced using AAFCO animal feeding trials rather than the formulation method used by many of the companies whose grain-free diets are associated with DCM.

Commercial Pet Food May Not Be the Best Option for all Dogs and Cats

Some pets refuse to eat a commercial diet. This refusal may be the result of pet owners feeding their own food to their pets when they are eating, and that becomes the expectation of those pets when they want food. This situation may also occur as a result of food aversion caused by an underlying disease, or for other reasons. Some pets have multiple health problems for which available commercials diets are not appropriate. Some pet owners also enjoy making their own pets' food, and feeding a commercial diet may not fulfill this desire. For these patients, feeding a homemade diet formulated by a board-certified veterinary nutritionist[24] may be the best option.

There are also some healthy dogs and cats that refuse to eat a commercial diet. Although this is most often the result of learned behavior, it is the author's opinion that the owners should not be told that, if their pets get hungry enough, they will eat that diet. Not only is this not always true, but it is not in the best interest of any dog or cat to starve, and cats are also at risk of developing hepatic lipidosis if they refuse to eat. Even in healthy pets, starvation has adverse effects. Telling the clients to let their pets starve until they eat the diet the owners want them to eat also has the potential to disrupt the veterinary-client relationship. It also ignores the human-animal

Box 5
Timeline of United States Food and Drug Administration investigation of diets associated with dilated cardiomyopathy

2017. Veterinary cardiologists began to notice an increased incidence of DCM in golden retrievers and other breeds of dogs, including breeds that typically are not at risk of developing primary DCM.[85,86]

As veterinary cardiologists and others in the veterinary community investigated factors that these cases shared in common, they discovered that most were consuming grain-free diets.[81,82] These cases were also unusual because many of the cases seemed to be consistent with secondary (nutritional) DCM, and not primary DCM. Dramatic improvement or reversal of DCM in some dogs occurred when the owners changed the dog's diet to a grain-containing diet, often combined with taurine and/or L-carnitine supplementation, as well as appropriate cardiac medications. A concurrent diagnosis of taurine deficiency was made in some dogs with DCM, but this was not a consistent finding.

Members of the veterinary community notified the FDA about these cases and their concern about this problem.

July 12, 2018. The FDA formally announced they were conducting an investigation into the potential connection between diet and cases of canine heart disease.[86] They asked pet owners and veterinary professionals to report cases of DCM to them.

June 27, 2019. The FDA published an update on this investigation.[89] The FDA reported that 91% of the patients with DCM reported to them were consuming grain-free diets, 93% of the diets contained peas and/or lentils, and 89% contained peas. There are numerous breeds of dogs involved with this problem, most of which are not breeds predisposed to primary DCM. The FDA issued the following statement: "Based on the data collected and analyzed thus far, the agency believes that the potential association between diet and DCM in dogs is a complex scientific issue that may involve multiple factors."[89]

Sept 29, 2020. The FDA updated the findings of their investigation at a scientific forum.[84] As of July 20, 2020, more than 1100 cases of dogs with DCM and more than 20 cats with DCM have been reported to the FDA.

Data from a subset of approximately 150 dogs with DCM were presented in greater detail. Group 1 consists of 121 dogs reported to them from January 2018 to April 2019. One-hundred and seven of 121 dogs in this group have had full or partial recovery of the heart disease. Two of 107 cases of full or partial recovery did not have enough information to determine the type of diet these dogs were consuming at the time of their diagnosis. Of the remaining 105 dogs, the following are the characteristics of the diets the dogs were consuming at the time of the diagnosis.

- 98 of 105 (93%) were consuming grain-free diets.
- 95 of 105 (90%) were consuming a grain-free diet exclusively.
- 7 of 105 were consuming grain-containing diets.
  - 4 of 7 were consuming a vegan diet with whole peas as the first ingredient.
  - 2 of 7 were consuming chicken or lamb and rice diets containing split peas.
  - 1 of 7 was consuming a lamb meal and rice diet.
- 100 of 103 (97%) were consuming diets containing whole-pulse ingredients.
- 0% of cases were exposed to diets with meat by-products or poultry by-products.

All dogs with DCM in group 1 that fully recovered consumed a different diet from the one they were consuming when the diagnosis of DCM was made.

- 96% consumed a grain-containing diet during the recovery period.
  - 3 consumed hydrolyzed protein diets (2 contained corn starch and 1 contained brewers rice).
  - Peas were reported as the top ingredient in 8% of diets; 4% contained whole peas.
  - None of the recovery diets contained lentils.
  - Meat by-products or poultry by-products were contained in 42% of recovery diets.
  - Lamb meal was present in 8% of recovery diets.

Group 2 consisted of 40 dogs with DCM reported to the FDA from November 2019 to July 2020. To date, 12% recovered fully, 75% have had partial recovery, and 13% had no recovery.

- Diet changes were made in all dogs diagnosed with DCM. The FDA did not provide a breakdown of the diets that group 2 dogs were changed to.

- Key take home points from the FDA's most recent reports include from group 1 dogs include:
  - Most dogs diagnosed with DCM have secondary DCM because dogs are making either full or partial recovery.
  - Most dogs were consuming grain-free diets containing whole-pulse ingredients and no meat by-products or poultry by-products at the time DCM was made.
  - All dogs that have fully recovered were changed to diets containing grains during the recovery period.
  - The association between dogs consuming grain-free diets and developing secondary DCM is clear, and consuming grain-containing diets is an important component in the treatment of dogs that fully recover.
  - The cause of dogs developing DCM while consuming grain-free diets is still unknown; however, there are numerous grain-containing diets not associated with this problem. Veterinarians should reconsider recommending grain-free diets to their clients.

bond that exists, where food often plays an important role in that relationship. Instead, owners should be given advice on how best to transition to a new diet. Sometimes pets do not like the specific brand of food the owner is feeding, so trying a different brand of food results in some pets consuming a commercial diet. Sometimes, a gradual transition, slowly adding more and more of the commercial food while decreasing the alternative diet, can promote acceptance.

SUMMARY

Commercial pet food has existed for nearly 100 years in the United States. That industry now consists of a diverse range of diets made by a diverse range of companies with varying degrees of expertise. The plethora of misinformation about commercial pet food available on the Internet, through advertising, social media, and other sources has led to many pet owners feeling overwhelmed and confused about what is the best diet to feed their dogs or cats. However, veterinarians are still the most trusted source of information about nutrition for pet owners, and it is important that veterinarians include nutrition as part of routine visits. The commercial pet food industry continues to grow not only in sales but also in the number of companies making commercial diets. As a result, marketing is a way for some companies to distinguish their products from those of their competitors. However, marketing claims are not always supported by research, which can lead to untoward problems, such as what is being seen with grain-free diets and their association with DCM in dogs. Both the commercial pet food industry and the human food industry are highly regulated in the United States, to ensure that both pet food and human food is safe to eat. Although recalls of commercial pet food occasionally occur, they happen less frequently than recalls of human foods. Commercial pet foods are processed, as are essentially all the foods humans consume, and commercial pet food, which is a complete and balanced diet, currently does not fit well into the classification of ultraprocessed foods. These types of foods include candy, cake, and ice cream. In addition, the current definitions of processing are confusing, inconsistent, and do not necessarily correlate with the nutritional content of the food or its safety. Although commercial pet foods provide excellent nutrition and are still the most common type of food fed to pets in the United States, and pets continue to live longer, it is not the best option for all pets. If pet owners do not feed a commercial pet food, it is important that they feed a homemade diet formulated by a board-certified veterinary nutritionist.[24]

CLINICS CARE POINTS

- Veterinarians remain the most important source of nutritional advice for pet owners.
- Most pet owners want their veterinarians to recommend a diet for their pets, but only about a third of veterinarians routinely provide this information to their clients.
    - Include a discussion about pet nutrition at each pet owner visit.
    - Provide a list of specific pet diets or pet food companies that the practice is comfortable recommending.
    - Provide additional nutritional advice and resources through the clinic's webpage or as printed handouts.
- Be willing to discuss potential myths and misinformation pet owners may have if the pet owner is interested in hearing what your understanding of a particular topic is.
- New information about pet nutrition continues to increase, so it is important for veterinarians to provide current and accurate information to their clients.
    - Many opportunities exist to receive continuing education (CE) in the area of pet nutrition, but choose CE that is given by qualified individuals who support their recommendations with published scientific studies

DISCLOSURE

The author currently is receiving supplemental support from Nestle Purina in the form of cat food and cat litter for a study funded by the Human Animal Bond Research Institute (HABRI), and has previously received research funding from Hill's and Nestle Purina. The author has also lectured for Hill's Pet Nutrition, Royal Canin, and Nestle Purina.

REFERENCES

1. Crane SW, Crowell CS, Stout NP, et al. Commercial pet foods. In: Hand MS, Thatcher CD, Remillard RL, et al, editors. Small animal clinical nutrition. 5th edition. Topeka (KS): Mark Morris Institute; 2010. p. 157–90.
2. Pet Food Institute. History of Pet Food. Available at: https://www.petfoodinstitute.org/pet-food-matters/nutrition-2/history-of-pet-food/. Accessed July 10, 2020.
3. Petfood Industry. Survey: Dog owners have difficulty choosing pet food. Available at: https://www.petfoodindustry.com/articles/5407-survey-dog-owners-have-difficulty-choosing-pet-food. Assessed July 13, 2020.
4. Association of Pet Obesity Prevention. Pet Obesity survey results 2018. Available at: https://petobesityprevention.org/2018/#PetFoodSurvey. Accessed July 10, 2020.
5. Google search using the phrase "How safe is commercial pet food?". Available at: https://www.google.com/search?client=firefox-b-1-d&sxsrf=ALeKk02rLKZTscISz-6cKCmP6HdfG1vG5A%3A1594822896018&ei=8BAPX-FDi8v9Btznm9gJ&q=How+safe+is+commercial+pet+food%3F&oq=How+safe+is+commercial+pet+food%3F&gs_lcp=CgZwc3ktYWIQAzIFCCEQoAEyBQghEKsCMgUIIRCrAjIFCCEQqwI6BAgAEEdQ_7UBWP-1AWCXuQFoAHABeACAAWyIAWySAQMwLjGYAQCgAQGqAQdnd3Mtd2l6&sclient=psy-ab&ved=0ahUKEwjh-8ihus_qAhWLZd8KHdzzBpsQ4dUDCAs&uact=5. Accessed July 10, 2020.
6. Association of American Feed Control Official (AAFCO). Official Publication. Feed terms and definitions. 2020. Available at: https://www.aafco.org/Publications. Accessed July 12, 2020.

7. Petfood Industry. US pet food market report reveals pet humanization trend. Available at: https://www.petfoodindustry.com/articles/6694-us-pet-food-market-report-reveals-pet-humanization-trend. Accessed July 13, 2020.
8. Schleicher M, Cash SB, Freeman LM. Determinants of pet food purchasing decisions. Can Vet J 2019;60:644–50.
9. American Pet Products Association. Pet industry market size & ownership statistics. Available at: https://www.americanpetproducts.org/press_industrytrends.asp. Accessed July 10, 2020.
10. Number of dogs in the United States from 2000 to 2017 (in millions). Available at: https://www.statista.com/statistics/198100/dogs-in-the-united-states-since-2000/. Assessed September 23, 2020.
11. Number of cats in the United States from 2000 to 2017 (in millions). Available at: https://www.statista.com/statistics/198102/cats-in-the-united-states-since-2000/. Assessed September 23, 2020.
12. Veterinary Practice News. Vet care spending tops $13 Billion in 2010. Available at: https://www.veterinarypracticenews.com/vet-care-spending-tops-13-billion-in-2010/. Assessed Sept 23, 2020.
13. Available at: https://www.pressreader.com/canada/vancouver-sun/20171016/281840053897777https:/www.aafco.org/Publications. Accessed September 21, 2020.
14. Calinoius LF, Vodnar DC. Whole grains and phenolic acids: a review on bioactivity, functionality, health benefits and bioavailability. Nutrients 2018;10:1615.
15. Laflamme DP, Abood SK, Fascetti AJ, et al. Pet feeding practices of dog and cat owners in the United States and Australia. J Am Vet Med Assoc 2008;232:687–94.
16. Banfield Pet Hospital. State of Pet Health 2013 Report. Available at: https://www.banfield.com/Banfield/media/PDF/Downloads/soph/Banfield-State-of-Pet-Health-Report_2013.pdf. Accessed July 10, 2020.
17. de Godoy MRC, Hervera M, Swanson KS, et al. Innovation in canine and feline nutrition: technologies for food and nutrition assessment. Annu Rev Anim Biosci 2016;4:311–33.
18. U.S. Bureau of Labor Statistics. Ahead of the pack: why are veterinary occupations growing much fast than average? Employment & Unemployment 2019;8. Available at: https://www.bls.gov/opub/btn/volume-8/veterinary-occupations-growing.htm#_edn11. Accessed August 18, 2020.
19. FDA. FDA's Regulation of Pet Food. Available at: https://www.fda.gov/animal-veterinary/animal-health-literacy/fdas-regulation-pet-food#FSMA. Accessed August 18, 2020.
20. AAFCO. The Role of AAFCO in Pet Food Regulation. Available at: https://talkspetfood.aafco.org/roleofaafco. Accessed August 18, 2020.
21. Barfworld. Available at: https://www.barfworld.com/. Accessed August 18, 2020.
22. Dogs naturally.10 Scary Truths About Your Dog's Food. Available at: https://www.dogsnaturallymagazine.com/dog-food-ten-scary-truths/. Accessed November 2, 2020.
23. Pets-N-More.Kickbacks to Vets…Is This True?. Available at: https://www.petsnmore.org/2015/05/kickbacks-to-vetsis-this-true.html. Accessed November 2, 2020.
24. American College of Veterinary Nutrition. Nutrition Consults. Available at: https://acvn.org/nutrition-consults/. Accessed August 1, 2020.
25. Dog Food Advisor. The Shocking Truth About Commercial Dog Food. Available at: https://www.dogfoodadvisor.com/dog-food-industry-exposed/shocking-truth-about-dog-food/. Accessed November 2, 2020.

26. Myths About Raw Feeding. Available at: http://rawfed.com/myths/vets.html. Accessed November 2, 2020.
27. Best Cat and Dog Food Nutrition (BCDN) by Roger Budick. Available at: http://www.bestcatanddognutrition.com/roger-biduk/kickbacks-from-pet-food-companies-to-veterinarians-and-vet-schools/. Accessed November 2, 2020.
28. Healthy Pets. Is This Pet Food Vilification Ever Justified, or Just a Bunch of Hot Air. Available at: https://healthypets.mercola.com/sites/healthypets/archive/2014/02/28/commercial-pet-food-fillers.aspx. Accessed November 2, 2020.
29. Stockman J, Fascetti AJ, Kass PH, et al. Evaluation of recipes of home-prepared maintenance diets for dogs. J Am Vet Med Assoc 2013;242:1500–5.
30. de Fornel-Thibaud P, Blanchard G, Escoffier-Chateau L, et al. Unusual case of osteopenia associated with nutritional calcium and vitamin D deficiency in an adult dog. J Am Anim Hosp Assoc 2007;43:52–60. Accessed August 17, 2020.
31. Baltzer W. Angular limb deformities in a giant-breed puppy. Clinician's Brief 2009;15–7.
32. Hutchinson D, Freeman LM, McCarthy R, et al. Seizures and severe nutrient deficiencies in a puppy fed a homemade diet. J Am Vet Med Assoc 2012;241:477–83.
33. Taylor MB, Geiger DA, Saker KE, et al. Diffuse osteopenia and myelopathy in a puppy fed a diet composed of an organic premix and raw ground beef. J Am Vet Med Assoc 2009;234:1041–8.
34. Dodd S, Barry M, Verbrugghe A. Abnormal bone mineralization in a puppy fed an imbalanced raw meat homemade diet diagnosed and monitored using dual-energy X-ray absorptiometry. J Am Physiol Nutr 2019;00:1–8.
35. Tal M, Parr JM, MacKenzie S, et al. Dietary imbalances in a large breed puppy, leading to compression fractures, vitamin D deficiency, and suspected nutritional secondary hyperparathyroidism. Can Vet J 2018;59:36–42.
36. Diquelou A, Chaput C, Benoit E, et al. Hypocalcemia due to nutritional calcium deficiency and hypothyroidism in an adult dog. Vet Rec 2005;156:45–8.
37. Niza MMRE, Vilelia CL, Freeman LMA. Feline pansteatitis revisited: hazards of unbalanced home-made diets. J Feline Med Surg 2003;5:271–7.
38. FDA Animal and Veterinary Recalls & Withdrawals. Available at: https://www.fda.gov/animal-veterinary/safety-health/recalls-withdrawals. Assessed August 1, 2020.
39. FDA Recalls, Market Withdrawals, & Safety Alerts. Food and Beverages. Available at: https://www.fda.gov/safety/recalls-market-withdrawals-safety-alerts. Accessed August 17, 2020.
40. United States Department of Agriculture Food Safety and Inspection Service. Recalls and Public health concerns. Available at: https://www.fsis.usda.gov/wps/portal/fsis/topics/recalls-and-public-health-alerts/current-recalls-and-alerts. Accessed August 17, 2020.
41. United States Department of Agriculture Food Safety and Inspection Service. Recall Case Archive 2020. Available at: https://www.fsis.usda.gov/wps/portal/fsis/topics/recalls-and-public-health-alerts/recall-case-archive/recall-case-archive-2020. Accessed August 17, 2020.
42. United States Department of Agriculture Food Safety and Inspection Service. Recall case Archive 2019. Available at: https://www.fsis.usda.gov/wps/portal/fsis/topics/recalls-and-public-health-alerts/recall-case-archive/recall-case-archive-2019. Accessed August 17, 2020.

43. Guidance for FDA Staff. Compliance Policy Guide Sec. 690.800 Salmonella in Food for Animals. Available at: https://www.fda.gov/media/86240/download. Accessed October 4, 2020.
44. Consumer Reports. Available at: https://www.consumerreports.org/media-room/press-releases/2013/12/consumer-reports-potentially-harmful-bacteria-found-on-97-percent-of-chicken-breasts-tested/. Potentially harmful bacteria found on 97 percent of chicken breasts tested. Accessed October 4, 2020.
45. Consumer Reports. Antibiotic-resistant salmonella in chicken sickens 92. Available at: https://www.consumerreports.org/cro/salmonella/antibiotic-resistant-salmonella-outbreak-raw-chicken. Accessed Oct 4, 2020.
46. Barf World. Processed Pet food – Why you should avoid it. Available at: https://www.barfworld.com/WhatIsBarf/DogFoodsToAvoid. Accessed August 20, 2020.
47. Healthy pets – with Dr. Karen Becker. FDA's Dire Warnings Create a Laughingstock. Available at: https://healthypets.mercola.com/sites/healthypets/archive/2016/04/04/pet-fresh-food-natural-diets.aspx. Accessed August 17, 2020.
48. U.S. Department of Agriculture. Available at: https://www.usda.gov/. Accessed August 20, 2020.
49. Weaver CM, Dwyer J, Fulgoni VL III, et al. Processed foods: contributions to nutrition. Am J Clin Nutr 2014;99:1525–42.
50. Fardet A, Rock E, Bassama J, et al. Current food classifications in epidemiological studies do not enable solid nutritional recommendations for preventing diet-related chornic diseases: the impact of food processing. Adv Nutr 2015;6:629–38.
51. Bleiweiss-Sande R, Chui K, Evans EW, et al. Robustness of food processing classification systems. Nutrients 2019;11:1344.
52. Poti JM, Mendex MA, Ng SW, et al. Is the degree of food processing and convenience linked with the nutritional quality of foods purchased by US households? Am J Clin Nutr 2015;101:1251–62.
53. Eicher-Miller HA, Fulgoni VI III, Keast DR. Contributions of processed foods to dietary intake in the US from 2003-2008: a report of the food and nutrition science solutions joint task force of the academy of nutrition and dietetics, American society for nutrition, institute of food technologists, and international food information council. J Nutr 2012;142:2065S–72S.
54. PetfoodIndustry.com. How processing affects pet food products, Part 1. Available at: https://www.petfoodindustry.com/articles/9392-how-processing-affects-pet-food-products-part-1. Accessed November 30, 2020.
55. PetfoodIndustry.com. How processing affects pet food products, Part 2. Available at: https://www.petfoodindustry.com/articles/9473-how-processing-affects-pet-food-products-part-2. Accessed November 30, 2020.
56. Singh S, Gamlath S, Wakeling L. Nutritional aspects of food extrusion: a review. Int J Food Sci Technol 2007;42:916–29.
57. Tran QD, Hendricks WH, van der Poel AFB. Effects of extrusion on nutrients in dry pet food. J Sci Food Agric 2008;88:1487–93.
58. Shelar G, Gaikwad ST. Extrusion in food processing: an overview. Pharma Innovation J 2019;8:562–8.
59. Miglio C, Chavaro E, Visconti A, et al. Effects of different cooking methods on nutritional and physicochemical characteristics of selected vegetables. J Agric Food Chem 2008;56:137–49.
60. Garcaia AL, Koebnick C, Dagnelie P, et al. Long-term strict raw food diet is associated with favourable plasma β–carotene and low plasma lycopene concentrations in Germans. Br J Nutr 2008;99:1293–300.

61. Prasanna KD, Gunathilake P, Somathilaka Ranaweera KKD, et al. Effect of different cooking methods on polyphenols, carotenoids and antioxidant activities of selected edible leaves. Antioxidants 2018;7:117.
62. Meade SJ, Reid EA, Gerrard JA. The impact of processing on the nutritional quality of food proteins. J Assoc Off Anal Chem 2005;88:904–22.
63. Carmody RN, Wrangham RW. The energetic significance of cooking. J Hum Evol 2009;57:379–91.
64. Boback SM, Cox CI, Ott BD, et al. Cooking and grinding reduces the cost of meat digestion. Comp Biochem Physiol A 2007;148:651–6.
65. Kerr KR, Vester Bolar BM, Morris CL, et al. Apparent total tract energy and macronutrients digestibility and fecal fermentative end-product concentrations of domestic cats fed extruded, raw beef-based, and cooked, beef-based diets. J Anim Sci 2012;90:515–22.
66. Wrangham R. Brain foods. In: Catching fire. How cooking made us human. New York (NY): 2009. p. 105–28.
67. Foodsafety.gov. Food Safety Charts. Available at: https://www.foodsafety.gov/food-safety-charts. Assessed August 20, 2020.
68. FDA. Food Safety A to Z Reference Guide. Available at: https://www.fda.gov/media/90663/download. Accessed August 20, 2020.
69. Finley R, Ribble C, Aramini J, et al. The risk of salmonellae shedding by dogs fed *Salmonella*-contaminated commercial raw food diets. Can Vet J 2007;48:69–75.
70. Parr JM, Remillard RL. Handling alternative dietary requests from pet owners. Vet Clin Small Anim 2014;44:667–88.
71. WSAVA Mission & Plan. Available at: https://wsava.org/about/mission-plan/. Accessed July 14. 2020.
72. WSAVA Global Nutrition Committee: Recommendations on Selecting Pet Foods. Available at: https://wsava.org/wp-content/uploads/2020/01/Selecting-the-Best-Food-for-your-Pet.pdf. Assessed July 12, 2020.
73. Dietary Guidelines 2015-2020. Chapter 1. Key elements of healthy eating patterns. Available at: https://health.gov/our-work/food-nutrition/2015-2020-dietary-guidelines/guidelines/chapter-1/a-closer-look-inside-healthy-eating-patterns/#callout-wholegrains. Assessed August 20, 2020.
74. Twomey LN, Pethick DW, Rowe JB, et al. The use of sorghum and corn as alternatives to rice in dog foods. J Nutr 2002;132:1704S–5S.
75. Golder C, Weemhoff JL, Jewell DE. Cats have increased protein digestibility as compared to dogs and improve their ability to absorb protein as dietary protein intake shifts from animal to plant sources. Animals 2020;10:541.
76. Moron B, Cebolla A, Manyani H, et al. sensitive detection of cereal fractions that are toxic to celiac disease patients by using monoclonal antibodies to a main immunogenic wheat peptide. Amer J Clin Nutr 2008;87:405–14.
77. Hall EJ, Batt RM. Dietary modulation of gluten sensitivity in a naturally occurring enteropathy of Irish setter dogs. Gut 1992;33:198–205.
78. Garden OA, Pidduck H, Laldani KH, et al. Inheritance of gluten-sensitive enteropathy in Irish Setters. Am J Vet Res 2000;61:462–8.
79. Lowrie M, Garden OA, Hadjivassiliou M, et al. The clinical and serological effect of a gluten-free diet in Border Terriers with epileptoid cramping syndrome. J Vet Intern Med 2015;29:1564–8.
80. PetfoodIndustry. The mother of all petfood trends: grain free. Available at: https://www.petfoodindustry.com/blogs/7-adventures-in-pet-food/post/4551-the-mother-of-all-petfood-trends-grain-free. Accessed August 20, 2020.

81. PetfoodIndustry. Riding the grain-free petfood wave. Available at: https://www.petfoodindustry.com/articles/4107-riding-the-grain-free-petfood-wave. Accessed August 20, 2020.
82. WSAVA Global Nutrition Committee. Frequently Asked questions & Myths. Available at: https://wsava.org/wp-content/uploads/2020/01/Frequently-Asked-Questions-and-Myths.pdf. Accessed August 10, 2020.
83. Laflamme D, Izquierdo O, Eirmann L, et al. Myths and misperceptions about ingredients used in commercial pet foods. Vet Clin Small Anim 2014;44:689–98.
84. Kansas State University Scientific Forum Exploring Causes of Dilated Cardiomyopathy in Dogs. FDA Updates on Dilated Cardiomyopathy: Fully and Partially Recovered Cases. Available at: https://www.ksvdl.org/resources/dilated-cardiomyopathy-dogs-forum.html. Accessed October 25, 2020.
85. Freeman LM, Stern JA, Fries R, et al. Diet-associated dilated cardiomyopathy in dogs: what do we know? (commentary). J Am Vet Med Assoc 2018;253:1390–4.
86. FDA. FDA Investigating Potential Connection Between Diet and Cases of Canine Heart Disease. Available at: https://www.fda.gov/animal-veterinary/cvm-updates/fda-investigating-potential-connection-between-diet-and-cases-canine-heart-disease. Accessed August 21, 2020.
87. Kaplan JL, Stern JA, Fascetti A, et al. Taurine deficiency and dilated cardiomyopathy in golden retrievers fed commercial diets. PLoS One 2018;13:e0209112.
88. Adin DD, DeFrancesco, Keene B, et al. Echocardiographic phenotype of canine dilated cardiomyopathy differs based on diet type. J Vet Cardiol 2019. https://doi.org/10.1016/j.jvc.2018.11.002.
89. FDA. FDA Investigation into Potential Link between Certain Diets and Canine Dilated Cardiomyopathy. Available at: https://www.fda.gov/animal-veterinary/outbreaks-and-advisories/fda-investigation-potential-link-between-certain-diets-and-canine-dilated-cardiomyopathy. Accessed August 21, 2020.

Insights into Commercial Pet Foods

Donna M. Raditic, DVM, CVA

KEYWORDS

- Pet food • Food processing • Home-prepared pet diet
- Advanced glycation end products

KEY POINTS

- Use a pet food processing categorization system that identifies pet foods as ultra-processed (UP) or minimally processed (MP) to discuss different commercial pet foods.
- Bacterial pathogen transmission has been documented from contaminated UP and MP commercial diets; therefore, universal education about safe pet food handling practices is needed or all diet types.
- Emerging research in dietary advanced glycation end products will impact the future of pet food industry.

PET FOOD DEFINITIONS

Pet food reviews have used "unconventional diets, alternative and raw meat-based diet" to identify pet foods that are not typical commercial extruded dry and retorted canned foods familiar to veterinarians.[1–4] These historic definitions do not clearly represent the different types of pet foods being fed today. It is important to clearly identify the type of pet food; therefore, the first pet food designation is whether the pet food is a commercial diet, that is, made by a pet food manufacturing company, or is a home-prepared diet, that is, made by an owner, breeder, or such, for a pet or pets. Commercial diets formulated to meet values in the Association of American Feed Control Official's (AAFCO) Dog or Cat Food Nutrient Profiles listed for adult maintenance, growth, and gestation-lactation, or for all life stages are considered nutritionally adequate in their final form. Commercial diets also include diets labeled for "intermittent or supplemental feeding only," which are not AAFCO complete and balanced, and "use under direct veterinarian supervision," which designates veterinary therapeutic diets, which may or may not be complete and balanced. Home-prepared diets should be evaluated by determining if the recipes were formulated by a qualified individual with advanced nutrition training, that is, Diplomate of the American College of Veterinary Nutrition or similar qualifications. Home-prepared

Nutrition and Integrative Medicine Consultants, 945 Creek Ridge Lane, Athens, GA 30606, USA
E-mail address: draditic@gmail.com

Vet Clin Small Anim 51 (2021) 551–562
https://doi.org/10.1016/j.cvsm.2021.01.013
vetsmall.theclinics.com

diets from recipes provided by an unqualified individual, that is, owner or breeder, or have an unknown formulator, are problematic.[5,6]

APPLYING FOOD PROCESSING CATEGORIZATION SYSTEM TO PET FOODS

A food categorization system is needed to define the vast array of commercial pet foods in the marketplace. Studies of dietary effects in the human nutrition literature often use 1 of 3 food processing categorizations systems: Nova, International Food Information Council, or University of North Carolina at Chapel Hill. These food processing categorizations systems were developed in response to the arrival of ultra-processed (UP) human foods, that is, fractionated recombined foods with added ingredients. Epidemiologic studies determined that populations consuming the highest amounts of UP foods exhibited higher prevalence of chronic disease. This finding prompted development of food classification systems according to the degree of processing, that is, minimally processed (MP), processed, and UP. For example, breakfast cereals are produced with multiple treatment steps, that is, mechanical, thermal, and extrusion cooking; therefore, they are considered "ultra-processed."[7–10] Dry pet food production is similar, with multiple processing steps using heat and pressure, whereas commercial canned pet foods also undergo multiple thermal processing with cooking and retorting.[11] As there is such a wide variety of types of foods now on the market, developing a categorization of pet foods by the level of processing is logical and relevant. In this review, pet food categories will be "minimally processed" (MP) and "ultra-processed" (UP), common to established human food processing category systems, in combination with the traditional pet food definitions of commercial, home-prepared, and nutritionally adequate or supplemental feeding where appropriate. Ultra-processed commercial diets (UPCD) are dry, canned, and any other pet foods that are manufactured using more than 1 thermal or pressure processing step to produce the final product. Minimally processed commercial diets (MPCD) previously defined as unconventional, alternative, raw meat–based diets, raw animal product, and so forth will include fresh, frozen, and any pet food manufactured with no or only 1 thermal or pressure processing step. Using a "pet food processing categorizations system" with these definitions is a starting point to provide veterinarians with neutral terminology to discuss pet diet types with owners. In the future, this pet food processing classification system can be expanded by veterinary and animal nutritionists.

PET FOODS AND EVIDENCE-BASED MEDICINE

This review presents the issues of both UP and MP commercial diets sold to consumers, as they are similarly held to pet food regulations and impact large populations. In veterinary medicine, evidence-based medicine (EBM), defined as the integration of the best research, clinical expertise, and client values, is used to determine standards of care and to make medical decisions. Best research evidence is considered systematic reviews of several trials (meta-analysis) and randomized, controlled clinical trials (RCCT). The problem in comparing UPCDs and MPCDs is the paucity of quality studies. Currently, there are no published peer-reviewed meta-analysis or RCCTs evaluating different types of pet foods, that is, UPCD compared with MPCD over a significant period measuring different whole-diet effects on the health, disease, and lifespan of a population of dogs or cats. In fact, published peer-reviewed studies evaluating whole-diet effects are scant and more often involve veterinary therapeutic diets.[12,13]

Pet Food Studies

There are a few studies that have compared UP and MP diets types in small populations over short time periods. Hamper and colleagues[14] reported on an AAFCO kitten growth trial with a canned UPCD control, MPCD group, and a third group fed a qualified formulator, complete and balanced, minimally processed home- prepared diet (MPHD) that was raw. No differences in body condition score, weight, height, or length measurements were noted, and the MPCD and the MPHD passed the AAFCO growth feeding trial criteria. In this RCCT and other studies, the digestibility of 2 MP diets compared with UPCD was higher, but long-term effects of diets with higher digestibility on health, disease, and longevity of dogs and cats are unknown.[15–17] Algya and colleagues[16] determined the apparent total macronutrient digestibility and microbiome in dogs consuming 3 commercial diets: dry UPCD, raw MPCD, and a mildly cooked MPCD. All study dogs remained healthy, and the 2 MPCD diets modified the fecal microbiome. Other studies have evaluated diet types and effects on gut microbiome, but whether changes in microbiome translate to better diets for pets is unknown. Furthermore, microbiome changes could be due to different levels of processing, different nutrient content, or some combination of these factors.[18–21] The most evidence-based statement that can be said about pet diet impact on health and longevity would be that dogs fed to maintain a lean body condition score result in statistically significant increased lifespan. This finding is based on a lifetime study of 48 Labrador retrievers fed a dry UPCD, which resulted in statistically significant longer lifespan in the diet-restricted group as compared with the control-fed dogs. Because all dogs ate the same UPCD, this study is not evidence that UPCDs are "best nutrition" but demonstrates the benefits of restricting caloric intake.[22]

Veterinarians should understand that stating UPCD is better nutrition than MPCD is not supported by published peer-reviewed studies. Similarly, the literature does not suggest MP diets represent better nutrition. EBM is the integration of the best research, clinical expertise, and client values, but when applied to UP and MP pet food comparisons, there is limited published research available. Veterinarians are integrating their clinical experiences when recommending UPCDs, but there is a need to add client values to EBM decision making, especially for owners interested in MPCDs. Recommending only UPCD as a nutritional standard of care may be eroding pet owner confidence in veterinarians. Surveys of pet owners feeding MP diets indicate they tend to obtain nutrition information from sources other than veterinarians and may view their veterinarian less favorably.[23–25] These surveys suggest determinants of pet food purchases more often involve humanization and the desire to feed healthy, quality diets that are less processed.[25–27] To improve pet owner confidence, today's veterinarians need to understand many owners are not looking to feed a wolf, but instead are trying to provide healthy, less processed diets to a family member.

PET FOOD HEALTH RISKS TO PETS AND HUMANS

It is difficult to compare the health risks of UPCDs and MPCDs using the published literature because studies often do not clearly state whether they are referring to commercial diets, home-prepared, or pet food ingredients.[3,28–37] Even veterinary organizations, such as American Veterinary Medical Association (AVMA), World Small Animal Veterinary Association (WSAVA), and American Animal Hospital Association (AAHA), have position statements that use the term "raw pet food" but are unclear whether this applies to MPCDs, MPHDs, or both. There is a need to apply a pet food categorization system to clearly define "pet diet/food" as (1) home prepared or commercial diet, (2) nutritionally adequate or supplemental/intermittent feeding, or

(3) UP or MP. For example, MPHDs that use MP human ingredients would be expected to contain bacterial contamination, as meats for human consumption are meant to be cooked; therefore, they are not required to be sterile. Veterinarians may perceive MP pet diets as unsafe; this paradigm is problematic if it includes complete and balanced MPCDs, which are held to the exact same pet food regulations as UPCDs.

The pet food categorization as discussed is applied in this review to provide veterinarians a comparison of reported and potential health risks from UP and MP commercial pet foods. In the comparison, pet food recalls can be used because the recalled brand can be identified as a UPCD or MPCD. These "contamination incidents" are reported by the Food and Drug Administration (FDA) Pet Food Recalls and/or publications. The author compiled the recall data shown in **Fig. 1**A (1998–2009) and **Fig. 1**B (2010–2020) as a summary shown by year using 4 categories: bacterial pathogens, nutritional imbalances, aflatoxins, and other toxic contaminations.[38] **Fig. 1**A has no MPCD recalls because there were few MPCDs on the market during this period of time. Even from 2010 to 2020, the sales of MPCD were less than UPCD, that is, US sales of more than $20 billion in 2015, whereas MP pet food sales were about $120 million that same year.

Bacterial Pathogens

That bacterial-contaminated pet foods are a risk to humans was exemplified by a large outbreak with Mars Petcare's dry UPCDs that was linked to 79 human infections with *Salmonella enterica* serotype *Schwarzengrund* from 2006 to 2008.[36,39,40] Another major outbreak occurred in 2012 with 53 persons infected with *S enterica* serotype *Infantis* that occurred across 21 states and 2 Canadian provinces from Diamond Pet Foods dry UPCDs.[41] Following these outbreaks, the Center for Veterinary Medicine's Veterinary Laboratory Investigation Response Network began testing UPCDs as well as MP diets, exotic animal feeds, and treats. In phase 1, 480 samples were tested with only 2 dry cat UPCDs positive, one for *Salmonella* and the other for *Listeria greyii*. During phase 2, tested were 576 samples with 15 MPCD positive for *Salmonella* and 32 MPCD positive for *Listeria monocytogenes*.[35] The Feed Contaminants Program (2002–2009) and Salmonella Assignment (2007–2009) reported testing of 2058 samples for *Salmonella* with 9.8% of dry UPCDs *Salmonella* positive.[42] As a result of these outbreaks and surveillances, in July 2013, FDA set forth Compliance Policy Guide Sec. 690.800 Salmonella in Food for Animals: "The policies in this guidance apply to finished animal feed and pet food and the ingredients used to manufacture these products. FDA believes regulatory action is warranted in cases involving pet foods contaminated with any *Salmonella* serotype, due to the heightened human health risk given

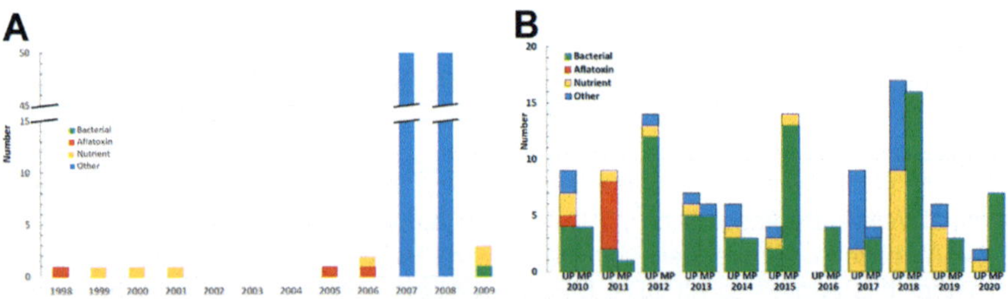

Fig. 1. (*A*) Pet food recalls from 1998 through 2009. UP foods only, as no reports of MP recalls. (*B*) Pet food recalls from 2010 to 2020.

the high likelihood of direct human contact with such food."[43] This policy essentially established a policy of zero tolerance for *Salmonella* in pet food, which is more stringent than policies for human food. When the FDA's Food Safety and Modernization Act was passed, it required all pet food manufacturing companies to have in place appropriate quality control measures to prevent bacterial contamination. Despite these regulations, in 2018, a *Salmonella* outbreak with 90 human illnesses was traced to an MPCD, while state product testing identified *Salmonella* contamination initiating a 2020 UPCD recall.[44,45] It should be understood, although FDA has the authority to initiate recalls, most recalls today are initiated voluntarily by pet food manufacturers.[46] Another concern with bacterial pathogens in pet foods is the antimicrobial resistance in pathogenic bacteria isolates that are reported in more recent studies and reviews of UPCDs and MPCDs.[30,34,47–50] Lambertini and colleagues[36] discuss risk profiles of bacterial pathogens in UPCDS and MP-type diets and concluded MP incurred higher risk, but also stated "none would be risk free." Based on FDA recalls for bacterial pathogens and documented reports of human and pet illness from *Salmonella* from both UPCD and MPCDs, veterinarians should communicate to owners that all pet food types can contain bacterial pathogens and may be a health concern for both humans and pets.

Nutritional Imbalances

Rumbeiha and Morrison[51] reported on UPCD recalls for nutritional imbalances from 1998 to 2008 that included IAMS and Golden Sun Feeds for excess vitamin D3 (7 deaths and 11 illnesses) and IAMS for excess methionine (21 illnesses). **Fig. 1**B shows UPCD recalls are predominantly for nutritional imbalances that include excess copper, thiamine deficiency, excess choline, and excess vitamin D. Most familiar to veterinarians will be the three 2019 recalls of Hills over-the-counter and veterinary therapeutic canned UPCD for excess vitamin D. To date, there has been 1 MPCD recall for thiamine deficiency.

Aflatoxin

The common mycotoxin, aflatoxin, in pet food has been reported as the primary cause of acute illness from pet food worldwide. Mycotoxins can be found in corn, rice, wheat, and other grains as ingredients; therefore, primarily UPCD dry foods are at risk.[52] Mycotoxins are relatively resistant to heat, chemical inactivation, and other types of processing. Aflatoxicosis in dogs and cats can present with signs of feed refusal, anorexia, vomiting, diarrhea, or more severe signs of melena, hematemesis, petechia, icterus, and death. Dogs can die within days of initial signs or have a protracted disease course depending on exposure. Diagnosis is based on history, clinical signs, postmortem changes in the liver, and laboratory testing of the suspect diet.[52,53] Reported in 1952 and described as "hepatitis X," aflatoxins in UPCDs resulted in 71 cases of illness and death in dogs.[54] In 1998, Doane UPCDs were recalled for aflatoxins with at least 25 dog deaths; then, in 2006, Diamond UPCDs were recalled with more than 100 pet deaths followed by 7 more in 2010 to 2011 (see **Fig. 1**A, B).[51,53–55] The concern for aflatoxin would seem overstated except for 2 recent 2020 UPCD recalls for potential aflatoxin.[56]

Other Health Risks in Commercial Diets

The biggest pet food recall began in March 2007, as seen in **Fig. 1**A, from contamination of UPCDs with melamine and cyanuric acid. This contamination was a deliberate contamination by an ingredient supplier for financial gain that resulted in about 53 million cans and pouches of dog and cat food and more than 100 brands of UPCDs recalled. Of the 586 cases of melamine-induced nephrotoxicity, 278 pets (171 cats and 107 dogs) were reported to have died. The melamine investigation also identified melamine poisoning in other countries.[53,57,58]

In 2017 and 2018, there were 7 recalls for thyroid hormone and 8 recalls for pentobarbital in canned UPCD (see **Fig. 1**B).

Pet Food Processing and Advanced Glycation End Products

Food processing is used to increase the taste, safety, shelf life, and bioavailability of nutritional components in foods. One of the adverse effects of thermal pet food processing is the denaturing of proteins. Protein denaturing during thermal food processing involves the Maillard reaction (MR), which is a spontaneous, "nonenzymatic reaction" that occurs between the carbonyl group of reducing sugars and the amino group of amino acids. MR forms compounds necessary for aroma, flavor, and color of food, but in addition, MR can result in dietary "advanced glycation end products" or AGEs.[59] AGEs are also formed in the body by in vivo glycation of tissue proteins, and these are termed "endogenous AGEs." Endogenous AGEs are produced and accumulate with the physiologic processes of aging and disease states. One of the first recognized endogenous AGE identified was hemoglobin A1c, a glucose-derived hemoglobin increased in diabetes mellitus. Both endogenous AGEs and dietary AGEs contribute to the body's AGE pool.[60] Studies implicate that dietary AGEs that add to the total body AGEs have a role in aging and the pathogenesis of chronic disease states.[59] AGE-associated diseases develop via 2 mechanisms: (i) structural alteration of intermolecular and intramolecular cross-linking of tissue proteins that change molecular properties and function, or (ii) by activation of cellular signaling pathways through receptor binding or direct activation to produce reactive oxygen species and an inflammatory response.[59,61] Receptors for AGEs termed RAGE are widely expressed on cells playing roles in oxidative stress, vasoconstriction, excessive collagen deposition, and inflammatory responses. RAGE activation, via AGE binding, may result in development of a chronic inflammatory state, which is observed in many disease states in both humans and dogs. Furthermore, dietary AGEs can impact the intestinal microbiota, compromise epithelial barrier functions, and cause immune stimulation resulting in diseases.[62] This absorption of AGEs from the diet and their accumulation into the AGE pool in the body may be one of the ways diets can impact age-related diseases in humans and animals.[62–66] AGEs have been associated with the cause of age-related diseases in humans, such as atherosclerosis, nephropathy, retinopathy, osteoarthritis, neurodegenerative diseases, and diabetes mellitus. These age-related diseases are also seen in dogs, showing many similarities to these human diseases. Elevated levels of AGEs in tissue proteins were observed in aging dogs with diabetes mellitus, cataracts, osteoarthritis, neurodegenerative diseases, vascular dysfunction, and atherosclerosis.[59,65,67,68]

To promote human public health and prevent chronic disease, it is recommended to limit the intake of UP foods containing high dietary AGEs.[69–72] As pets are now family members, some owners are looking to apply these same recommendations, avoiding UPCDs and instead purchasing MPCDs. As more is learned about the role of AGEs in processed foods, whether for human or pet consumption, food manufacturers will face the challenge to produce foods with lower AGE content while still being palatable, shelf stable, and safe.[59,73–75]

Advanced Glycations End Products Studies in Pet Food

Similar to human foods, UPCDs are subjected to thermal processing, which facilitates the MR and formation of AGEs. AGEs in pet foods may be derived in 3 ways: the pet food ingredients, the conditions of processing, and lysine reactions during coating and storage.[68,76–78] In a study examining different processed forms of dog and cat foods, the AGEs, fructoselysine (FL), carboxymethyllysine (CML), hydroxymethylfurfural (HMF), and lysinoalanine, were measured using Ultra high performance liquid chromatography- mass spectrometry (UHPLC-MS).[79] Based on dry matter analysis, it was found that canned pet foods contained the most FL, HMF, and CML followed by pelleted, and then extruded foods.[79] The investigators calculated that the content of CML and HMF that is present in commercial pet foods is, on average, within the range reported in processed human food products, and that the average daily intake (mg/kg body weight$^{0.75}$) of HMF was 122 times higher for dogs and 38 times higher for cats than the calculated average intake for adult humans. It was concluded that thermal processing used in manufacturing UPCD heavily influences AGE levels, and UPCDs are a significant source of AGEs for dogs and cats.[68,79] Another study determined AGE levels in dry and canned cat UPCDs and analyzed AGEs in urine from cats consuming these diets. Similar to human studies of dietary AGEs absorption and excretion, they reported an increase in urinary AGE excretion with increasing dietary intake of AGEs.[80] Another recent study evaluated urinary AGEs in privately owned dogs and cats consuming differently processed diets. Urinary AGEs in dogs consuming UPCDs were reported to be 2 to 3 times higher compared with dogs consuming raw MPCDs. Similarly, the cats consuming MPCD excreted less AGEs than cats consuming the can/dry or dry UPCDs.[81] A study of the canine plasma concentrations of CML and carboxy-ethyl-lysine (CEL), related to consumption of 4 diets, was done to determine if plasma AGE concentrations would differ between different processed diets: dry UPCD, canned UPCD, air-dried UPCD, and an MPCD. A Latin square design using 8 dogs consuming each diet for 4 weeks was conducted, and food and plasma samples were collected at the end of each feeding period. Samples were analyzed by UHPLC-MS with the UP canned, dry, and air-dried diets containing significantly more AGEs than MPCD. A significant difference in CML and CEL was found between diets and in plasma with higher plasma levels of AGEs reported when dogs consumed canned, dry, and air-dried UPCD as compared with MPCD. These initial studies in dogs, cats, UPCDs, and MPCDs demonstrate, similar to processed human foods, UPCDs contain higher levels of AGEs, and when consumed, result in higher plasma AGEs and urine excretion of AGEs. Future studies to determine the "effect and no effect levels" of AGEs in UPCDs are needed because, unlike humans who eat a variety of processed and unprocessed foods, UPCDs are often the primary source of nutrition for pets, and the majority will consume these diets for their entire lifespan.[68,78–82] It is this author's opinion that, similar to studies of the role of dietary AGEs in humans health and disease, a true benefit of feeding MPCD may be the fact that they contain lower levels of dietary AGEs as compared with UPCD.

CLINIC CARE POINTS

- The descriptive ultra-processed commercial diets for dry and can pet diets and for other less processed commercial diets, minimally processed commercial diets, can be used in veterinarian client discussions about the different types of commercial pet diets.
- Education about safe pet food handling practices should be discussed with clients for all commercial pet diets and treats.
- Veterinarians should be aware of historic and ongoing pet food recalls for health risks, such as nutritional imbalances, bacterial pathogens, aflatoxin, and toxic contaminations.

DISCLOSURES

The author has no commercial or financial conflicts of interest and no funding sources for this publication.

REFERENCES

1. Michel KE. Unconventional diets for dogs and cats. Vet Clin North Am Small Anim Pract 2006;36(6):1269–1281, vi-vii.
2. Freeman LM, Michel KE. Evaluation of raw food diets for dogs. J Am Vet Med Assoc 2001;218(5):705–9.
3. Freeman LM, Chandler ML, Hamper BA, et al. Current knowledge about the risks and benefits of raw meat-based diets for dogs and cats. J Am Vet Med Assoc 2013;243:1549–58.
4. Parr JM, Remillard RL. Handling alternative dietary requests from pet owners. Vet Clin North Am Small Anim Pract 2014;44(4):667–88.
5. Heinze CR, Gomez FC, Freeman LM. Assessment of commercial diets and recipes for home-prepared diets recommended for dogs with cancer. J Am Vet Med Assoc 2012;241(11):1453–60.
6. Wilson SA, Villaverde C, Fascetti AJ, et al. Evaluation of the nutritional adequacy of recipes for home-prepared maintenance diets for cats. J Am Vet Med Assoc 2019;254(10):1172–9.
7. Gibney MJ. Ultra-processed foods: definitions and policy issues. Curr Dev Nutr 2018;3(2):nzy077–.
8. Alam MS, Kaur J, Khaira H, et al. Extrusion and extruded products: changes in quality attributes as affected by extrusion process parameters: a review. Crit Rev Food Sci Nutr 2016;56(3):445–75.
9. Bleiweiss-Sande R, Chui K, Evans EW, et al. Robustness of food processing classification systems. Nutrients 2019;11(6):1344.
10. Monteiro CA, Cannon G, Moubarac JC, et al. The UN decade of nutrition, the NOVA food classification and the trouble with ultra-processing. Public Health Nutr 2018;21(1):5–17.
11. Lopez A, editor. A complete course in canning and related processes. Baltimore, MD: The Canning Trade Inc; 1987.
12. Davies M. Veterinary clinical nutrition: success stories: an overview. Proc Nutr Soc 2016;75(3):392–7.
13. de Godoy MR, Hervera M, Swanson KS, et al. Innovations in canine and feline nutrition: technologies for food and nutrition assessment. Annu Rev Anim Biosci 2016;4:311–33.
14. Hamper BA, Bartges JW, Kirk CA. Evaluation of two raw diets vs a commercial cooked diet on feline growth. J Feline Med Surg 2017;19(4):424–34.
15. Hamper BA, Kirk CA, Bartges JW. Apparent nutrient digestibility of two raw diets in domestic kittens. J Feline Med Surg 2016;18(12):991–6.
16. Algya KM, Cross TL, Leuck KN, et al. Apparent total tract macronutrient digestibility, serum chemistry, urinalysis, and fecal characteristics, metabolites and microbiota of adult dogs fed extruded, mildly cooked, and raw diets. J Anim Sci 2018. https://doi.org/10.1093/jas/sky235.
17. Kerr KR, Vester Boler BM, Morris CL, et al. Apparent total tract energy and macronutrient digestibility and fecal fermentative end-product concentrations of domestic cats fed extruded, raw beef-based, and cooked beef-based diets. J Anim Sci 2012;90(2):515–22.

18. Sandri M, Dal Monego S, Conte G, et al. Raw meat based diet influences faecal microbiome and end products of fermentation in healthy dogs. BMC Vet Res 2017;13(1):65.
19. Herstad KMV, Gajardo K, Bakke AM, et al. A diet change from dry food to beef induces reversible changes on the faecal microbiota in healthy, adult client-owned dogs. BMC Vet Res 2017;13(1):147.
20. Bermingham EN, Young W, Kittelmann S, et al. Dietary format alters fecal bacterial populations in the domestic cat (Felis catus). Microbiologyopen 2013;2(1): 173–81.
21. Young W, Moon CD, Thomas DG, et al. Pre- and post-weaning diet alters the faecal metagenome in the cat with differences in vitamin and carbohydrate metabolism gene abundances. Sci Rep 2016;6:34668.
22. Lawler DF, Larson BT, Ballam JM, et al. Diet restriction and ageing in the dog: major observations over two decades. Br J Nutr 2008;99(4):793–805.
23. Morelli G, Bastianello S, Catellani P, et al. Raw meat-based diets for dogs: survey of owners' motivations, attitudes and practices. BMC Vet Res 2019;15(1):74.
24. Connolly KM, Heinze CR, Freeman LM. Feeding practices of dog breeders in the United States and Canada. J Am Vet Med Assoc 2014;245(6):669–76.
25. Morgan SK, Willis S, Shepherd ML. Survey of owner motivations and veterinary input of owners feeding diets containing raw animal products. PeerJ 2017;5: e3031.
26. Viegas FM, Ramos CP, Xavier RGC, et al. Fecal shedding of Salmonella spp., Clostridium perfringens, and Clostridioides difficile in dogs fed raw meat-based diets in Brazil and their owners' motivation. PLoS One 2020;15(4):e0231275.
27. Schleicher M, Cash SB, Freeman LM. Determinants of pet food purchasing decisions. Can Vet J 2019;60(6):644–50.
28. Bojanic K, Midwinter AC, Marshall JC, et al. Isolation of campylobacter spp. from client-owned dogs and cats, and retail raw meat pet food in the Manawatu, New Zealand. Zoonoses Public Health 2017;64(6):438–49.
29. Bottari B, Bancalari E, Barera A, et al. Evaluating the presence of human pathogens in commercially frozen, biologically appropriate raw pet food sold in Italy. Vet Rec 2020. https://doi.org/10.1136/vr.105893.
30. Davies RH, Lawes JR, Wales AD. Raw diets for dogs and cats: a review, with particular reference to microbiological hazards. J Small Anim Pract 2019;60(6): 329–39.
31. Hellgren J, Hasto LS, Wikstrom C, et al. Occurrence of Salmonella, Campylobacter, Clostridium and Enterobacteriaceae in raw meat-based diets for dogs. Vet Rec 2019;184(14):442.
32. Hinney B. The trend of raw meat-based diets: risks to people and animals. Vet Rec 2018;182(2):47–9.
33. Strohmeyer RA, Morley PS, Hyatt DR, et al. Evaluation of bacterial and protozoal contamination of commercially available raw meat diets for dogs. J Am Vet Med Assoc 2006;228(4):537–42.
34. van Bree FPJ, Bokken G, Mineur R, et al. Zoonotic bacteria and parasites found in raw meat-based diets for cats and dogs. Vet Rec 2018;182(2):50.
35. Nemser SM, Doran T, Grabenstein M, et al. Investigation of Listeria, Salmonella, and toxigenic Escherichia coli in various pet foods. Foodborne Pathog Dis 2014; 11(9):706–9.
36. Lambertini E, Buchanan RL, Narrod C, et al. Transmission of bacterial zoonotic pathogens between pets and humans: the role of pet food. Crit Rev Food Sci Nutr 2016;56(3):364–418.

37. Mehlenbacher S, Churchill J, Olsen KE, et al. Availability, brands, labelling and Salmonella contamination of raw pet food in the Minneapolis/St. Paul area. Zoonoses Public Health 2012;59(7):513–20.
38. FDA Recalls Withdrawals 2020. Available at: https://www.fda.gov/animal-veterinary/safety-health/recalls-withdrawals.
39. Behravesh CB, Ferraro A, Deasy M 3rd, et al. Human Salmonella infections linked to contaminated dry dog and cat food, 2006-2008. Pediatrics 2010;126(3): 477–83.
40. Kukanich KS. Update on Salmonella spp contamination of pet food, treats, and nutritional products and safe feeding recommendations. J Am Vet Med Assoc 2011;238(11):1430–4.
41. Imanishi M, Rotstein DS, Reimschuessel R, et al. Outbreak of Salmonella enterica serotype Infantis infection in humans linked to dry dog food in the United States and Canada, 2012. J Am Vet Med Assoc 2014;244(5):545–53.
42. Li X, Bethune LA, Jia Y, et al. Surveillance of salmonella prevalence in animal feeds and characterization of the salmonella isolates by serotyping and antimicrobial susceptibility. Foodborne Pathog Dis 2012;9(8):692–8.
43. Compliance Policy Guide Sec. 690.800 Salmonella in Food for Animals. U.S. Department of Health and Human Services Food and Drug Administration; Center for Veterinary Medicine Office of Regulatory Affairs; July 2013.
44. Milanov D, Aleksic N, Vidakovic S, et al. Salmonella spp. in pet feed and risk it poses to humans. Food and Feed Research 2019;46(1):137–45.
45. Available at: https://www.fda.gov/safety/recalls-market-withdrawals-safety-alerts/sunshine-mills-inc-issues-voluntary-recall-natures-menur-super-premium-dog-food-blend-real-chicken. Accessed October 8, 2020.
46. Dzanis DA. Anatomy of a recall. Top Companion Anim Med 2008;23(3):133–6.
47. Baede VO, Broens EM, Spaninks MP, et al. Raw pet food as a risk factor for shedding of extended-spectrum beta-lactamase-producing Enterobacteriaceae in household cats. PLoS One 2017;12(11):e0187239.
48. Nilsson O. Hygiene quality and presence of ESBL-producing Escherichia coli in raw food diets for dogs. Infect Ecol Epidemiol 2015;5:28758.
49. Nüesch-Inderbinen M, Treier A, Zurfluh K, et al. Raw meat-based diets for companion animals: a potential source of transmission of pathogenic and antimicrobial-resistant Enterobacteriaceae. R Soc Open Sci 2019;6:191170.
50. Wu Y, Fan R, Wang Y, et al. Analysis of combined resistance to oxazolidinones and phenicols among bacteria from dogs fed with raw meat/vegetables and the respective food items. Sci Rep 2019;9(1):15500.
51. Rumbeiha W, Morrison J. A review of class I and class II pet food recalls involving chemical contaminants from 1996 to 2008. J Med Toxicol 2011;7(1):60–6.
52. Boermans HJ, Leung MC. Mycotoxins and the pet food industry: toxicological evidence and risk assessment. Int J Food Microbiol 2007;119(1–2):95–102.
53. Bischoff K, Rumbeiha WK. Pet food recalls and pet food contaminants in small animals: an update. Vet Clin North Am Small Anim Pract 2018;48(6):917–31.
54. Leung MCK, Díaz-Llano G, Smith TK. Mycotoxins in pet food: a review on worldwide prevalence and preventative strategies. J Agric Food Chem 2006;54(26): 9623–35.
55. Newman S, Smith J, Stenske K, et al. Aflatoxicosis in nine dogs after exposure to contaminated commercial dog food. J Vet Diagn Invest 2007;19:168–75.
56. FDA. Sunshine Mills, Inc. issues voluntary recall of certain dog food products due to potentially elevated levels of aflatoxin. In: FDA, editor. 2020. Available at: https://www.fda.gov/safety/recalls-market-withdrawals-safety-alerts/sunshine-

mills-inc-issues-voluntary-recall-certain-dog-food-products-due-potentially-elevated-levels. Accessed October 8, 2020.
57. Bischoff K, Rumbeiha WK. Pet food recalls and pet food contaminants in small animals. Vet Clin North Am Small Anim Pract 2012;42(2):237–250, v.
58. Rumbeiha WK, Agnew D, Maxie G, et al. Analysis of a survey database of pet food-induced poisoning in North America. J Med Toxicol 2010;6(2):172–84.
59. Uribarri J, del Castillo MD, de la Maza MP, et al. Dietary advanced glycation end products and their role in health and disease. Adv Nutr 2015;6(4):461–73.
60. Poulsen MW, Hedegaard RV, Andersen JM, et al. Advanced glycation endproducts in food and their effects on health. Food Chem Toxicol 2013;60:10–37.
61. Delgado-Andrade C. Maillard reaction products: some considerations on their health effects. Clin Chem Lab Med 2014;52(1):53–60.
62. Teodorowicz M, Hendriks WH, Wichers HJ, et al. Immunomodulation by processed animal feed: the role of Maillard reaction products and advanced glycation end-products (AGEs). Front Immunol 2018;9:2088.
63. Gentzel JB. Does contemporary canine diet cause cancer?; a review. Vet World 2013;6(9):632–9.
64. Teissier T, Boulanger É. The receptor for advanced glycation end-products (RAGE) is an important pattern recognition receptor (PRR) for inflammaging. Biogerontology 2019;20(3):279–301.
65. Hudson BI, Lippman ME. Targeting RAGE signaling in inflammatory disease. Annu Rev Med 2018;69:349–64.
66. Vlassara H, Uribarri J. Advanced glycation end products (AGE) and diabetes: cause, effect, or both? Curr Diab Rep 2014;14(1):453.
67. Chaudhuri J, Bains Y, Guha S, et al. The role of advanced glycation end products in aging and metabolic diseases: bridging association and causality. Cell Metab 2018;28(3):337–52.
68. van Rooijen C, Bosch G, van der Poel AF, et al. The Maillard reaction and pet food processing: effects on nutritive value and pet health. Nutr Res Rev 2013;26(2):130–48.
69. Kim Y, Keogh JB, Deo P, et al. Differential effects of dietary patterns on advanced glycation end products: a randomized crossover study. Nutrients 2020;12(6):1767.
70. AL N, Carbonero F. Impact of Maillard reaction products on nutrition and health: current knowledge and need to understand their fate in the human digestive system. Crit Rev Food Sci Nutr 2019;59(3):474–87.
71. Sharma C, Kaur A, Thind SS, et al. Advanced glycation end-products (AGEs): an emerging concern for processed food industries. J Food Sci Technol 2015;52(12):7561–76.
72. Uribarri J, Woodruff S, Goodman S, et al. Advanced glycation end products in foods and a practical guide to their reduction in the diet. J Am Diet Assoc 2010;110(6):911–6.e12.
73. Cooke J. Dietary reduction of advanced glycation end products: an opportunity for improved nutrition care. J Ren Nutr 2017;27(4):e23–6.
74. Lin JA, Wu CH, Yen GC. Perspective of advanced glycation end products on human health. J Agric Food Chem 2018;66(9):2065–70.
75. Wautier MP, Tessier FJ, Wautier JL. Advanced glycation end products: a risk factor for human health. Ann Pharm Fr 2014;72(6):400–8.
76. Williams PA, Hodgkinson SM, Rutherford SM, et al. Lysine content in canine diets can be severely heat damaged. J Nutr 2006;136:1998S–2000S.

77. Rutherford SM, Rutherford-Marwick KJ, Moughan PJ. Available (ileal digestible reactive) lysine in selected pet foods. J Agric Food Chem 2007;55:3517–22.
78. van Rooijen C, Bosch G, van der Poel AF, et al. Reactive lysine content in commercially available pet foods. J Nutr Sci 2014;3:e35.
79. van Rooijen C, Bosch G, van der Poel AF, et al. Quantitation of Maillard reaction products in commercially available pet foods. J Agric Food Chem 2014;62(35): 8883–91.
80. van Rooijen C, Bosch G, Butré CI, et al. Urinary excretion of dietary Maillard reaction products in healthy adult female cats. J Anim Sci 2016;94(1):185–95.
81. Palaseweenun P, Hagen-Plantinga EA, Schonewille JT, et al. Urinary excretion of advanced glycation end products in dogs and cats. J Anim Physiol Anim Nutr (Berl) 2020;105(1):149–56.
82. Bridglalsingh S. Influence of four differently processed diets on plasma levels of advanced glycation end products (AGEs), serum levels of receptors for advanced glycation end products (RAGE), serum and urine metabolome, and fecal microbiome in healthy dogs [PhD dissertation]. Athens (GA): University of Georgia; 2020.

Sustainability and Pet Food

Is There a Role for Veterinarians?

Heather L. Acuff, MS[1], Amanda N. Dainton, MS[1], Janak Dhakal, DVM, PhD[2], Samuel Kiprotich, MS[1], Greg Aldrich, PhD*

KEYWORDS

• Sustainability • Pet food • Life-cycle assessment • Carbon footprint • Waste

KEY POINTS

- Sustainability is defined here as the conscientious management of resources and waste necessary to meet the physiologic requirements of companion animals without compromising the ability of future generations to meet their environmental, social, or economic needs.
- Life-cycle analysis of pet foods has identified that the most significant impact category to the environment is climate change (quantified as kg CO_2 eq), with wet foods tending to have a greater impact than dry foods, and dogs having a greater impact than cats.
- Opportunities for improvement in sustainability exist at all phases of the pet food life cycle, including formulation, ingredient selection, manufacturing processes, packaging materials, transportation methods, reduction of food and packaging wastes, and proper disposal of pet waste.
- Veterinarians have a central role as a resource for clients on diet selection, feeding management, and proper pet waste disposal practices, as well as the sustainable farming of livestock animals.
- The advancement of sustainable practices in companion animal care will require a collaborative effort between pet food industry stakeholders, veterinarians, and pet owners.

INTRODUCTION

The overuse of resources has become a concern as world populations increase. The environmental footprint of pet ownership and provision of necessary supplies and food for pets on the use of natural resources, emissions, and waste are also growing. The questions regarding the size of that impact and where opportunities for

Department of Grain Science and Industry, Kansas State University, Manhattan, KS 66502, USA
[1] Present address: 1301 Mid Campus Drive, 201 Shellenberger Hall, Manhattan, KS 66506.
[2] Present address: Integrated Life Science Building, 1981 Kraft Drive, Blacksburg, VA 24060.
* Corresponding author. 1301 Mid Campus Drive, 201 Shellenberger Hall, Manhattan, KS 66506.
E-mail address: aldrich4@ksu.edu

Vet Clin Small Anim 51 (2021) 563–581
https://doi.org/10.1016/j.cvsm.2021.01.010 **vetsmall.theclinics.com**

improvement exist begin with the pet owner and the general public's perception of the topic regarding sustainability and move upstream to the raw material suppliers, food manufacturing companies, packaging producers, and transportation sectors. Overcoming barriers to sustainability will require the implementation of successful intervention strategies, and the pet owner will need to assign value to this effort, as sustainable products are likely to cost more at retail. The following objectives are critical to the discussion of sustainability of pet food: (1) to define sustainability and its importance to veterinary practitioners; (2) to describe the life-cycle analysis (LCA) of the pet food industry and identify areas for improvement; (3) to determine how food process, product type, nutrient composition, and ingredient selection might influence the sustainability of pet foods; and (4) to provide veterinarians information about the pet food LCA in order to educate pet owners in areas where they can influence sustainability.

CURRENT KNOWLEDGE

Environmental Impact of Dog and Cat Ownership

According to recent US pet ownership statistics, two-thirds of US households are estimated to own at least 1 pet across nearly 85 million homes.[1] Companion animals enrich the lives of their owners in numerous ways, such as increasing physical activity, lowering blood pressure, and reducing risks of certain heart diseases.[2] Pet ownership has also been associated with psychological benefits, including increased self-esteem in children, reduced risk of depression, and increased social engagement and cohesion.[2–4]

Despite the many rewards of pet ownership, our pet-centric way of life may take a toll on the environment. The growing populations of urbanized pets have been linked to loss of wildlife biodiversity because of predation and disturbance, as well as a greater consumption of goods and services.[5,6] Driven largely by humanization and concern for their pet's well-being, owners serve generous portions of food and treats and supply products that support a comfortable and stimulating environment. Many pets receive regular veterinary care and participate in a variety of vocational and social activities. It is estimated that the cumulative US pet industry expenditures reached $95.7 billion in 2019, with pet food and treats making up the largest sales segment (38%), followed by veterinary care and product sales (31%), and then supplies and other services.[1] All of these place a demand, either directly or indirectly, on the consumption of natural resources and energy and generation of waste into the environment.

Pet excrement (urine and feces) is perhaps the most widely scrutinized contributor to impact the environment. Dog and cat feces present a public health risk because of the potential for pathogenic, parasitic, or antibiotic-resistant microorganism transmission through direct contact or contamination of municipal waterways, especially in urban areas where human and animal populations are dense.[7] Abandoned pet waste carried into nearby streams or lakes by stormwater also contains nutrients that can encourage excessive algae growth and release ammonia, which can be toxic to fish and other aquatic wildlife.[8] Alternative methods of disposal of pet feces include passage through sanitary sewage lines (eg, flushing) or in municipal solid waste channels (eg, landfill). The latter is the preferred method recommended by the Environmental Protection Agency (EPA); however, decaying fecal material results in greenhouse gas (GHG) emissions in the form of CO_2, NH_3, CH_4, and N_2O.[8] Researchers estimate 5.62×10^6 US tons of total (cat and dog) fecal matter are produced annually in the United States.[9] This amount is comparable to the amount of landfill waste generated annually by the state of Indiana (population 6.73 million in 2019).[10]

Several researchers have also evaluated the environmental impact of dogs and cats based on annual pet food consumption, with results ranging from 27 to 1444 kg CO_2 eq per year for dogs (**Table 1**), and 43 to 228 kg CO_2 eq per year for cats (**Table 2**). Because pet excrement is a direct product of food intake, it could be argued that pet food production and consumer purchasing behaviors should shoulder the responsibility of environmental stewardship. Thus, considering sustainability as it relates to all aspects of pet food allows for a broader understanding of the environmental impact of our pets.

Defining Sustainability in the Pet Food Industry

Sustainability has previously been defined as practices that ensure the current population meets their requirements without compromising the ability of future generations to meet their needs.[2] The EPA defines sustainability as a harmonious and productive system in which humans and nature could exist, permitting the fulfilment of social, economic, and other requirements of the present generation without jeopardizing the needs and requirements of future generations.[11] From the perspective of pet food production, sustainability has been defined as the ability to produce pet food in adequate amounts while providing the sufficient essential nutrients required to maintain optimum health and viability now and in the future with the smallest environmental footprint.[12] Here, the authors propose a broader definition for sustainability that incorporates the stewardship of companion animals: the conscientious management of resources and waste necessary to meet the physiologic requirements of companion animals without compromising the ability of future generations to meet their environmental, social, or economic needs.

Quantifying Carbon Footprints with Pet Food Life-Cycle Analysis

The environmental impact of a food system can be quantified by analyzing all material inputs (energy and natural resources) and outputs (waste and emissions) and their associated costs, a process known as LCA. Following ISO 14044:2006 standards, LCA serves as a globally recognized model framework to study the environmental impact categories associated with a product or process such as climate change (biogenic and land use and transformation), ozone depletion, human toxicity risk (cancerous and noncancerous), particulate matter, ionizing radiation, photochemical ozone formation, acidification, eutrophication (terrestrial, freshwater, and marine), freshwater ecotoxicity, and natural resource use.[13]

The LCA of dog and cat foods is highly complex considering the variety of raw materials, manufacturing technologies, and packaging options that exist today. The environmental impact of food and agricultural systems can differ considerably.[14–16] Geographic location also influences the environmental burden of agricultural products, in terms of both production and transportation. In addition to raw material extraction, manufacturing technology (eg, extrusion, canning, baking, freeze-drying), nutritional composition of product (eg, moisture and protein level), packaging specifications, distribution channel, and storage and usage requirements are additional factors interlinked with a product's carbon footprint.

Despite these many complexities, in 2018 the European Commission adopted the Product Environmental Footprint Category Rules (PEFCRs) as a standardized model for calculating environmental impacts for the full life cycle of prepared pet foods for dogs and cats. The model development consists of 4 LCA studies of complete pet foods sold in Europe representing cat and dog foods, kibble, and canned foods. Dog food (wet and dry) collectively had a greater environmental impact than cat food because of higher consumption volume of dog food. The estimated impact of wet food also exceeded dry food because of the high use of natural resources for

Table 1
Summary of climate change impact (CO_2 eq) estimations of dog ownership

Sector	Functional Unit	Assumptions	Footprint Estimation	Geographic Area	Source
Wet dog food	Annual impact for 1 pet	Only includes products sold and consumed in the European Union Average dog weighs 15 kg Excludes impact of use stage	464 kg CO_2 eq	European Union	FEDIAF,[17] 2018
Dry dog food	Annual impact for 1 pet	Only includes products sold and consumed in the European Union Average dog weighs 15 kg Excludes impact of use stage	139 kg CO_2 eq	European Union	FEDIAF,[17] 2018
Companion dogs consuming dry food	Annual impact for 1 pet	Average dog weight of 10–20 kg; per capita dry food consumption of 61–247 kg per year	317–1292 kg CO_2 eq	Netherlands	Martens et al,[75] 2019
Companion medium-sized dogs consuming dry food	Annual impact for 1 pet	Average dog weight of 10–20 kg; per capita dry food consumption of 19–123 kg per year	115–754 kg CO_2 eq	Japan	Martens et al,[75] 2019; Su and Martens,[76] 2018
Companion dogs consuming dry food	Annual impact for 1 pet	Average dog weight of 10–20 kg; per capita dry food consumption of 48–243 kg per year	284–1444 kg CO_2 eq	China	Martens et al,[75] 2019
Companion small-sized dogs consuming dry food	Annual impact for 1 pet	Average dog weight of 1.5–10 kg; per capita dry food consumption of 5–61 kg per year	27–372 kg CO_2 eq	Japan	Martens et al,[75] 2019

Companion large-sized dogs consuming dry food	Annual impact for 1 pet	Average dog weight of 25–59 kg; per capita dry food consumption of 96–498 kg per year	109–191 kg CO_2 eq	Japan	Martens et al,[75] 2019
Average-sized dogs consuming wet food	Annual impact for 1 pet[a]	Average dog weight of 15 kg and average life expectancy of 13 y; per capita wet food consumption of 348 kg per year	631 kg CO_2 eq	European Union	Yavor et al,[77] 2020
Large-sized dogs consuming wet food	Annual impact for 1 pet[a]	Average dog weight of 30 kg and high life expectancy of 18 y; per capita wet food consumption of 365 kg per year	1056 kg CO_2 eq	European Union	Yavor et al,[77] 2020
Small-sized dogs consuming wet food	Annual impact for 1 pet[a]	Average dog weight of 7.5 kg and short life expectancy of 8 y; per capita wet food consumption of 199 kg per year	375 kg CO_2 eq	European Union	Yavor et al,[77] 2020

[a] Annual impact for 1 pet for was calculated as lifetime impact CO_2 eq/life span for each dog size scenario.

Table 2
Summary of climate change impact (CO_2 eq) estimations of cat ownership

Sector	Functional Unit	Assumptions	Footprint Estimation	Geographic Area	Source
Wet cat food	Annual impact for 1 pet	Only includes products sold and consumed in the European Union Average cat weighs 4 kg Excludes impact of use stage	141 kg CO_2 eq	European Union	FEDIAF,[17] 2018
Dry cat food	Annual impact for 1 pet	Only includes products sold and consumed in the European Union Average cat weighs 4 kg Excludes impact of use stage	43 kg CO_2 eq	European Union	FEDIAF,[17] 2018
Companion cats consuming dry food	Annual impact for 1 pet	Average cat weight of 2–6 kg; per capita dry food consumption of 20–33 kg per year	136–228 kg CO_2 eq	Netherlands	Martens et al,[75] 2019
Companion cats consuming dry food	Annual impact for 1 pet	Average cat weight of 2–6 kg; per capita dry food consumption of 18–31 kg per year	110–191 kg CO_2 eq	Japan	Martens et al,[75] 2019; Su & Martens,[76] 2018
Companion cats consuming dry food	Annual impact for 1 pet	Average cat weight of 2–6 kg; per capita dry food consumption of 20–34 kg per year	128–215 kg CO_2 eq	China	Martens et al,[75] 2019

packaging production (tin plating). Overall, the most relevant impact categories for pet food were determined to be climate change, eutrophication (freshwater, marine, terrestrial), land use, and natural resource depletion (water, mineral, and fossil).[17] Although the PEFCRs were developed using data sets for EU energy reporting, pet food production in the United States follows a similar life cycle (**Fig. 1**), and thus, the principles of the PEFCRs could be applied to the US pet food systems.

Pet Food Life-Cycle Analysis by Segment

Diet selection and nutritional composition

There are 2 defining attributes that influence the path of a pet food product's life cycle. Diet selection, which dictates the intended species, life stage, food format, and inclusion or exclusion of specific ingredients, and nutritional composition, which determines the level of raw materials needed to achieve the desired nutrient levels, both of which have a direct impact on the resources required to construct a product.

Protein is the most expensive and ecologically demanding macronutrient, yet is a key factor for the selection of pet food products by pet owners.[18–20] Pets require a moderate level of protein in their diets, with Association of American Feed Control Officials minimums set at 18% for adult dogs and 26% for adult cats on a dry matter (DM) basis.[21,22] However, high-protein formulas (>30% crude protein on a DM basis) are commonly marketed for both species, as more protein may be needed to maintain lean body mass and support the needs of older dogs and cats, and working dogs, as examples. The idea that protein levels in excess of an animal's requirement are beneficial is debatable and adds strain to the increasing global demand for protein for humans, agricultural animals, and companion animals.[9,20]

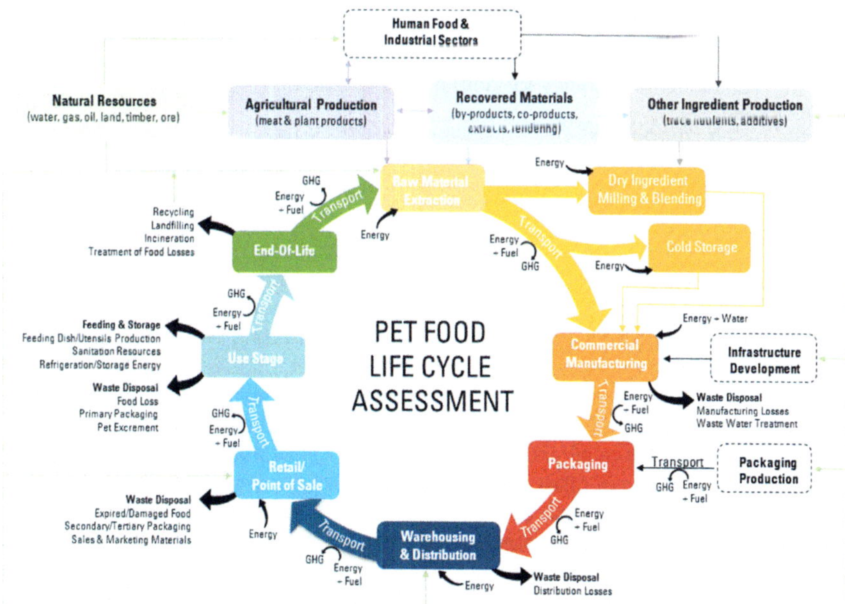

Fig. 1. A generic LCA for commercially prepared pet food beginning with raw material extraction and tracing through manufacturing, packaging, distribution, retail, usage, and end-of-life disposal.

There is a belief, shared by 29.4% of dog owners and 21.7% of cat owners, that raw diets are healthier for their pets; however, only 3.9% of veterinary professionals agree with this.[23] One in 5 pet owners also report following raw feeding practices originating from online resources rather than published references or seeking veterinary advice, which may exacerbate nutritional or safety risks associated with raw feeding.[24] With regard to sustainability, raw pet foods are thought to compete with the human food chain because of the high inclusion of edible ingredients.[25] In addition, the handling and storage of the leftover raw pet food can become a safety concern to pet owners because of the high risk of exposure to pathogens.[26] The American Veterinary Medical Association (AVMA) also discourages feeding pets raw animal-based foods, especially those that have not gone through pathogen elimination steps during processing.[27]

Raw Material Selection

Animal-based protein sources

Much of the protein in pet foods originates from animal sources, and there is a trend for increasing both quality and quantity of meat in pet foods.[9] Dog and cat owners generally prefer meat as a source of protein for their pets compared with alternative sources, such as insect proteins, vegetable proteins, or laboratory-grown meats.[23] Animal-based ingredients are considered to be a high-quality source of dietary protein, containing a complete profile of essential amino acids dogs and cats require. However, these tend to have a greater ecological footprint as compared with plant-based proteins (**Table 3**).[28]

Antibiotic-free protein sources, especially poultry, have become increasingly popular in both human food and pet food. This popularity is attributed to a widely accepted belief that antibiotic-free products are healthier and safer; however, there are no scientific data to support the nutritional superiority of the antibiotic-free animal tissues.[29,30] Antibiotic-free animal production, in turn, has potentially adverse effects on the sustainability aspects of the food chain because of compromised animal health, reduced production efficiency, and increased costs of production.[31] The AVMA recommends the judicious use of medically important antimicrobials in animal production in order TO sustain their utility for both man and animal.[32]

Animal-based coproducts

A by-product, by regulatory definitions, is merely the secondary product produced from manufacturing the primary product. Critics would suggest this presumes the secondary product has little value. The authors' way of thinking should probably shift to that of a "coproduct," in which the entire value proposition is considered. Presuming that there will be meat consumption by the North American human population for the foreseeable future, the proper use of all the available resources, including animal by-products, is necessary.[11] Average carcass yield, or dressing percentage, ranges between 50% and 74% of live animal weight for red meat, pork, and poultry products in the United States, leaving behind a significant portion of animal-derived material that does not enter the human food system.[33] When managed responsibly, producers can lessen the environmental effects of organic waste disposal and help recover valuable nutrients.[34] Clean animal offals, for example, provide good-quality protein and higher levels of trace minerals, such as iron, zinc, calcium, and copper, in comparison to muscle tissues and can be incorporated into pet foods in raw, dried, or rendered forms.[35,36] According to the National Renderers Association, 56 billion pounds of renderable raw material is diverted from landfills and recycled into useable fat, oil, and protein products annually in North America.[37] Rendering also avoids at least 90% of potential GHG emissions when compared with industrial composting, which is equivalent to removing more than 12 million cars from the road.[38]

Table 3
Average global warming potential estimates of select insect-, animal-, and plant-origin ingredients with applications in US pet foods

Ingredient	LCA Study Location[1]	Carbon Footprint (kg CO_2 Eq/kg Functional Unit)	Reference
Insect, origin			
Black soldier fly larvae[a]	DEU	1.36–15.1	Smetana et al,[78] 2016
Animal, origin			
Plains, ranched beef[b]	USA	20.4–23.2	Rotz et al,[79] 2019
Pasture, finished beef[c]	USA	19.2	Pelletier et al,[80] 2010
Feedlot beef[c]	USA	14.8	Pelletier et al,[80] 2010
Grassland, grazed lamb[b]	NZL	19	Ledgard et al,[81] 2011
Hillside, raised lambs[c]	ENG	17.9	Jones et al,[82] 2014
Lowland, raised lambs[c]	ENG	10.9	Jones et al,[82] 2014
Organic farmed salmon[c]	CAN	2.7	Pelletier and Tyedmers,[83] 2007
Farmed salmon[c]	CAN	2.1	Pelletier and Tyedmers,[83] 2007
Pork[c]	USA	2.01–3.02	Thoma et al,[84] 2015
Chicken[c]	USA	1.99	Putman et al,[85] 2017
Poultry by-product meal	PRT	0.73	Campos et al,[86] 2020
Poultry fat	PRT	0.67	Campos et al,[86] 2020
Hydrolyzed feather meal	PRT	0.60	Campos et al,[86] 2020
Rendered animal protein	GBR	0.15	Ramirez et al,[87] 2012
Rendered animal fat	GBR	−0.77 to 0.15	Ramirez et al,[87] 2012
Plant, origin			
Rice	USA	1.41–1.88	Johnson et al,[88] 2016
Potato	FRA	0.10–0.11	Godard et al,[89] 2012
Sorghum	USA	0.60–1.24	Johnson et al,[88] 2016
Wheat	USA	0.45–1.32	Johnson et al,[88] 2016
Soybean	USA	0.34–0.70	Johnson et al,[88] 2016
Oats	FRA	0.31	Wilfart et al,[90] 2016
Corn	USA	0.30–1.68	Johnson et al,[88] 2016
Spring peas	FRA	0.29	Wilfart et al,[90] 2016
Rainfed legumes	ESP	0.23	Aguilera et al,[91] 2015

[a] Functional unit = 1 kg insect protein meal.
[b] Functional unit = 1 kg carcass weight.
[c] Functional unit = 1 kg live weight.
[1] CAN = Canada; DEU = Germany; ENG = England; ESP = Spain; FRA = France; GBR = United Kingdom; NZL = New Zealand; PRT = Portugal; USA = United States of America

Plant-based ingredients

Exchanging protein sources of animal origin with those of plant origin has been proposed to improve the sustainability of pet foods by using fewer natural resources and maintaining a smaller carbon footprint.[39] Animal-based proteins are widely perceived as superior in quality for dogs and cats compared with plant-based proteins; however, the relative digestibility has been reported to be similar between both sources.[40] Plant-based proteins generally contain a limited amount of 1 or 2 essential amino acids, which reduces their overall protein quality. However, by combining complementary ingredients, those that provide an abundance of the limiting amino acids of the other, the overall quality of plant-based protein can be at least as good as that from animal-source proteins.[41] Dogs, being omnivores, are well adapted for a plant-based diet; however, cats are obligate carnivores, so are not able to meet their nutritional requirements from unsupplemented plant-based diets alone.[42]

In addition to providing bioavailable protein, fat, and energy to pets (**Table 4**), plant-based ingredients and their coproducts possess food-functional properties as well. An ingredient that is currently underutilized but has substantial availability includes distillers dried grains with solubles (DDGS) derived from ethanol production. For instance, 50 kg of corn yields approximately 20.8 L of ethanol, which reduces the dependence on fossil fuels and generates 13.9 kg of DDGS. DDGS contain moderate levels of protein and fermentable fiber and improve palatability in pet food applications.[43] Plant-based coproduct inclusion in foods for pets supports environmental sustainability by using every aspect of the respective crop and supports economic sustainability by increasing the number of competitively priced ingredients available to pet food formulators.

Meat analogues are emerging sources of dietary protein that imitate the texture, appearance, or flavor of animal muscle tissues.[44] Dried texturized vegetable protein is an example of a modern meat analogue that can be made from extruded defatted soy meal, soy protein concentrates, or wheat gluten.[45,46] Plant-based proteins with elastic or spongy textures, such as wheat gluten and soy protein, also offer versatility in structural formation, and texturized soy proteins can produce meatlike textural attributes with high nutritional quality.[47–50] These components have been used with success in canned, frozen, or dried pet foods.

Alternative ingredients

Alternative ingredients, such as single-cell organisms (SCO: yeast, fungi, and algae) and insects, are being evaluated as potential meat or plant substitutes.[51] The idea behind use of SCO and insects is that they can be grown on carbon sources that might otherwise be considered unrecoverable in the food production system. For example, a recent LCA of microbial protein produced using a potato wastewater system reported an 87% lower impact on the ecosystem compared with traditional soybean meal production.[52] Microbial proteins are currently being used as a source of high-quality protein and essential fatty acids in aquaculture and are reported to contain higher levels of crude protein compared with conventional animal or plant sources.[53] Insects, such as black soldier fly (*Hermetia illucens*) larvae, housefly (*Musca domestica*), and mealworm (*Tenebrio molitor*), are a major protein source in many countries in Asia, Africa, and Latin America, but are less common in the United States because of negative public perceptions.[54] Application of insect protein as a key ingredient in pet food formulation has gained interest; however, there are few data regarding nutritional quality, and regulatory approvals are pending.[55–57]

Commercial Manufacturing

The greatest potential for sustainability improvement within the commercial manufacturing sectors are cropland, energy, and water usage.[58] Total annual production of dog and cat food in the United States is estimated to be 9.8 million metric tons.[59] Through LCA, the environmental impact translates to roughly 851 gha of cropland, 14 TJ of energy, and 686,821 KL of water used to produce 1 metric ton of pet food.[58] There is room for improvement, but the impacts made by producing food for dogs and cats are estimated to be lower than many human food product industries.[58]

Impacts on cropland are not directly affected by processing, but energy usage and water could be decreased with operational planning, such as installing more energy

Table 4
Proximate composition (as-is basis) of select pet food ingredients and coproducts

Ingredient	DM, %	CP, %	Fat, %	TDF, %	Ash, %	Reference
Beef, MSM	40.6	15.0	23.5	0.0	2.1	NRC,[92] 2006
Beef liver	31.0	20.0	3.9	0.0	1.3	NRC,[92] 2006
Beef heart	24.4	17.1	3.8	0.0	1.0	NRC,[92] 2006
Beef kidney	23.0	16.6	3.1	0.0	1.1	NRC,[92] 2006
Beef tripe	18.6	14.6	4.0	0.0	0.4	NRC,[92] 2006
Animal fat	99.0	0.0	98.0	NR	NR	Batal et al,[93] 2016
Meat & bone meal	92.0	45.0	8.5	NR	37.0	Batal et al,[93] 2016
Chicken, whole carcass	33.9	18.5	12.0	NR	NR	Kadim et al,[94] 2005
Chicken, meat & skin	38.2	17.6	20.3	0.0	1.0	NRC,[92] 2006
Chicken gizzard	23.8	18.2	4.2	0.0	0.9	NRC,[92] 2006
Chicken liver	26.4	18.0	3.9	0.0	1.2	NRC,[92] 2006
Poultry fat	99.0	0.0	98.0	NR	NR	Batal et al,[93] 2016
Chicken meal	95.9	64.2	12.2	NR	14.7	Donadelli et al,[96] 2019
Poultry by-product meal	93.5	59.0	13.5	NR	16.0	NRC,[92] 2006
Feather meal	93.0	85.0	4.0	NR	3.9	Batal et al,[93] 2016
Dried whole egg	96.6	47.2	41.1	0.0	3.6	NRC,[92] 2006
Eggshell meal	99.6	6.6	0.0	NR	53.6	Ode et al,[95] 2016
SD egg white	91.1	76.0	0.1	NR	4.9	Donadelli et al,[96] 2019
SD inedible whole egg	93.5	45.8	34.9	NR	3.9	Donadelli et al,[96] 2019
Corn meal, whole kernel	89.7	8.1	3.6	7.3	1.1	NRC,[92] 2006
Corn starch	91.7	0.3	0.1	0.9	0.1	NRC,[92] 2006
Corn germ meal	90.1	28.4	6.0	45.0	3.9	de Godoy et al,[97] 2009
Corn gluten meal	89.1	55.2	1.1	NR	1.2	Donadelli et al,[96] 2019
Corn protein concentrate	91.4	72.1	2.3	NR	0.8	Donadelli et al,[96] 2019
Corn fiber	90.9	11.0	6.0	71.4	0.9	de Godoy et al,[97] 2009
DDGS	90.2	26.8	9.0	NR	4.7	NRC,[92] 2006
Soybean flour, full fat	96.2	38.1	21.9	NR	5.9	NRC,[92] 2006
Soybean meal, expeller	89.0	42.0	3.5	NR	6.0	Batal et al,[93] 2016
Soy protein isolate	95.0	84.6	0.6	NR	3.8	Donadelli et al,[96] 2019
Soybean hulls	90.9	12.6	2.4	NR	4.4	NRC,[92] 2006
Wheat flour, whole grain	89.7	13.7	1.9	12.2	1.6	NRC,[92] 2006
Wheat flour, white	88.1	10.3	1.0	2.7	0.5	NRC,[92] 2006
Wheat germ meal	89.0	25.0	7.0	NR	5.3	Batal et al,[93] 2016
Wheat gluten	93.3	75.6	0.8	NR	0.8	Tomás-Vidal et al,[98] 2017
Wheat middlings	89.5	16.6	4.0	NR	4.5	NRC,[92] 2006
Wheat bran	89.0	14.8	4.0	NR	6.4	Batal et al,[93] 2016

Abbreviations: MSM, mechanically separated meat; NR, not reported; SD, spray-dried; TDF, total dietary fiber.

efficient equipment or reducing the amount of water used during extrusion or retort processing. A tuna canning plant for pet food in Thailand reduced their water consumption by 32% by switching to hot water and reducing water usage when cleaning cans, cooling cans with pressurized spray nozzles, and teaching employees about the importance of using less water and how they could make a difference.[60] Many such decisions could be considered when new pet food manufacturing facilities are built.

Food Packaging

Food packaging serves many important functions, including protecting food from spoilage and nutritional degradation, improving efficiencies in distribution and storage, and serving as a source of information to feed regulators and pet owners. Pet food bags and containers are commonly constructed from layers of plastic (polyethylene and its derivatives), paper and paperboard, or metals (aluminum, tin, or steel). Most pet food packages are also designed for single use and nonrecyclable, leaving pet owners few options besides disposal.[61] Food containers and packaging waste are estimated to make up just under one-third of all municipal solid waste in the United States.[62] Packaging developers face many challenges with regards to sustainability. In order for sustainable packaging to be effective, it must reduce food waste, preserve food quality, and prevent food contamination. It must also address the issue of plastic waste accumulation in the environment. In addition, the materials must also be nontoxic for humans and animals, and cost-effective for feasibility of use.[63]

The next generation of sustainable food packaging research is focusing on the use of renewable starting materials to develop biodegradable polymeric films. For example, dairy-based films are currently being explored as an alternative to petroleum-based packaging by the Agricultural Research Service.[64] Biopolymers from cornstarch, chitosan, carrot processing waste, cellulose, and other agricultural products also show promise for biodegradable film construction in the effort to reduce plastic wastes accumulation in the environment.[65–67] However, the cost and performance of ecofriendly and lower-barrier packaging compared with synthetic alternatives may still impede their widespread adoption.

Transportation and Distribution

The transportation of material between each phase of the pet food life cycle is an integral part of today's modern food system; however, it contributes directly to fossil fuel consumption and GHG emissions. The EPA estimates a total 6677 million metric tons of GHG emissions were produced in the United States in 2018, of which transportation was the largest contributor at 29%, followed by electricity (27%), industry (22%), commercial and residential (13%), and agriculture (10%).[68] The concept of "food miles" is an important consideration because many raw materials, packaging, and finished products embark on global transport through its life cycle. Reduction of pet food's carbon footprint through sourcing local or regional raw materials is a marketing strategy that has gained popularity.

In addition to geographic distance traveled, the method of transport has an impact on GHG emissions from fossil fuel combustion. The US Department of Transportation estimates that the largest share of total GHG emissions by vehicle type are passenger vehicles and light-duty trucks (59%), medium and heavy-duty trucks (23%), aircraft (9%), ships and boats (3%), rail (2%), and buses, motorcycles, and pipelines (4%).[69] Many of the early pet food life-cycle phases use bulk transportation of dry ingredients, which minimizes the number of vehicles required, and thus the environmental burden. However, when transportation of high-moisture commodities, such as fresh or frozen animal or plant products, is required, the use of refrigerated trucks can exacerbate energy consumption. Consumer shopping behaviors, such as transportation method, trip length, and trip frequency, also play an important role in the "last mile" of the pet food life cycle.[70] Direct-to-consumer models are estimated to have a net carbon footprint similar to traditional brick-and-mortar retailers because of expedited shipping methods, an increase in lightweight parcel delivery vehicles routing to pet owner residences, and inefficient transit packaging to protect the product from damage in shipping.[71]

APPLICABILITY TO VETERINARY PRACTITIONERS

An overwhelming majority of US dogs and cats are taken to their veterinarian at least once a year.[18] Veterinarians are regarded as reliable sources of information on pet food and pet nutrition and have influence over the foods owners purchase.[72,73] During annual visits, veterinarians have the opportunity to educate owners on the importance of pet foods and ingredients, as well as guidance on diet selection, feeding quantities, and waste management strategies, thus influencing the environmental impact of their clients and patients.

Veterinarians also play a central role in the sustainable farming of livestock animals.[74] Because veterinarians are a trusted source of information for livestock producers, communicating about animal welfare, judicious use of antibiotics, and the search for alternative and sustainable sources of food for livestock are a few key factors in which veterinarians can take a lead. Furthermore, veterinary professionals serve as educators of food safety, food quality, food security, and biodiversity maintenance. Because of the nature of veterinary professionals' daily duties and their regular interaction with both livestock producers and pet owners, the hands-on sharing of information has become critical for a client to begin considering sustainability in the food selections they make for their animals.

SUMMARY

Sustainability in the pet food industry can be summarized as those practices and beliefs that can continue indefinitely for future generations. Key opportunities for the improvement to sustainability of pet foods involve sustainable ingredient selection, avoiding nutritional and feeding excesses, and optimizing resource and waste management. Progress will depend on the collective efforts of suppliers, manufacturers, personnel, availability of ingredients, and consumer purchasing choices. There are many aspects of the pet food industry that are sustainable, such as using coproducts from the human food industry and decreasing energy and natural resources used during production. In fact, pet food production is more sustainable than many human food processing industries in terms of cropland, energy, and water usage. However, the pet food industry's ability to adopt some of these practices is limited by negative perceptions of coproducts and novel ingredients, as well as expectations for increasingly rapid product delivery. It also appears that pet owners may not fully understand the direct impacts purchasing decisions have on sustainability. Veterinarians are uniquely positioned to educate pet owners when they bring their animals in for examinations. This education could be in the form of providing more information about the benefits of coproducts discussed here and how to decrease the impact of their pets on the sustainability of pet food. Pet food companies respond to the values of pet owners, and an increase in pet owner awareness and interest in sustainability will encourage the pet food industry to continue improving in this area.

CLINICS CARE POINTS

- Veterinarians have an opportunity to cultivate sustainable practices by educating clients on proper waste disposal, conscientious food selection, and optimal feeding management.

- Veterinarians can help socially conscious pet owners manage their pet's diet in a sustainable manner by encouraging a modest level of protein and the use of conventional ingredients.
- Evidence provided by life-cycle analysis indicates that plant-origin ingredients tend to have a lower carbon footprint compared with animal-origin ingredients, and that poultry, fish, and rendered animal proteins have a lower carbon footprint compared with large ruminant proteins.
- The carbon footprint of pet ownership in the United States is trivial compared with that of the human waste, transportation, and industrial sectors.

DISCLOSURE

The authors have nothing to disclose.

REFERENCES

1. American Pet Products Association (APPA). Pet industry market size and ownership statistics. 2020. Available at: http://www.americanpetproducts.org/pubs_survey.asp. Accessed July 23, 2020.
2. Swanson KS, Carter RA, Yount TP, et al. Nutritional sustainability of pet foods. Adv Nutr 2013;4(2):141–50.
3. Allen KM, Blascovich J, Tomaka J, et al. Presence of human friends and pet dogs as moderators of autonomic responses to stress in women. J Pers Soc Psychol 1991;61(4):582–9.
4. Serpell J. Beneficial effects of pet ownership on some aspects of human health and behaviour. J R Soc Med 1991;84(12):717–20.
5. Reed SE, Merenlender AM. Efectos del manejo de perros domésticos y recreación sobre carnívoros en areas protegidas en el norte de California. Conserv Biol 2011;25(3):504–13.
6. Kitts-Morgan SE. Sustainable ecosystems: domestic cats and their effect on wildlife populations. J Anim Sci 2015;93:848–59.
7. Cinquepalmi V, Monno R, Fumarola L, et al. Environmental contamination by dog's faeces: a public health problem? Int J Environ Res Public Health 2013;10(1):72–84.
8. Paillat JM, Robin P, Hassouna M, et al. Predicting ammonia and carbon dioxide emissions from carbon and nitrogen biodegradability during animal waste composting. Atmos Environ 2005;39(36):6833–42.
9. Okin GS. Environmental impacts of food consumption by dogs and cats. PLoS One 2017;12(8). https://doi.org/10.1371/journal.pone.0181301.
10. United States Census Bureau. Annual estimates of the resident population for the United States, Regions, states, and Puerto Rico: April 1, 2010 to July 1, 2019 2019. Available at: https://www.census.gov/data/tables/time-series/demo/popest/2010s-state-total.html. Accessed 23 July 2020.
11. Fiksel J, Tarsha E, Frederickson H. A framework for sustainability indicators at EPA. 2012; 4-5. Environmental Protection Agency (EPA) Office of Research and Development. Available at: https://www.epa.gov/sites/production/files/2014-10/documents/framework-for-sustainability-indicators-at-epa.pdf. Accessed July 23, 2020.
12. Meeker DL, Meisinger JL. Rendered ingredients significantly influence sustainability, quality, and safety of pet food. J Anim Sci 2015;93:835–47.

13. International Standardization Organization (ISO). ISO 14044:2006 environmental management – life cycle assessment – requirements and guidelines. 2006. Available at: https://www.iso.org/standard/39498. Accessed July 23, 2020.
14. McCarthy D, Matopoulos A, Davies P. Life cycle assessment in the food supply chain: a case study. Int J Logist Res Appl 2015;18(2):140–54.
15. Cucurachi S, Scherer L, Guinée J, et al. Life cycle assessment of food systems. One Earth 2019;1(3):292–7.
16. Eady S, Carre A, Grant T. Life cycle assessment modelling of complex agricultural systems with multiple food and fibre co-products. J Clean Prod 2012;28: 143–9.
17. European Pet Food Industry Federation (FEDIAF); C&D Foods; FACCO, Chambre Syndicale des Fabricants d'Aliments pour Chiens, Chats, Oiseaux et autres Animaux Familiers (the French Pet Food Association for Dogs, Cats, Birds and Other Domestic Pets); Mars PetCare Europe; Nestlé Purina PetCare Europe; Saturn Petcare GmbH, and Quantis. Product environmental footprint category rules (PEFCRs): prepared pet food for cats and dogs, final version; European Commission: Brussels, Belgium. 2018. Available at: https://ec.europa.eu/environment/eussd/smgp/pdf/PEFCR_PetFood_FinalPEFCRs_2018-05-09.pdf. Accessed July 23, 2020.
18. Laflamme DP, Abood SK, Fascetti AJ, et al. Pet feeding practices of dog and cat owners in the United States and Australia. J Am Vet Med Assoc 2008;232(5): 687–94.
19. Berardy A, Johnston CS, Plukis A, et al. Integrating protein quality and quantity with environmental impacts in life cycle assessment. Sustainability 2019;11(10): 2747.
20. Nijdam D, Rood T, Westhoek H. The price of protein: review of land use and carbon footprints from life cycle assessments of animal food products and their substitutes. Food Policy 2012;37(6):760–70.
21. Association of American Feed Control Officials (AAFCO). AAFCO dog food nutrient profiles based on dry matter. In: Lueders D, editor. 2020 Official Publication. West Lafayette (IN): Association of American Feed Control Officials Inc; 2020. p. 158.
22. Association of American Feed Control Officials (AAFCO). AAFCO cat food nutrient profiles based on dry matter. In: Lueders D, editor. 2020 Official Publication. West Lafayette (IN): Association of American Feed Control Officials Inc; 2020. p. 168.
23. Association for Pet Obesity Prevention (APOP). 2018 pet obesity survey results. 2018. Available at: https://petobesityprevention.org/2018. Accessed July 23, 2020.
24. Morgan SK, Willis S, Shepherd ML. Survey of owner motivations and veterinary input of owners feeding diets containing raw animal products. PeerJ 2017; 2017(3):1–16.
25. Famula TR. Domestication of animals. In: Van Alfen NK, editor. Encyclopedia of agriculture and food systems. Second edition. Waltham (MA): Elsevier Inc.; 2014. p. 462–73.
26. Freeman LM, Chandler ML, Hamper BA, et al. Current knowledge about the risks and benefits of raw meat-based diets for dogs and cats. J Am Vet Med Assoc 2013;243(11):1549–58.
27. American Veterinary Medical Association (AVMA). Raw or undercooked animal-source protein in cat and dog diets. 2012. Available at: https://www.avma.org/

resources-tools/avma-policies/raw-or-undercooked-animal-source-protein-cat-and-dog-diets. Accessed July 23, 2020.
28. Pimentel D, Pimentel M. Sustainability of meat-based and plant-based diets and the environment. Am J Clin Nutr 2003;78(3):660S–3S.
29. Newman L, Mehlhorn J, Tewari R, et al. Consumer perception of antibiotic-free and hormone-free meat products. J Food Stud 2020;9(1):80.
30. Smith-Spangler C, Brandeau ML, Hunter GE, et al. Are organic foods safer or healthier than conventional alternatives? Ann Intern Med 2012;157(5):348–66.
31. Cervantes HM. Antibiotic-free poultry production: is it sustainable? J Appl Poult Res 2015;24(1):91–7.
32. American Veterinary Medical Association (AVMA). Raising food animals without antibiotics: is it sustainable? 2018. Available at: https://www.avma.org/blog/raising-food-animals-without-antibiotics-it-sustainable. Accessed July 23, 2020.
33. Knight R. Livestock & meat domestic data: all meat statistics. Washington, DC: United States Department of Agriculture Economic Research Service; 2020. Available at: https://www.ers.usda.gov/data-products/livestock-meat-domestic-data/. Accessed October 10, 2020.
34. Gooding CH, Meeker DL. Review: comparison of 3 alternatives for large-scale processing of animal carcasses and meat by-products. Prof Anim Sci 2016;32(3):259–70.
35. Murray SM, Patil AR, Fahey GC Jr, et al. Raw and rendered animal by-products as ingredients in dog diets. J Anim Sci 1997;75(9):2497–505.
36. Biel W, Czerniawska-Piatkowska E, Kowalczyk A. Offal chemical composition from veal, beef, and lamb maintained in organic production systems. Animals 2019;9(8):489–99.
37. National Renderers Association. Rendering is recycling infographic. 2014. Available at: https://renderingisrecycling.com/2014/07/02/infographic1/. Accessed July 23, 2020.
38. Meeker DL, Hamilton CR. An overview of the rendering industry. In: Meeker DL, editor. Essential rendering : all about the animal by-products industry. Arlington (VA): National Renderers Association; 2006. p. 1–16.
39. Knight A, Leitsberger M. Vegetarian versus meat-based diets for companion animals. Animals 2016;6(9):57.
40. Golder C, Weemhoff JL, Jewell DE. Cats have increased protein digestibility as compared to dogs and improve their ability to absorb protein as dietary protein intake shifts from animal to plant sources. Animals 2020;10(3):541–52.
41. Li P, Wu G. Composition of amino acids and related nitrogenous nutrients in feedstuffs for animal diets. Amino Acids 2020;52(4):523–42.
42. Legrand-Defretin V. Differences between cats and dogs: a nutritional view. Proc Nutr Soc 1994;53(1):15–24.
43. Silva JR, Sabchuk TT, Lima DC, et al. Use of distillers dried grains with solubles (DDGS), with and without xylanase, in dog food. Anim Feed Sci Technol 2016;220:136–42.
44. Ismail I, Hwang Y-H, Joo S-T. Meat analog as future food: a review. J Anim Sci Technol 2020;62(2):111–20.
45. Asgar MA, Fazilah A, Huda N, et al. Nonmeat protein alternatives as meat extenders and meat analogs. Compr Rev Food Sci Food Saf 2010;9(5):513–29.
46. Kumar P, Chatli MK, Mehta N, et al. Meat analogues: health promising meat substitutes. Crit Rev Food Sci Nutr 2017;57(5):923–32.

47. Orcutt MW, McMindes MK, Chu H, et al. Textured soy protein utilization in meat and meat analog products. In: Riaz MN, editor. Soy applications in food. New York: CRC Press; 2006. p. 155–584.
48. Stein HH, Berger LL, Drackley JK, et al. Nutritional properties and feeding values of soybeans and their coproducts. In: Johnson LA, White PJ, Galloway R, editors. Soybeans: chemistry, production, processing, and utilization. Urbana (IL): AOCS Press; 2008. p. 613–60.
49. Featherstone S. Ingredients used in the preparation of canned foods. In: Featherstone S, editor. A complete course in canning and related processes. 4th edition. Oxford (England): Woodhead; 2015. p. 147–211.
50. Sha L, Xiong YL. Plant protein-based alternatives of reconstructed meat: science, technology, and challenges. Trends Food Sci Technol 2020;102:51–61.
51. Food and Agriculture Organization (FAO) of the United Nations. Edible insects. Future prospects for food and feed security. 2013. Available at: http://www.fao.org/3/i3253e/i3253e.pdf. Accessed July 23, 2020.
52. Spiller M, Muys M, Papini G, et al. Environmental impact of microbial protein from potato wastewater as feed ingredient: comparative consequential life cycle assessment of three production systems and soybean meal. Water Res 2020; 171:115406.
53. Matassa S, Boon N, Pikaar I, et al. Microbial protein: future sustainable food supply route with low environmental footprint. Microb Biotechnol 2016;9(5):568–75.
54. Kim TK, Yong HI, Kim YB, et al. Edible insects as a protein source: a review of public perception, processing technology, and research trends. Food Sci Anim Resour 2019;39(4):521–40.
55. McCusker S, Buff PR, Yu Z, et al. Amino acid content of selected plant, algae and insect species: a search for alternative protein sources for use in pet foods. J Nutr Sci 2014;3. https://doi.org/10.1017/jns.2014.33.
56. Mouithys-Mickalad A, Schmitt E, Dalim M, et al. Black soldier fly (*Hermetia illucens*) larvae protein derivatives: potential to promote animal health. Animals 2020;10(6):941.
57. Bosch G, Zhang S, Oonincx DGAB, et al. Protein quality of insects as potential ingredients for dog and cat foods. J Nutr Sci 2014;3:E29.
58. Egilmez G, Kucukvar M, Tatari O, et al. Supply chain sustainability assessment of the U.S. food manufacturing sectors: a life cycle-based frontier approach. Resour Conserv Recycl 2014;82:8–20.
59. Institute of Feed Education & Research (IFEEDER). Pet food production and ingredient analysis. 2020. Available at: http://ifeeder.org/wp-content/uploads/200218-Pet-Food-Report.pdf. Accessed July 23, 2020.
60. Uttamangkabovorn M, Prasertsan P, Kittikun AH. Water conservation in canned tuna (pet food) plant in Thailand. J Clean Prod 2005;13(6):547–55.
61. Nemat B, Razzaghi M, Bolton K, et al. The potential of food packaging attributes to influence consumers' decisions to sort waste. Sustain 2020;12(6). https://doi.org/10.3390/su12062234.
62. United States Environmental Protection Agency (EPA). Facts and figures about materials. Waste and recycling: containers and packaging. 2017. Available at: https://www.epa.gov/facts-and-figures-about-materials-waste-and-recycling/containers-and-packaging-product-specific-data. Accessed July 23, 2020.
63. Pauer E, Wohner B, Heinrich V, et al. Assessing the environmental sustainability of food packaging: an extended life cycle assessment including packaging-related food losses and waste and circularity assessment. Sustain 2019;11(3). https://doi.org/10.3390/su11030925.

64. Agricultural Research Service. Improving the sustainability and quality of food and dairy products from manufacturing to consumption via process modeling and edible packaging. Research project #428714. United States Department of Agriculture. 2020. Available at: https://www.ars.usda.gov/research/project/?accnNo=428714. Accessed July 23, 2020.
65. Dorado AA, Peralta EK, Carpio EV, et al. Biodegradable corn starch/silica nanocomposite sheets for food packaging applications. Mater Sci Forum 2017;894 MSF:66–71.
66. Miteluţ AC, Tănase E, Popa VI, et al. Sustainable alternative for food packaging: chitosan biopolymer - a review. Agrolife Sci J 2015;4(2):52–61.
67. Otoni CG, Lodi BD, Lorevice MV, et al. Optimized and scaled-up production of cellulose-reinforced biodegradable composite films made up of carrot processing waste. Ind Crops Prod 2018;121:66–72.
68. United States Environmental Protection Agency (EPA). Inventory of U.S. Greenhouse gas emissions and Sinks: 1990-2018. 2020. Available at: https://www.epa.gov/ghgemissions/inventory-us-greenhouse-gas-emissions-and-sinks. Accessed July 23, 2020.
69. United States Department of Transportation. Transportation GHG emissions and trends. 2004. Available at: https://www.transportation.gov/sustainability/climate/transportation-ghg-emissions-and-trends. Accessed July 23, 2020.
70. van Loon P, Deketele L, Dewaele J, et al. A comparative analysis of carbon emissions from online retailing of fast moving consumer goods. J Clean Prod 2015;106:478–86.
71. Shahmohammadi S, Steinmann ZJN, Tambjerg L, et al. Comparative greenhouse gas footprinting of online versus traditional shopping for fast-moving consumer goods: a stochastic approach. Environ Sci Technol 2020;54(6):3499–509.
72. Boya UO, Dotson MJ, Hyatt EM. A comparison of dog food choice criteria across dog owner segments: an exploratory study. Int J Consum Stud 2015;39(1):74–82.
73. Sprinkle D. Pet owners trust veterinarians for food purchasing advice revealed. Pet food forum 2018 personal communication. Available at: https://www.petfoodforumevents.com/news/pet-owners-trust-veterinarians-food-purchasing-advice-revealed-petfood-forum-2018-speaker/. Accessed July 23, 2020.
74. Cáceres SB. The roles of veterinarians in meeting the challenges of health and welfare of livestock and global food security. Vet Res Forum Int Q J 2012;3(3):155–7.
75. Martens P, Su B, Deblomme S. The ecological paw print of companion dogs and cats. Bioscience 2019;69(6):467–74.
76. Su B, Martens P. Environmental impacts of food consumption by companion dogs and cats in Japan. Ecol Indic 2018;93:1043–9.
77. Yavor KM, Lehmann A, Finkbeiner M. Environmental impacts of a pet dog: an LCA case study. Sustain 2020;12(8):3394–406.
78. Smetana S, Palanisamy M, Mathys A, et al. Sustainability of insect use for feed and food: life cycle assessment perspective. J Clean Prod 2016;137:741–51.
79. Rotz CA, Asem-Hiablie S, Place S, et al. Environmental footprints of beef cattle production in the United States. Agric Syst 2019;169:1–13.
80. Pelletier N, Pirog R, Rasmussen R. Comparative life cycle environmental impacts of three beef production strategies in the Upper Midwestern United States. Agric Syst 2010;103(6):380–9.
81. Ledgard SF, Lieffering M, Coup D, et al. Carbon footprinting of New Zealand lamb from the perspective of an exporting nation. Anim Front 2011;1(1):40–5.

82. Jones AK, Jones DL, Cross P. The carbon footprint of lamb: sources of variation and opportunities for mitigation. Agric Syst 2014;123:97–107.
83. Pelletier N, Tyedmers P. Feeding farmed salmon: is organic better? Aquaculture 2007;272(1–4):399–416.
84. Thoma G, Matlock M, Putman B, et al. A life cycle analysis of land use in US pork production. A comprehensive report. Pork Checkoff and University of Arkansas Division of Agriculture Center for Agricultural and Rural Sustainability; 2015. Available at: http://research.pork.org/FileLibrary/ResearchDocuments/13-208-Thoma-UofARK.pdf. Accessed September 9, 2020.
85. Putman B, Thoma G, Burek J, et al. A retrospective analysis of the United States poultry industry: 1965 compared with 2010. Agric Syst 2017;157:107–17.
86. Campos I, Pinheiro Valente LM, Matos E, et al. Life-cycle assessment of animal feed ingredients: poultry fat, poultry by-product meal and hydrolyzed feather meal. J Clean Prod 2020;252:119845.
87. Ramirez AD, Humphries AC, Woodgate SL, et al. Greenhouse gas life cycle assessment of products arising from the rendering of mammalian animal byproducts in the UK. Environ Sci Technol 2012;46(1):447–53.
88. Johnson MD, Rutland CT, Richardson JW, et al. Greenhouse gas emissions from U.S. grain farms. J Crop Improv 2016;30(4):447–77.
89. Godard C, Boissy J, Suret C, et al. LCA of Starch Potato from Field to Starch Production Plant Gate. In: 8th International Conference on LCA in the Agri-Food Sector. October 2-4 2012; Rennes, France.
90. Wilfart A, Espagnol S, Dauguet S, et al. ECOALIM: a dataset of environmental impacts of feed ingredients used in French animal production. PLoS One 2016; 11(12):1–17.
91. Aguilera E, Guzmán G, Alonso A. Greenhouse gas emissions from conventional and organic cropping systems in Spain. I. Herbaceous crops. Agron Sustain Dev 2015;35(2):713–24.
92. National Research Council. Proximate analysis of select feed ingredients (as-fed). In: Nutrient requirements of dogs and cats. Washington, DC: The National Academies Press; 2006. p. 320–3. https://doi.org/10.17226/10668.
93. Batal A, Dale N, Farms S. Feedstuffs ingredient analysis table: 2016 edition. In: Feedstuffs; November 2015;11:7-8. Available at: https://feedstuffs.farmcentric.com/mdfm/Feeess50/author/427/2015/11/Feedstuffs_RIBG_Ingredient_Analysis_Table_2016.pdf. Accessed October 16, 2020.
94. Kadim IT, Mahgoub O, Al-Marzooqi W, et al. Prediction of crude protein, extractable fat, calcium and phosphorus contents of broiler chicken carcasses using near-infrared reflectance spectroscopy. Asian-Australas J Anim Sci 2005;18(7): 1036–40.
95. Ode C, Addass P, Dim N. Effect of diets containing graded levels of eggshell meal on bone parameters, organ weights and by-products of growing West African dwarf goats. Amer J Food Sci Health 2016;2(4):55–9.
96. Donadelli RA, Aldrich CG, Jones CK, et al. The amino acid composition and protein quality of various egg, poultry meal by-products, and vegetable proteins used in the production of dog and cat diets. Poult Sci 2019;98(3):1371–8.
97. De Godoy MRC, Bauer LL, Parsons CM, et al. Select corn coproducts from the ethanol industry and their potential as ingredients in pet foods. J Anim Sci 2009;87(1):189–99.
98. Tomás-Vidal A, Monge-Ortiz R, Jover-Cerdá M, et al. Apparent digestibility and protein quality evaluation of selected feed ingredients in Seriola dumerili. J World Aquac Soc 2019;50(4):842–55.

Nutrition for Pocket Pets (Ferrets, Rabbits, and Rodents)

Lindsey E. Bullen, DVM[a,b,*]

KEYWORDS

• Nutrition • Ferret • Rabbit • Rodent • Pocket pet • Small mammal • Diet

KEY POINTS

- Ferrets, rabbits, and rodents are increasingly common pets that may present for veterinary evaluation.
- The anatomy and physiology of each species is as different as their physical appearances, resulting in unique nutritional needs and dietary idiosyncrasies.
- Illness in small mammals is often associated with poor husbandry and/or inappropriate nutrition.
- Although there are species-specific, commercial products available, there is limited information regarding the exact nutritional needs for many pocket pets.

INTRODUCTION

Over the past several decades, ownership of pocket pets has been increasing.[1] Although exotic-focused practices have also increased, canine-focused and feline-focused clinicians may still be presented with a pocket pet. Although education before obtaining a pocket pet would be ideal, many clients do not first seek professional advice. Lack of general knowledge may ultimately result in nutrient imbalances and severe illness. Thus, veterinary practitioners must be able to provide routine preventive care and counsel, which not only includes husbandry but also encompasses a full nutritional assessment (including dietary history; **Box 1**), and subsequent recommendations. It should be noted that all species/groups of species have unique idiosyncrasies emphasizing specialized nutritional and environmental requirements.[1–10]

Significant progress in nutrition-focused research for small mammals occurred in the early 2000s; most advances revolved around optimizing production (ie, furs/meat) or laboratory uses, rather than companion animal needs. Despite limited knowledge of precise nutritional needs for many pocket pets, there are several

[a] Clinical Nutrition Service, Veterinary Specialty Hospital of the Carolinas, 6405 Tryon Road Suite 100, Cary, NC 27518, USA; [b] Private Veterinary Nutrition Consultant, Apex, NC 27502, USA
* Clinical Nutrition Service, Veterinary Specialty Hospital of the Carolinas, 6405 Tryon Road Suite 100, Cary, NC 27518.
E-mail address: lindsey.bullen@bluepearlvet.com

Vet Clin Small Anim 51 (2021) 583–604
https://doi.org/10.1016/j.cvsm.2021.01.001

Box 1
Dietary history questions

- What commercial products are fed? (Includes pellets, hays/forage, and treats.)
  - Full name, flavor, form (when in doubt, evaluate label).
  - How much is fed and how often (for each product)?
  - Request standard units (ie, tablespoon or grams).
- What human foods are fed?
  - How much is fed and how often (for each food type)?
  - Request standard units (ie, tablespoon or gram).
- If receiving medications, what foods/treats are used for administration?
  - How much and how often?

species-specific commercial diets that seem to provide adequate nutritional support. Although many practitioners are not true pocket-pet experts, using the knowledge at hand, recommendations tailored to the patients' species and individual needs must be provided.

DOMESTIC FERRETS

Background and Husbandry

Domestic ferrets (*Mustela putorius furo*) live up to their order classification (Carnivora) by showing traits of a true obligate carnivore.[4–6] Furthermore, as a member of the phylogenetic family Mustelidae (which also includes mink, weasels, badgers, and otters), ferrets represent just 1 of the diverse and adaptable species classified therein. Ferrets initially were used for hunting small game and rodent control; however, over time, their uses extended to the fur trade and biomedical research.[2,4,5] Because of their small size, endearing and inquisitive nature, and ease of care, ferrets have become increasingly popular as companion animals.[10]

At birth, ferrets are both blind and deaf, weighing approximately 6 to 10 g. Although they can eat soft solids by 21 days, true weaning is typically around 6 to 8 weeks of age.[2,4] Adulthood occurs between 8 and 12 months, and life expectancy is approximately 8 to 12 years.[2,5] Although seasonal variations of 30% to 40% are considered normal, neutered adults typically weigh between 0.8 and 1.2 kg.[2,4–6] Other than neonatal or lone juvenile kits, ferrets tolerate cold temperatures well, with the optimal being between 4°C and 18°C (39°F–64°F). However, because of poorly developed sweat glands, temperatures hotter than 30°C (86°F) are not tolerated.[5] Environmental enrichment is critical to the well-being of domesticated ferrets. Although there are many different options, mental stimulation can be associated with feeding.[2] Examples include:

- Alternating feeding times/locations
- Hiding food
- Variety (form, flavor, and so forth)
- Choices

Although territorial behaviors are possible, ferrets are social creatures, making them ideal for research and companion animals.[5]

Anatomic and Physiologic Considerations

Ferrets are obligate carnivores whose natural diet predominantly consists of small, whole prey (eg, birds, mammals, eggs, amphibians). They rely extensively on sense of smell, developing an olfactory preference to food during their first few months of life. Young kits exposed to a variety of food textures, tastes, smells, and so forth early on are likely to be more flexible to dietary changes as adults.[2,10] Ferrets' oral anatomy also supports their carnivorous lifestyle, with dentition consisting of few molars and large canines and their well-developed muscle of mastication contributing to a strong/unrelenting bite.[2,3,6]

The ferrets' striated esophagus terminates in the stomach without a true sphincter allowing them to vomit (although they routinely do not, even when obstructed).[2] The gastric capacity of ferrets is considerable (50mL/kg)[2]; however, they preferentially eat multiple small meals throughout the day rather than intermittent gorging.[1–5,11] Compared with other carnivore species, ferrets have a short small intestine, which contributes to their extremely short gastrointestinal (GI) transit time (3–4 hours for meat-based diets), ultimately decreasing their digestive and absorptive efficiencies,[1–4,6] which should be considered before fasting because a ferret's stomach should be appropriately empty within a 3-hour period. Prolonged fasting can result in significant and severe hypoglycemia in both juvenile kits and ferrets with insulinomas.[2,4,6] In addition, the fast GI transit increases the frequency of defecation, resulting in a need for multiple available litter boxes to avoid fecal messes.[2]

Ferret digestive abilities are also affected by low concentrations of brush border enzymes. Although total proteolytic activity is high, in general, digestive enzyme activity (eg, amylase, lipase, peptidase, and sucrase) is numerically lower compared with other species.[3,6] Furthermore, the GI microbiome of the domestic ferret is presumed to be unsophisticated, having a minimal functionality and reduced number of populations. Contrary to other species, the author is unaware of any studies examining either the ferret microbiome itself or the dietary effect on the ferret microbiome.[3,4]

Nutrition

Requirements

The exact nutrient and caloric needs depend on environmental and physiologic factors; however, the estimated caloric needs of adult ferrets are between 200 and 300 kcal of metabolizable energy (ME) per kilogram of body weight (BW) per day. Growth, reproduction, and lactation can increase those needs by up to 3-fold, but variation between individuals should be expected.[1–3,5,6,12] In addition, although the exact water needs of ferrets is largely unknown, it is estimated that approximately 60 mL/kg_{BW}/d is sufficient.[4,6,13] Because ferrets love water play, multiple sources of fresh, potable water daily in a heavy, nontippable bowl, are recommended. Although sippers can be used, several sources state that bowls are ferrets' preference.[2,4,6]

Historically, ferrets had been successfully raised on whole prey or a freeze-dried carnivore diet. Although the stool of the ferret is often low in odor and volume on these diets, this feeding method is not considered feasible or desirable for many modern ferret owners, thus resulting in the use of commercial diets.[1,6,10] Although the exact nutrient requirements for ferrets are unknown, their needs seem to be successfully met using data extrapolated from both mink and feline research.[1–4,10,12,14,15]

Although there are several products designed and marketed specifically for ferrets (**Table 1**), commercial mink and feline diets are often considered.[1,2,6] The author cautions against using such products without first carefully evaluating the nutrient profile and ingredient list. Mink diets may meet ferrets' nutritional needs; however, they are often fish based, which is undesirable to ferrets' palates and olfaction.[4,6] Regarding feline diets, a highly digestible and high-quality kitten diet often more than meets ferrets' nutritional needs. However, a less-costly, poorer-quality feline diet often results in poor haircoat, poor reproduction, and failure to thrive.[1,2,4,6] In general, the quality and

Table 1
[a,b]Commercial ferret diets versus recommended intake of select nutrients[1,2,6]

Nutrient	Recommended	Product A[c]	Product B[d]	Product C[e]
Crude Protein (%)	30–35	38.8	43.2	44.4
Crude Fat (%)	15–20	20	23.3	22.2
Crude Fiber (%)	<5	4.4	4.6	3.3
Taurine (%)	undefined	Added, unquantified	0.28	0.17

All numbers expressed in percentage of dry matter (DM).
[a] Product information converted from guaranteed analysis to estimated percentage of DM.
[b] The diets listed in this table are not intended to be an exhaustive list.
[c] Marshall Select Chicken Formula (product information: https://www.marshallferrets.com/store/product/select-chicken-formula-ferret-diet/).
[d] Mazuri Ferret Diet (product information: https://www.mazuri.com/mazuri/small-animal/ferret/ferret-diet-25lb?viewState=DetailView&cartID=&portalUser=&store=&cclcl=en_US).
[e] ZuPreem Ferret Diet (product information: https://www.zupreem.com/products/ferret-small-animal/premium-ferret-diet/).

order of the ingredients on the label is more important that the protein content in the diet. Not only are plant-based proteins often less concentrated in essential amino acids (EAAs), their use has also been linked to a highly alkaline urine and struvite urolithiasis.[1,2,10,12] To reduce the risk of EAA deficiency and urolithiasis, the literature recommends that the diet contain a total protein level of 30% to 35% dry matter (DM) and that animal meat/protein be the first 3 ingredients on the product label; however, commercial products containing more than 35% seem to be well tolerated.[2,3,6,10]

It is presumed that ferrets have the same EAA needs as other carnivores.[4] Like felids, whose urea cycle relies on arginine for the conversion of ammonia to blood urea nitrogen, ferrets fed an arginine-deficient meal show hyperammonemia and encephalopathy within a matter of hours.[3,4,10,16] Methionine, which is considered to be a limiting amino acid in both cats and mink, is presumed to also be limiting in ferrets.[3,4,10] It is also presumed that taurine, a beta-aminosulfonic acid, may be essential in ferrets because both dilated cardiomyopathy and retinal degeneration have been diagnosed. Although these disease processes have not been definitively linked to taurine deficiency in ferrets, because they have been linked in other species, the addition of taurine to commercial diets is considered an appropriate safeguard.[3,4,10]

Ferrets are efficient at using dietary fat for energy. To support adult maintenance, their diet should contain approximately 15% to 20% DM. Because their exact essential fatty acid needs are not known, dietary sources of linoleic, linolenic, and arachidonic acids are recommended.[1,2,4,5,15] In addition, ferrets likely maintain high levels of gluconeogenesis and do not obligately require an external source of carbohydrates.[1,2,4] It is suspected that, like cats, they have reduced glucokinase activity as well. Despite their carnivorous nature, healthy ferrets seem to tolerate diets containing approximately 25% to 35% digestible carbohydrates. Regarding fiber, the natural source for wild ferrets is from the gut content of ingested whole prey. Given their large intestine is simple and their microbiome unsophisticated, ferrets are unable to engage in significant fermentation activities.[2–5,10] Compounded with their inefficient digestive and absorptive abilities, a low-fiber and highly digestible diet is ideal.[1,2,4]

As with most other nutrients, vitamin and mineral requirements are estimated based on extrapolations from mink and cat studies. Based on their identical clinical signs associated with calcium (Ca) deficiency, it is presumed that ferrets require a Ca to phosphorus (P) ratio of 1 to 2:1 (Ca/P).[4] Although ferrets' conversion of B-carotene to vitamin A (retinol) is considered more efficient than that of cats and mink, it is still inefficient and thus is supplemented in many, if not all, commercial products.[5,12,14,15,17]

Feeding method

Although dry kibble tends to be the preferred diet form chosen by most ferret owners, this comes with its own set of issues. Ferrets' teeth did not evolve to eat hard kibble, thus increased wear can be seen in captivity.[3,18,19] Although dry kibble can be left out, this is neither stimulating nor enriching for the pet. However, predominately soft diets may be problematic, unless medically necessitated, because they may increase plaque accumulation.[4]

A diet composed primarily of dry ferret kibble with intermittent and varied snacks can help to maintain dietary enrichment as well as dietary flexibility (**Box 2**). However, although their anatomy and physiology is primed for fresh, raw ingredients, if the provided ingredient is not truly fresh, it poses a risk of the development of pathogenic illness such as *Escherichia coli*, *Salmonella* spp, and *Campylobacter* spp.[2,4] In addition, although ferrets prefer sweet foods (eg, sugary cereals), they are not recommended, because they may not only affect dietary flexibility but may also contribute to disease of the pancreatic beta cells.[2] Regardless of feeding plan, it is essential to (1) not provide excess calories, and (2) not provide excessive treat calories (which may unbalance the diet).[2]

Select Diet-Responsive Disease Management

Insulinomas

The most common functional tumor in small animals, but especially ferrets, is insulinoma.[6,20–23] Whether benign or malignant, insulinomas are most often functional (~94%), insulin-secreting beta-cell tumors.[20,23] Although the associated masses typically have a much lower metastatic rate compared with those in dogs (4%–50%, respectively), insulinomas can still be deadly[20,24] because of the profound hypoglycemia that can occur from the continuous production and secretion of insulin.[4,6,20–23] Typically, a diagnosis is made based on the combination of clinical signs (**Box 3**), a low fasting blood glucose level, and a positive response to sugar administration.[20,24] However, to obtain a definitive diagnosis, histopathologic evaluation of the masses is needed.[20]

Treatment options include surgical excision, medical management, or ideally both.[20,23,25] It should be noted that most ferrets have multiple pancreatic nodules

Box 2
Example ferret feeding schedule[1,4,10]

- Ferret kibble daily
  - Varied times/locations
- Canned kitten food 3 times per week
- Whole prey once per week (eg, small poultry/birds)
- Treats (<10% of total caloric intake)
  - Organ meat[a]
  - Chicken meat
  - Eggs
  - Fruit

[a]Caution using liver because of high vitamin A levels.

Box 3
[a]Hypoglycemia-related clinical signs in ferrets[6,20–23]

- Ptyalism plus or minus pawing at mouth
- Weight loss
- Weakness/lethargy
- Collapse/ataxia
- Vomiting/nausea
- Twitching/trembling/convulsions/seizures
- Abnormal behavior/mentation/disorientation/confusion
- Loss of consciousness

[a]Patient may have any combination of these.

rather than a solitary tumor and that surgery is often not curative[23]; although surgery can slow progression of the disease, up to 40% of ferrets see recurrence by 10 months after surgery.[20] When surgical intervention is declined, medical management is indicated, beginning with a diet change to a high-protein, high-fat, low (and ideally complex)-carbohydrate diet. This diet helps to avoid high spikes in postprandial glucose (and insulin) level, thus aiding in glycemic control.[20,23] Such diets could include feline diabetic diets (**Table 2**). It is important to either free feed the patient (a premeasured amount) or enlist the aid of an automatic feeder, providing food at a minimum of every 4 hours. In addition, it is essential that the client discontinues all high-sugar treats or foods.[20,23] If diet alone fails to successfully manage the patient's disease, the use of prednisone should be considered, because it can stimulate both hepatic glycogenolysis and gluconeogenesis. However, the combination of surgery, medical management, and dietary management yields the longest disease-free interval and survival time.[20,23,25] Despite the potential for recurrent hypoglycemia, the

Table 2
Select feline diabetic diets[20,23]

	Product A[b]			Product B[c]			Product C[d]	
Trait	**Stew**	**Can**	**Dry**	**Stew**	**Can**	**Dry**	**Can[a]**	**Dry[a]**
Protein (%)	51.8	52.1	52.5	59.0	56.9	56.9	57.4	46.2
Fat (%)	25	24.8	21.8	32.5	24.4	18.1	16.4	12.1
Carbohydrates (%)	15.9	13.1	15.1	13.7	7.1	17.0	15.3	25.3
Crude Fiber (%)	1.0	2.7	4.3	0.6	3.5	1.17	5.3	4.8
Caloric Density (kcal ME/g)	0.95	1.11	3.98	1.11	1.13	4.22	0.72	3.51
Caloric Density (kcal/can or cup)	78	172	463	173	176	605	61	423

Except for caloric density (expressed as as fed, caloric), all numbers are expressed as percentage DM.

[a] Product information converted from as fed, caloric to percentage DM.
[b] Hill's Feline m/d GlucoSupport (product information is available via 2018 product guide).
[c] Purina Feline DM Dietetic Management (product information is available via 2020 product guide).
[d] Royal Canin Feline Glycobalance (product information is available via 2018 product guide).

prognosis and quality of life for ferrets is often markedly better compared with that in cats and dogs.[20,24]

Inflammatory bowel disease

Inflammatory bowel disease (IBD) is a common problem observed in domestic ferrets.[18,26] Although it is speculated that current commercial ferret diets may predispose to this illness,[6] the author is unaware of any active or past studies investigating this potential association. However, IBD can be challenging to initially diagnose, because associated clinical signs can mimic other enteric diseases.[18,26] Ideally, full-thickness biopsies should be obtained to definitely diagnose the disease[18]; however, it is the author's opinion that diagnostics, such as abdominal ultrasonography and serum B-vitamin levels, could be used to support a provisional diagnosis of IBD. Furthermore, successful long-term response without evidence of disease progression could provide further support.

Similarly to one treatment type for canine and feline IBD, a novel or hydrolyzed diet to minimize antigenic stimulation is often recommended.[27] Because many commercial ferret diets are chicken based, it is advised to avoid this protein source. However, in order to determine the best possible elimination diet, a full dietary history is needed (see **Box 1**). Although there are several chicken-free, over-the-counter ferret products available, the author is unaware of their efficacy and quality control measures being validated. Many clinicians instead choose a novel or hydrolyzed feline product (**Tables 3** and **4**) that has not only been tested for feline efficacy but whose manufacturer practices strict quality control measures.[18] Most elimination diet trials are performed for 8 to 12 weeks, although clinical improvement is often observed sooner.

Table 3
Select feline novel-protein diets[18,27]

	Product A[b]		Product B[c]		Product C[d]		Product D[e]		Product E[f]	
Trait	Can	Dry	Can	Dry	Can[a]	Dry[a]	Can[a]	Dry[a]	Can[a]	Dry[a]
Protein (%)	38.1	34.5	37.3	34.5	43.1	32.7	40.8	33.1	37.3	32.7
Primary Source	Duck	Duck	Venison	Venison	Duck	Duck	Rabbit	Rabbit	Venison	Venison
Fat (%)	29.1	21.3	30.4	21.3	27.9	13.3	24.5	13.5	23.3	13.3
Carbohydrates (%)	22.3	32.7	21.1	32.7	20.9	37.3	15.6	38.7	27.5	35.7
Crude Fiber (%)	4.5	4.7	4.6	4.7	1.2	3.8	0.7	3.6	1.9	3.7
Caloric Density (kcal ME/g)	1.21	3.84	1.26	3.87	1.12	3.50	0.99	3.53	0.91	3.45
Caloric Density (kcal/can or cup)	189	468	197	472	189	329	167	332	146	324

Except for caloric density (expressed as as fed, caloric), all numbers are expressed as percentage DM.

[a] Product information converted from as fed, caloric to percentage DM.
[b] Hill's Feline d/d Duck (product information is available via 2018 product guide).
[c] Hill's Feline d/d Venison (product information is available via 2018 product guide).
[d] Royal Canin Feline Selected Protein Adult PD (product information is available via 2018 product guide).
[e] Royal Canin Feline Selected Protein Adult PR (product information is available via 2018 product guide).
[f] Royal Canin Feline Selected Protein Adult PV (product information is available via 2018 product guide).

Table 4
Comparison of select feline hydrolyzed-protein diets[18,27]

	Product A[b]		Product B[c]	Product C[d]	Product D[e]
Trait	**Can**	**Dry**	**Dry**	**Dry[a]**	**Dry[a]**
Protein (%)	34.6	34.5	34.0	25.7	26.8
Fat (%)	17.1	15.2	11.7	16.5	19.3
Carbohydrates (%)	40.9	40.7	44.5	40.4	34.2
Crude Fiber (%)	1.6	3.2	2.1	3.5	3.4
Caloric Density (kcal ME/g)	1.10	NA	3.79	3.76	3.91
Caloric Density (kcal/can or cup)	171	408	323	334	328

Except for caloric density (expressed as as fed, caloric), all numbers are expressed as percentage DM.

Abbreviation: NA, not available

[a] Product information converted from as fed, caloric to percentage DM.
[b] Hill's Feline z/d (product information is available via 2018 product guide).
[c] Purina Feline HA Hydrolyzed (product information is available via 2020 product guide).
[d] Royal Canin Feline Ultamino (product information is available via 2018 product guide).
[e] Royal Canin Feline Hydrolyzed Protein Adult HP (product information is available via 2018 product guide).

DOMESTICATED RABBITS

Background and Husbandry

The domestic rabbit is phylogenetically classified in the order Lagomorpha and subclassified in the family Leporidae.[7,9] Leporidae contains 8 different genera, including the European rabbit (*Oryctolagus cuniculus*), of which the domestic rabbit is directly descended.[9] Starting between the fifth and tenth centuries, rabbits were kept and bred for the purpose of food.[7] Since that time, their uses have expanded to both biomedical research and the fur trade.[7,9,28]

Weighing approximately 50 g at birth, rabbits are considered altricial.[7] In contrast with many other mammalian species, neonatal rabbits nurse for approximately 3 to 5 minutes only once per 24-hour period.[1,29] In addition to seeing and hearing, by day 7 to 10, infant rabbits begin to eat components of their nesting material, including their mother's fecal pellets.[7] This act helps to colonize a normal cecal microbiome, with the population numbers and concentration of colonies rapidly increasing daily.[29,30]

Although captive neonatal rabbits may nurse up to 5 to 10 weeks, in general, neonates begin consuming solids by about day 18; full weaning occurs between 5 and 8 weeks of age.[7,8,31] In contrast, wild rabbits have been observed abandoning their young by week 3 to 4 after birth.[7] Although the following traits are breed dependent, most rabbits reach sexual maturity by 3 to 8 months and weigh between 2.5 and 7 kg.[7] Although their wild cousins can expect to live no more than 5 or 6 years, captive rabbits often live between 9 and 10 years, with some anecdotally living more than 18 years.[7,32]

Rabbits can tolerate a range of temperatures (10°C–30°C [50°F–86°F]), although they do best in colder or more mild climates; they are most comfortable at approximately 20°C (68°F).[7] For waste elimination, wild rabbits use latrines or closets close to, but outside of, their burrows; to the delight of rabbit owners, indoor rabbits can be litter trained. To optimize mental and physical health, rabbits require daily exercise, which can be accomplished by allowing supervised roaming for several hours a day; it is essential that the space be rabbit proofed before allowing the pet to exercise.[7,32] In addition, because rabbits are naturally prey animals, hiding places should always be provided in case they become frightened.[32,33]

Rabbits are social creatures. Studies have shown that having a companion can improve quality of life and reduce untoward/destructive behaviors; thus, it is recommended that pet owners ideally have at least 2 at one time.[9] However, unless they are either family or previous companions, slow and careful introductions are needed to ensure that the rabbits respond favorably to, and do not injure, each other. Even then, a 2-male duo are more likely to fight than any other combination.[7,9,33] Although companionship is important, additional enrichment is recommended to optimize the pets' well-being. Examples include:[33]

- Viewing platform
- Hiding spaces
- Gnawing material
- Hay
- Toys
  - Toys may pose a foreign body risk
- Mirrors
  - Helps in absence from rabbit companion
- Leash walks
- Gentle, routine human interactions
  - Reduces fearfulness

Despite numerous resources describing how to support their pets physically and mentally, many clients are not aware of pet rabbits' needs.[7,34]

Anatomic and Physiologic Considerations

The use of rabbits in biomedical research has enabled the collection of a vast wealth of knowledge pertaining to their anatomy and physiology.[7,29,32] Rabbits are monogastric, hindgut-fermenting herbivores.[29,32,33] Although the jaws of rabbits are large, their mouths are small, with a long and narrow oral cavity.[7,9] They cannot see directly beneath their mouths; therefore, feed selection is based primarily on their olfactory and tactile senses.[32] Rabbit dentition comprises paired upper and lower incisors (2 and 1, respectively), paired upper and lower premolars (3 and 2 respectively), and paired upper and lower molars (3 and 3 respectively).[7] The incisors are responsible for cutting the foliage, and the check teeth (premolars and molars) horizontally masticate the ingested material.[7,29] In order to optimize digestive efficiencies, rabbits thoroughly chew their food at a rate of approximately 120 to 200 jaw movements per minute.[7,10,29,32] All teeth are long crowned (hypsodont); additionally, they are continuously growing (at varying rates) and possess no anatomic roots (elodont).[7,9,10,32,33] Rabbit teeth are uniquely aradicular, allowing for growth in tooth size as the animal grows and matures into adulthood.[7]

The contents of rabbits' long GI tract make up anywhere from 10% to 20% of its BW.[7] The lower esophagus terminates in a massive muscular sphincter into the well-developed cardia, which results in a rabbit's inability to vomit.[7,10,29,32] The simple stomach is the largest (relative to body size) of any monogastric mammal, containing approximately 15% of all ingested foods and materials.[7,9,29,32] Acting as a storage vessel, the stomach is never empty in healthy rabbits.[9,10,32] Although the normal gastric emptying time is 3 to 6 hours, even after 24 hours of starving, food and fecal pellets may still be found.[29] The pylorus is also well developed but easily compressed by the duodenum, gastric gas distention, or organomegaly, which can result in pyloric outflow obstruction.[7,35] Because of a highly acidic pH (~2), the stomach and proximal small intestine are essentially sterile in the adult rabbit.[7,29,31,32] In contrast, nursing neonates are highly susceptible to enteric pathogens and subsequent diarrhea because of their less acidic gastric pH (5–6.5).[7,29,32,36] Although diet is discussed in more detail later, note that fiber is especially important in early postweaned kits to help reduce digestive issues.[9,37]

Domestic rabbits' small intestines are short compared with other species, making up only 12% of total GI tract length. The small intestine is the major site of nutrient absorption; however, because of the significant fiber content in their diet, a large portion of nutrient intake is from the consumption of cecotropes (also called cecotrophs; discussed in more detail later).[29,36] The large intestine is composed of the cecum and the colon.[1,32,33] The cecum is the largest organ in the abdominal cavity, holding approximately 40% of the ingesta.[1,7,10,29,32] It is a biological fermentation vat that provides an optimal anaerobic environment for the highly complex populations of autochthonous microorganisms to break down fiber and starch.[1,8,29,32] The fusi coli is at the termination of the transverse colon, regulating GI motility and being responsible for separating fiber and nonfiber digesta, which ultimately regulates the elimination of hard versus soft fecal pellets (two-thirds to one-third, respectively).[9,32,38]

Cecotrophy

The production of 2 types of fecal pellets optimizes rabbits' ability to efficiently use nutrients.[7,32] Hard pellets contain the indigestible fiber component and are eliminated as single pellets outside the burrow or nest. In contrast, soft pellets (cecotropes or night feces), which are rich in protein, short-chain fatty acids (SCFAs), (volatile fatty acids; include acetate, propionate, and butyrate), B vitamins, water, and electrolytes, are excreted in a small cluster and are ingested directly from the anus.[1,7,9,29,32] The nutrients and microbes in the cecotropes are able to be used after ingestion because of the mucus barrier's protection from the extreme acidity of the stomach.[7,32] **Table 5** provides a comparison of the average nutrient profile of hard and soft feces. Although the quantity of cecotropes eaten is directly related to the protein and fiber content in the diet, cecotrophy is not a result of nutrient imbalances; this pseudorumination shows a specialized digestive strategy.[8,10,29,31] This characteristic is essential to communicate to new owners because they may mistake cecotropes for diarrhea.[7]

Nutrition

Requirements

Although there is extensive research regarding the husbandry and nutrition of both production and laboratory rabbits, because of their often iatrogenically shortened

Table 5
Average nutrient content of hard and soft feces[32]

Trait	Hard Feces	Soft Feces
Crude Protein (%)	15.4	34.0
Crude Fiber (%)	30.0	17.8
Ash (%)	13.7	15.2
Carbohydrate, Nitrogen-free Extract (%)	37.9	36.7
Energy (kcal ME/g)	4.35	4.54

All numbers expressed as DM.

lifespans, the subsequent conclusions may not always be applicable to their longer-living domesticated brethren.[33,35] As such, it has been suggested that the data extrapolated from these studies should be considered minimum standards only. Furthermore, although observing rabbits in their natural environment can provide a plethora of vital information, these conditions should not necessarily represent their ideal state of being.[33]

In general, rabbits have a high metabolic rate. Although there are several equations to calculate energy needs, adults need approximately 100 kcals per kg (BW)^0.75, and growing kits and reproducing females require significantly more energy per unit BW (**Table 6**).[10,29] Although the guidelines in **Table 6** are considered accurate, it is essential to feed the patients as individuals, recognizing they may need more or less based on the environment, activity level, life stage and physical examination parameters.[29] Occasionally, rabbit dietary nutrient information is provided in the form of digestible energy (DE), whereas caloric needs are calculated as ME. DE calculations tend to overestimate energy content in both protein-rich and fiber-rich diets, as well as to underestimate energy content in fat-rich diets. Although there has been some discussion in replacing DE with ME, most of the available information has been originally acquired as DE. As such, it has been estimated that ME is approximately 95% of DE.[31]

At 50 to 150 $mL/kg_{BW}/d$, the water requirements of rabbits are extremely high compared with other animals.[7,9,33,39] To meet these demands, it is essential that fresh, potable water be available always. Although it is reported that rabbits' clear preference is for open water dishes,[33] drinking bottles or sippers are easier to keep clean and may reduce the risk of developing dewlap dermatitis.[29] If the pet is reluctant to try a sipper bottle, applying corn syrup or molasses to the spout can help increase trainability.[29]

Typically, rabbits eat in the early mornings and evenings, with coprophagy beginning approximately 3 to 8 hours after each meal.[1,7,29,32,38] The total GI transit time is approximately 19 hours; this rapid rate allows high feed intake while increasing total energy consumed and minimizing the need to store fiber.[7,29,32,40] By nature, rabbits are selective feeders, preferentially eating tender and succulent plant parts as most their diet and coarse roughage as a minor component.[7,29,33] However, because of convenience, most rabbit owners choose to feed a complete and balanced pelleted feed. Although some commercial rabbit feeds may be appropriate, using them as the sole source of nutrition is not recommended.

Although all nutrients are important, fiber is arguably the most important for the rabbit. Insoluble fibers aid in regulating motility and controlling GI transit time, whereas

Table 6
Estimated caloric needs of rabbits[1,31]

Life Stage	Energy Requirement (kcals ME/d)[a]
Adult	100 ($kgBW^{0.75}$)
Growth	200 ($kgBW^{0.75}$)
Gestation: early	135 ($kgBW^{0.75}$)
Gestation: mid	200 ($kgBW^{0.75}$)
Gestation: late	300 ($kgBW^{0.75}$)

[a] Variation between individuals' needs should be expected.

more fermentable fibers directly feed the GI microflora, and indirectly, via cecotrophy, the rabbit.[10,29,32,36] Higher fiber levels have also been shown to be protective against enteritis[37] and aid in maintaining normal occlusion of teeth.[7,10] In addition to optimizing both GI and dental health, fiber may also help prevent behavioral and destructive issues, and reduces the risk of obesity by encouraging normal foraging behaviors.[10,29,32] Although the minimum crude fiber requirement is 12% to 16% DM,[10] a level of 20% to up to 32% DM is considered optimal.[1,29,32,33]

Rabbits have similar EAA needs to other mammalian species.[28] Their primary sources of protein are their forage and cecotropes.[8,29] A range of 12% to 16% DM is considered an appropriate dietary goal. Excessive levels are not recommended because they not only lead to the reduced ingestion of cecotropes but also may cause cecal dysbiosis because of increased ammonia production.[1,10,29,35] Dysbiosis and enterotoxemia can also be associated with excessive levels of simple carbohydrates, especially in the young. If a grain must be fed, a low-energy grain such as unprocessed oats is advised.[29,35] Fat is often added to pelleted feed to provide energy, improve palatability, and to reduce dust.[29] Although there is minimal fat associated with rabbits' natural diet (and sources indicate that exogenous fat is not essential), a level of 2.5% to 4% has been deemed ideal.[1,10,29] High-fat diets are contraindicated because they can predispose pets to obesity and hepatic lipidosis during times of starving.[29] **Table 7** shows the recommended nutrient levels for adult maintenance compared with available commercial products.

Rabbits are relatively self-sufficient when it comes to vitamins. They can synthesize vitamin C endogenously, although they may have a higher requirement under periods of illness or stress. In addition to providing B vitamins via cecotropes, cecal microbes likely provide sufficient quantities of vitamin K as well.[28,31,35] However, because the vitamin K requirements are unknown, it is often added to commercial diets as a safeguard.[10] Vitamin A requirements for domestic rabbits are also unknown.[9] Although

Table 7
[a,b]Commercial rabbit diets versus recommended intake of select nutrients[35]

Trait	Recommended	Product A[c]	Product B[d]	Product C[e]
Protein (%)	12–16	15.9	15.6	15.9
Fat (%)	2.5–4	1.7	2.2	1.7
Crude Fiber (%)	13–20	20.5–25	27.8–32.2	22.7–28.4
Base	—	Timothy	Timothy	Timothy
Ash (%)	—	10.2	NA	
Calcium (%)	—	0.9–1.4	0.4–0.8	0.4–0.97
Caloric Density (kcal ME/g)	—	2.60	2.13	NA

Except for caloric density (expressed as as fed, caloric), all numbers are expressed as percentage DM.

[a] All product information converted from guaranteed analysis to estimated percentage DM.
[b] The diets listed in this tables are not intended to be an exhaustive list.
[c] Mazuri Rabbit Diet (product information: https://www.mazuri.com/small-animal/small-wildlife/rabbit-diet-with-timothy-hay-530q?viewState=DetailView&cartID=&portalUser=&store=&cclcl=en_US).
[d] Oxbow Essentials- Adult Rabbit Food (product information: https://www.oxbowanimalhealth.com/our-products/fortified-food/essentials-adult-rabbit-food/).
[e] ZuPreem Timothy Naturals Rabbit Food (product information: https://www.zupreem.com/products/ferret-small-animal/timothy-naturals-rabbit/).

fresh forages provide sufficient vitamin A, because of rapid degradation over time, deficiency can be seen in companion rabbits when forage has been stored for longer than 6 months; thus vitamin A is often supplemented in commercial products.[1,10]

Like many other herbivorous species, rabbits can synthesize vitamin D from sunlight. However, because many captive rabbits are not regularly exposed to sunlight, it is added to commercial diets.[10] An interesting rabbit idiosyncrasy is that GI absorption of calcium is not vitamin D dependent.[8,29,41] Although calcium is absorbed via passive and active transport, and the carrier protein is synthesized in response to vitamin D, parathyroid hormone and calcitonin prevent dangerous levels of hypercalcemia.[8,29,31,35] Despite these mechanisms, rabbits fed a calcium-rich diet may have a higher total serum calcium level and higher urinary fractional excretion of calcium.[8,32,35,41] However, total ionized calcium levels are often comparable with other mammals.[32]

Feeding method

Commercial rabbit feed is available as either homogeneous pellets or as a mixed ration. Although mixed rations can be visually appealing to clients, they are not recommended because rabbits selectively eat the sweetest, less fibrous ingredients. Selective feeding can result in multiple nutrient deficiencies that have the potential to cause severe disease. Although pelleted feeds are a better option than mixed rations, they should not comprise most of rabbits' diets.[29,33] Specific feeding recommendations are given in **Box 4**. Regardless, careful attention to protein and fiber content is recommended to ensure the diet is ideal for the pet. If the pet does not have free access to grass for grazing, dried forage or hay should be available ad libitum.[10,29,33,42]

The provision of fresh, leafy green (low oxalate) vegetables is also recommended.[1,10,29,33] Fruit or root vegetables can be used as a source of environmental enrichment or as a treat but should not be a main component of the pet's dietary routine.[1,29] As with any species, but especially in rabbits, a gradual introduction to new foods is recommended to allow the GI microbes time to adapt. In addition, careful monitoring of the pet's weight and body condition is essential to ensuring the pet is neither overfed nor underfed.

Select Diet-Responsive Disease Management

Fiber-associated disease states

Obesity. Because of the dramatic shift in lifestyle and food source, pet rabbits are predisposed to obesity.[9,33,35] Rabbits are normally very active and a caged lifestyle can dramatically reduce energy.[10] The inappropriate use of energy-concentrated commercial products can compound metabolic issues by resulting in overfeeding.[1,29] It can be challenging to effectively diagnose obesity in rabbits because of their dense and/or long hair and the presence of dewlaps in females. In addition, there is no

Box 4
Rabbit feeding recommendations[1,29,32]

- One-quarter cup of pellets per 2.3kg$_{BW}$ (~25–30 g diet/kg$_{BW}$) twice daily
- From 1 to 2 cups (237 mLs [8 fl oz]) cups of fresh, green vegetables per 2.3kg$_{BW}$/d
  - Examples: collards, mustard, dandelion greens, carrot tops, beet tops, broccoli tops, alfalfa sprouts and clover, parsley, cilantro, basil
- No more than 1 to 2 tablespoons of fruit or other vegetables per 2.3 kg$_{BW}$ several times per week

validated body condition scoring system in rabbits.[10] Obese rabbits are prone to a plethora of physiologic impairments that can, and often do, negatively affect quality of life. Examples include:[7,33,35]

- Grooming difficulties
- Sludgy urine
- Cystitis
- Ulcerative pododermatitis
- Hepatic steatosis and subsequent hepatic lipidosis

In addition, many obese rabbits cannot reach their anus, which hinders the consumption of cecotropes, potentially resulting in nutritional deficiencies.[33]

To treat, and ideally prevent, obesity in rabbits, dried forage should always be available to increase fiber and decrease calorie intake. In addition, pellets should be fed as directed earlier and the diet should have a fat level no more than 4% DM. In addition, to address overfeeding, the calories provided should be decreased by 10% every 2 weeks until an ideal calorie intake is achieved. Despite these measures, successful weight loss in rabbits can be extremely challenging because of poor client compliance.[10]

Malocclusion. Malocclusion of the teeth is the result of consuming a diet low in crude fiber.[10,35] Although natural vegetation promotes normal wear by encouraging horizontal chewing, nontraditional foodstuffs (hard pellets, carrots, grains, and so forth) promote vertical chewing (and reduced wear) instead.[7] Typically the incisors are the most effected; however, cheek teeth can become maloccluded. Common clinical signs include:[10]

- Anorexia
- Bruxism
- Facial swelling
- Potentially nasal discharge

Although affected teeth can be trimmed or filed, and, if needed, extracted, the best course of action is prevention with a high-fiber diet.

Gastrointestinal stasis (plus or minus trichobezoars). GI stasis is one of the most common disorders in domestic rabbits and, like obesity and malocclusion, is associated with an inappropriate diet.[35,43] A dietary fiber content less than 12.5% can reduce normal GI peristalsis, leading to GI stasis and hair retention in the stomach.[10,35,43] With the addition of reduced or absent fecal pellets, clinical signs can mimic those of malocclusion, which is why a complete and thorough physical examination and history is necessary for every case. GI stasis is considered emergent if lasting more than 24 hours, because rabbits can rapidly develop hepatic lipidosis and multiorgan failure.[35,43]

Patients with GI stasis should be treated aggressively with fluids, analgesics, and increased fiber intake until they begin eating and defecating on their own.[35] Select examples of higher-fiber, critical-care diets include Emeraid Intensive Care Herbivore (product information: https://emeraid.com/vet/emeraid-herbivore/), Oxbow Critical Care Herbivore (product information: https://www.oxbowanimalhealth.com/our-products/professional-line/critical-care/), and Supreme Science Selective Recovery (product information: https://supremepetfoods.com/products/science-selective-recovery/). When necessary, gastric decompression with a nasogastric tube should be considered. If needed, prokinetics such as metoclopramide or cisapride can be used in the absence of obstruction.[35] Trichobezoars that are unresponsive to medical management may require surgical intervention.[10]

Urolithiasis

The cause and pathophysiology behind urolithiasis in rabbits is not clearly understood and, like other animals, is presumed to be multifactorial.[33,35] Although rabbits are markedly different regarding their calcium homeostasis, it is still hypothesized that excessive dietary calcium levels could predispose to calcium carbonate urolithiasis; nevertheless, this information is extrapolated from anecdotal case reports rather than prospective studies.[31,35] The treatment of urolithiasis is similar to other domestic animals, consisting of a urocystotomy, stone analysis and culture, encouraging an increase in water intake, and reduction of calcium content in the diet.[33,35,44] Although not considered a first-line therapy, thiazide diuretics could be considered in certain cases.

SMALL RODENTS

Background and Husbandry

The order Rodentia comprises more than 1700 species, making up more than half of the total mammalian species. Rodents are further subclassified into 3 suborders: Hystricomorpha contains guinea pigs and chinchillas (infraorder Caviomorpha); Sciuromorpha are squirrel-like rodents; and Myomorpha contains mice, rats, hamsters, and gerbils.[10,45] Guinea pigs and chinchillas both originated in South America.[46,47] The former were domesticated approximately 2000 years ago as a source of food, remaining a significant source to this day. A wealth of information is available on guinea pigs because of their use in research.[46] The latter have been domesticated for significantly less time and, in the wild, were hunted almost to extinction for their fur.[10,46] Nutrient requirements for chinchillas are often extrapolated from those of guinea pigs because of insufficient published data. Both caviomorphs are small, gentle, and docile, making them good pets.[46]

Mice, rats, gerbils, and hamsters originated from different regions of Asia. Gerbils tend to be the hardiest of the small rodents, hamsters the least, and mice and rats in between. In general, small rodents can make excellent pets. Rats are especially good for children, because they are calm, large enough to handle, intelligent, interactive, and rarely bite. Because of their small size, high activity level, and speed of movements, mice and gerbils are better pets for older (>10 years) children.[45] Hamsters can be gentle but are nocturnal and startle easily. They are particularly known for their ability to escape via chewing and are prone to stress-induced proliferative ileitis.[10,45]

Although there are likely species variations, in general, caviomorphs give birth to precocial young and have longer lifespans, whereas myomorphs give birth to altricial young and have shorter lifespans. In addition, the caviomorphs discussed are significantly larger than the myomorphs.[10,45–47] **Table 8** presents biological characteristics of each rodent species discussed in this article. Although both gerbils and hamsters hail from dry, arid regions, they and other rodents neither sweat nor pant, which reduces their tolerance to ambient heat.[45] Guinea pigs and chinchillas are the least tolerant, having come from higher elevations. They both do well at temperatures between 18°C and 27°C (65°F and 80°F) with low humidity, although they are most comfortable at 10°C to 16°C (50°F–60°F).[10,46] Hamsters also do well at a temperature between 18°C and 21°C (65°F–70°F), but they are able to tolerate low to moderate humidity levels. Interestingly, at temperatures less than 5°C (41°F), hamsters may enter a deep sleep because they are permissible hibernators.[10,45] As desert dwellers, gerbils are more heat tolerant, being comfortable at 18°C to 29°C (65°F–85°F); however, they are still not tolerant of excessive heat and humidity levels.[10]

Table 8
Average biological characteristics of select rodents[10,45–47]

Trait	Guinea Pig	Chinchilla[a]	Hamster[a]	Gerbil	Rats	Mice
Birth Weight (g)	45–115	30–50	1.5–3	2.5–3.5	4–6	1–1.5
Adult Weight (g)	700–1200	400–600[b]	85–130[b]	50–130	225–500	20–60
Solid food introduction (d)	NA	7	1	2	1.5	2
Weaning (wk)	3	6–8	2.5–3	3–4	3–4	3
Puberty (mo)	2–3	8 (average)2–14	1.5–2	2–4	4–5	1.5
Life Span (y)	5–6[a]	10[c]	1.5–3	2–3	2–4	1–3

[a] Anecdotally 12+ years.
[b] Females are larger than males.
[c] Sources varied from 4 to 20 years.

All rodents must be housed in an enclosure that provides safety and space to explore and exercise. Rodents are prey animals and are subject to stress associated with external stimuli; as such, hiding boxes must be incorporated into their enclosures.[46] Chinchillas are very active and have a larger space requirement than other rodent species. Chinchillas are also unique in that they require dust baths to keep their fur clean of lipid and dirt buildup. Ideally, a dust bath is provided 4 to 7 times per week for up to 1 hour at a time.[10,46] Enrichment is also essential to optimizing pet health. Examples of rodent enrichment include, but are not limited to[45]:

- Exercise wheels
- Hide boxes
- Hidden treats
- Human interactions
- Shredding material

Both guinea pigs and chinchillas are social creatures; the former often live in group of 5 to 10, seeking physical contact when housed together, although the latter often live in groups of more than 100.[10,46,47] Rats are social as well, with multiple males and females being successfully housed in the same enclosure.[45] Gerbils are social within their families, but can show aggressive and territorial behaviors leading to the death and cannibalization of strangers.[45] Mice are the least social and do well in solitude.[45]

Anatomic, Physiologic, and Species Considerations

Although all rodent incisors are elodont, caviomorph dentition is most similar to that of rabbits in that their cheek teeth are also elodont. In contrast, myomorph cheek teeth are anelodont, making them less likely to have malocclusion.[10,45–47] Although the rodents in this article are all monogastric hindgut fermenters, they each have unique digestive characteristics.[10,45,47] For example, guinea pigs have a gastric pH of 2.9, a GI transit time of 20 hours, and a large cecum containing 44% of large intestine DM content. Chinchillas have a long GI tract but a GI transit time of 12 to 15 hours; additionally, the cecum is smaller than a guinea pig's, only holding 23% of all large intestinal DM content.[10,46,47] Hamsters have large cheek pouches that can carry either food or their young. In addition, they have a distinct, microbe-containing forestomach with a high pH contributing to energy production in the form of SCFAs. Gerbils have the unique ability to lengthen their GI tracts in response to increased dietary fiber.[10,45–47] Despite these differences, all rodents are coprophages, practicing some degree of cecotrophy.[10,45,48] For more information, please see discussion of cecotrophy, presented earlier.

Nutrition

Requirements

The nutrient requirements for all but chinchillas have been well defined because of their time in biomedical research. Extensive nutritional information and requirement estimates have been published by the National Research Council.[10,45,48,49] With the exception of being placentophagic, both chinchillas and guinea pigs are herbivores.[46,47] Small rodents are omnivorous, naturally having a diet composed of grass, seeds, grain, and invertebrates.[45,47] Rodents have an extremely high metabolic rate, thus preoperative starving is neither required nor recommended.[45,48] Like any group of species, energy and nutrient requirements depend on a variety of factors. Compounded by rodents' innate instinct to hoard food, it can be challenging to estimate their energy needs.[45] **Table 9** presents estimated caloric needs of rodents for different life stages.

Quantitative water requirements have been investigated; however, each individual pets' needs depend on species, life stage, reproductive status, and ambient temperature.[48] Water can be provided via bowls or sippers. Guinea pigs are noted to be slovenly, often defecating in and upturning water bowls. Although water sippers can help, guinea pigs can also regurgitate ingesta into the sipper. If sippers are used, they should be evaluated for functionality and cleaned regularly.[45] The following are water requirements for select rodents:

- Guinea pigs: 10 mL/100g_{BW}/d[10]
- Gerbils: 4 to 10 mL/100g_{BW}/d[47]

Regardless of the method, fresh, potable water should be available ad libitum and provided daily.[10,46]

With the exception of a select few nutrients, it seems that most rodents have similar nutritional needs.[47] Historically, sources noted that rodents did not need fiber; however, it is now known that caviomorphs need a significant quantity.[10,46–48] In addition, although the omnivorous rodents may not need fiber to the same extent, moderate levels optimize their GI health and reduce diarrhea.[10] Protein and fat needs are similar throughout rodent species, although the concentrations in commercial products vary slightly.[1,10,45] Note that gerbils are susceptible to developing hypercholesterolemia

Table 9
Estimated caloric requirements of rodents[1,10,47,48]

Life Stage	Guinea Pigs	Chinchilla	Hamsters	Gerbils[c]	Mice	Rats
Adult	$110\ BW_{kg}^{3/4}$ [a]	21g diet/ 100 g_{BW}	$110\ BW_{kg}^{3/4}$ [b]	5–8 g diet/ 100 g_{BW}	$110\ BW_{kg}^{3/4}$ [d]	$110\ BW_{kg}^{3/4}$ [e]
Growth/ Gestation	$145\ BW_{kg}^{3/4}$	NA	$145\ BW_{kg}^{3/4}$	$110\ BW_{kg}^{3/4}$	$145\ BW_{kg}^{3/4}$	$145\ BW_{kg}^{3/4}$
Lactation	$165\ BW_{kg}^{3/4}$	NA	$330\ BW_{kg}^{3/4}$	$110\ BW_{kg}^{3/4}$	$440\ BW_{kg}^{3/4}$	$440\ BW_{kg}^{3/4}$

[a] Pelleted diet, ~6 g/100 g_{BW}.
[b] Pelleted diet, ~15 to 20 g/100 g_{BW}.
[c] True needs unknown; presumed to be analogous to rats and mice.
[d] Pelleted diet, ~4-5 g/100 g_{BW}.
[e] Pelleted diet, ~10 g/100 g_{BW}.

secondary to high fat intake; however, the use of a quality gerbil diet should address this.[10,45] Also note that, unlike other rodents, guinea pigs lack sufficient L-gulonolactone oxidase activity and so cannot synthesize vitamin C, making it an essential component to their diets.[10,46,49] **Box 5** provides estimated nutrient needs for small rodents.

Feeding method

As with other pocket pets, disease can manifest as a result of inappropriate nutrition. Education is essential because many owners are not aware of the availability of specialized diets.[50] Both caviomorphs develop food preference early in life and can be reluctant to change. It is recommended to introduce them to a variety of foodstuffs from a young age to decrease picky behaviors.[10,46] The rodent diet should consist of[10,46,47]:

- Species-appropriate pellets (premeasured, but readily available)
  - See **Table 9** for estimated caloric needs
- Fresh forage (with the exception of gerbils)
  - Examples include alfalfa (caution is needed because of calcium content), orchard grass, timothy, and blue grasses
- Fresh vegetables
  - Examples include mixed greens (kale, parsley, beet greens), broccoli, carrots, zucchini, green beans
- Treats should be intermittent to rare (exceeding no more than 10% of calories)
  - Examples include apples, berries, kiwi

Select Diet-Responsive Disease Management

Rodents are similar to rabbits regarding presentation, pathophysiology, and management of many potential medical problems and diseases requiring nutritional intervention. For example, inappropriately low fiber intake in rodents also results in dental malocclusion, obesity, GI stasis, and dysbiosis.[51,52] In addition, like rabbits, not only is the primary urolith type in caviomorphs calcium carbonate but the diagnostic and treatment approach is also essentially the same.[51–53] However, as mentioned earlier, guinea pigs are unique in their requirement for vitamin C. Diets that contain insufficient levels can result in hypovitaminosis C (scurvy) within a matter of weeks. Without an essential constituent, collagen cannot form or function appropriately, resulting in gingivitis, joint deformities and pain, anorexia, poor haircoat, and eventually death.[10,51]

Box 5
Average requirements of select nutrients for adult rodents[10,45–49]

- Protein: ~16% to 20%[a]
- Fat: ~2% to 5%
- Fiber: ≥15%[b]
- Calcium: ~0.6%
- Phosphorus: ~0.35%
- Vitamin C: ~200 mg/kg[c]

[a]Guinea pigs, 16% maximum.[b]Gerbils, 10% maximum.[c]Applies only to guinea pigs.

DISCUSSION

Although small mammals have been used in research for decades (some hundreds of years), few advances pertaining specifically to domestic pocket pets have come to light since the mid-1990s to late 1900s. Because of this loss of momentum in pocket-pet research, most of the available information is in the form of review articles, rather than prospective, primary research articles. There is a vast wealth of nutritional information available on small mammals; however, many nutritional recommendations are still based on extrapolation from other species, showing that there is still much that can be learned. Without active, progressive research, the true potential for small mammal nutrition will never be attained. As with any animal, scientific research is key to clinician comprehension, clinician comprehension is key to client education, and client education is key to optimizing the health and well-being of the pocket pets.

CLINICS CARE POINTS

- Many clients find pocket pets appealing but are often uneducated in their unique husbandry and nutrition needs. It is essential that, when presented with a captive small mammal, clinicians be able to provide the necessary guidance and support.
- Poor nutrition and husbandry can manifest as severe clinical illness. To optimize the quality and quantity of life, pocket pets should be fed based on their specialized needs. Ferrets are obligate carnivore, rabbits and caviomorphs are cecotrophic herbivores, and myomorphs are cecotrophic omnivores.
- Each species has select disease states that may be diet responsive. A thorough medical history, dietary history, and physical examination are essential to making a correct diagnosis and, thus, optimal nutritional recommendations.

DISCLOSURE

The author has nothing to disclose.

REFERENCES

1. Kupersmith DS. A practical overview of small mammal nutrition. Semin Avian Exot Pet Med 1998;7(3):141–7.
2. Powers LV, Brown SA. [Ferrets] Basic anatomy, physiology, and husbandry. In: Quesenberry KE, Carpenter JW, editors. Ferrets, rabbits, and rodents: clinical medicine and surgery. 3rd edition. Philadelphia: Saunders; 2012. p. 1–12.
3. Fox JG, Schultz CS, Vester Boler BM. Nutrition of the Ferret. In: Fox JG, Marini RP, editors. Biology and diseases of ferrets. 3rd edition. John Wiley and Sons, Inc; 2014. p. 123–43.
4. Bell JA. Ferret nutrition. Vet Clin North Am Exot Anim Pract 1999;2(1):169–92.
5. Mayer J, Marini RP, Fox JG. Biology and diseases of ferrets. In: Fox JG, Anderson LC, Otto G, et al, editors. Laboratory animal medicine. 3rd edition. Amsterdam (Netherlands): Elsevier; 2015. p. 577–622.
6. Johnson-Delaney CA. Ferret nutrition. Vet Clin North Am Exot Anim Pract 2014;17(3):449–70.
7. Vella D, Donnelly TM. [Rabbits] Basic anatomy, physiology, and husbandry. In: Quesenberry KE, Carpenter JW, editors. Ferrets, rabbits, and rodents: clinical medicine and surgery. 3rd edition. Philadelphia: Saunders; 2012. p. 157–73.
8. Irlbeck NA. How to feed the rabbit (*Oryctolagus cuniculus*) gastrointestinal tract. J Anim Sci 2001;79(E. Suppl):343–6.

9. Nowland MH, Brammer DW, Garcia A, et al. Biology and diseases of rabbits. In: Fox JG, Anderson LC, Otto G, et al, editors. Laboratory animal medicine. 3rd edition. Amsterdam (Netherlands): Elsevier; 2015. p. 411–61.
10. Carpenter JW, Wolf KN, Kolmstetter C. Feeding Small Pet Mammals. In: Hand MS, Thatcher CD, Remillard RL, et al, editors. Small animal clinical nutrition. 5th edition. Topeka(KS): Mark Morris Institute; 2010. p. 1215–36.
11. Johnson-Delaney CA. Anatomy and Physiology of the Gastrointestinal System of the Ferret and Selected Exotic Carnivores. In: Proceedings for Association of Avian Veterinarians San Antonio(TX); 2006:30–38.
12. Bell J. Ensuring Proper Nutrition in Ferrets. Vet Med 1996;91:1098–103.
13. Quesenberry KE, Orcutt C. [Ferrets] Basic approach to veterinary care. In: Quesenberry KE, Carpenter JW, editors. Ferrets, rabbits, and rodents: clinical medicine and surgery. 3rd edition. Philadelphia: Saunders; 2012. p. 13–26.
14. Committee on Animal Nutrition, National Research Council. Nutrient requirements of mink and foxes. 2nd edition. National Academy Press; 1982.
15. Ad Hoc Committee on Dog and Cat Nutrition, Committee on Animal Nutrition, National Research Council. Nutrient requirements of dogs and cats. Washington, DC: National Academy Press; 2006.
16. Deshmukh DR, Shope TC. Arginine requirement and ammonia toxicity in ferrets. J Nutr 1983;113:1664–7.
17. Lederman JD, Overton KM, Hofmann NE, et al. Ferrets (*Mustela putorius furo*) Inefficiently Convert β-carotene to Vitamin A. J Nutr 1998;128:271–9.
18. Hoefer HL, Fox JG, Bell JA. [Ferrets] Gastrointestinal diseases. In: Quesenberry KE, Carpenter JW, editors. Ferrets, rabbits, and rodents: clinical medicine and surgery. 3rd edition. Philadelphia: Saunders; 2012. p. 27–45.
19. Church RR. The impact of diet on the dentition of the domesticated ferret. Exot DVM 2007;9(2):30–9.
20. Rosenthal KL, Wyre NR. [Ferrets] Endocrine diseases. In: Quesenberry KE, Carpenter JW, editors. Ferrets, rabbits, and rodents: clinical medicine and surgery. 3rd edition. Philadelphia: Saunders; 2012. p. 86–102.
21. Chen S. Advanced diagnostic approaches and current medical management of insulinomas and adrenocortical disease in ferrets (*Mustela putorius furo*). Vet Clin North Am Exot Anim Pract 2010;13:439–52.
22. Lurye JC, Behrend EN. Endocrine Tumors. Vet Clin North Am 2001;31(5): 1083–110.
23. Meleo K, Peterson M. Treatment of insulinoma in dogs, cats, and ferrets. In: Bonagura JD, Twedt DC, editors. Current veterinary therapy 15. Philadelphia: Saunders Elsevier; 2014. p. e130–4.
24. Antinoff N, Williams BH. [Ferrets] Neoplasia. In: Quesenberry KE, Carpenter JW, editors. Ferrets, rabbits, and rodents: clinical medicine and surgery. 3rd edition. Philadelphia: Saunders; 2012. p. 103–21.
25. Weiss CA, Williams BH, Scott MV. Insulinoma in the ferret: clinical findings and treatment comparison of 66 cases. J Am Hosp Assoc 1998;34:471–5.
26. Watson MK, Cazzini P, Mayer J, et al. Histology and immunohistochemistry of severe inflammatory bowel disease versus lymphoma in the ferret (*Mustela putorius furo*). J Vet Diagn Invest 2016;28(3):198–206.
27. Davenport DJ, Remillard RL, Jergens AE. Inflammatory bowel disease. In: Hand MS, Thatcher CD, Remillard RL, et al, editors. Small animal clinical nutrition. 5th edition. Topeka(KS): Mark Morris Institute; 2010. p. 1065–77.

28. Subcommittee on Rabbit Nutrition, Committee on Animal Nutrition, National Research Council. Nutrient requirements of rabbits. 2nd edition. Washington, DC: National Academy Press; 1977.
29. Campbell-Ward ML. [Rabbits] Gastrointestinal physiology and nutrition. In: Quesenberry KE, Carpenter JW, editors. Ferrets, rabbits, and rodents: clinical medicine and surgery. 3rd edition. Philadelphia: Saunders; 2012. p. 183–92.
30. Combes S, Michelland RJ, Monteils V, et al. Postnatal development of the rabbit caecal microbiota composition and activity. FEMS Microbiol Ecol 2011;77:680–9.
31. De Blas C, Wiseman J, editors. Nutrition of the rabbit. 2nd edition. Wallingford (Oxfordshire): CAB International; 2010.
32. Jenkins JR. Feeding recommendations for the house rabbit. Vet Clin North Am Exot Anim Pract 1999;1(2):143–51.
33. Clauss M, Hatt JM. Evidence-based rabbit housing and nutrition. Vet Clin North Am Exot Anim Pract 2017;20:871–84.
34. News and Reports. Survey reveals lack of knowledge of rabbit husbandry. Vet Rec 2010;166:543.
35. Maftoum L, Mayer J. Prescription diets for rabbits. Vet Clin North Am Exot Anim Pract 2014;17:485–502.
36. Gidenne T. Dietary fibres in the nutrition of the growing rabbit and recommendations to preserve digestive health: a review. Animal 2015;9(2):227–42.
37. Carabaño R, Badiola I, Chamorro S, et al. New trends in rabbit feeding: influence of nutrition on intestinal health. Spanish J Agric Res 2008;6(special issue):15–25.
38. Ehrlein HJ, Reich H, Schwinger M. Colonic motility and transit of digesta during hard and soft faeces formation in rabbits. J Physiol 1993;338:75–86.
39. Ciek LJ. Relationship between food and water ingestion in the rabbit. Am J Physiol 1961;201:557–66.
40. De Blas C, Wiseman J, editors. The nutrition of the rabbit. Wallingford (Oxfordshire): CAB International; 1998.
41. Clauss M, Burger B, Liesegang A, et al. Influence of diet on calcium motabolism, tissue calcification and urinary sludge in rabbits (*Oryctolagus cuniculus*). J Anim Physiol Anim Nutr (Berl) 2012;96:798–807.
42. McNitt JI, Lukefahr SD, Cheeke PR, et al, editors. Rabbit production. 9th edition. Wallingford (Oxfordshire): CAB International; 2013. p. 88–105.
43. Oglesbee BL, Jenkins JR. [Rabbits] Gastrointestinal Diseases. In: Quesenberry KE, Carpenter JW, editors. Ferrets, rabbits, and rodents: clinical medicine and surgery. 3rd edition. Philadelphia: Saunders; 2012. p. 193–204.
44. Kamphues J. Calcium metabolism of rabbits as an etiological factor for urolithiasis. J Nutr 1991;121:S95–6.
45. Lennox AM, Bauck L. [Rodents] Basic anatomy, physiology, husbandry, and clinical technique. In: Quesenberry KE, Carpenter JW, editors. Ferrets, rabbits, and rodents: clinical medicine and surgery. 3rd edition. Philadelphia: Saunders; 2012. p. 339–53.
46. Quesenberry KE, Donnelly TM, Mans C. Biology, husbandry, and clinical techniques of guinea pigs and chinchillas. In: Quesenberry KE, Carpenter JW, editors. Ferrets, rabbits, and rodents: clinical medicine and surgery. 3rd edition. Philadelphia: Saunders; 2012. p. 279–94.
47. Grant K. Rodent Nutrition. Vet Clin North Am Exot Anim Pract 2014;17:471–83.
48. Knapka JJ. Nutrition of Rodents. Vet Clin North Am Exot Anim Pract 1999;1(2): 153–67.

49. Subcommittee on Laboratory Animal Nutrition, Committee on Animal Nutrition, Board on Agriculture, National Research Council. Nutrient requirements of laboratory animals. *4th* edition. Washington, DC: National Academy Press; 1995.
50. Brown C, Donnelly TM. Disease problems of small rodents. In: Quesenberry KE, Carpenter JW, editors. Ferrets, rabbits, and rodents: clinical medicine and surgery. 3rd edition. Philadelphia: Saunders; 2012. p. 354–72.
51. Hawkins MG, Bishop CR. Disease problems of guinea pigs. In: Quesenberry KE, Carpenter JW, editors. Ferrets, rabbits, and rodents: clinical medicine and surgery. 3rd edition. Philadelphia: Saunders; 2012. p. 295–310.
52. Mans C, Donnelly TM. Disease problems of chinchillas. In: Quesenberry KE, Carpenter JW, editors. Ferrets, rabbits, and rodents: clinical medicine and surgery. 3rd edition. Philadelphia: Saunders; 2012. p. 311–25.
53. Hawkins MG, Ruby AL, Drazenovich TL, et al. Composition and characteristics of urinary calculi from guinea pigs. J Am Vet Med Assoc 2009;234(2):214–20.

The Gut Microbiome of Dogs and Cats, and the Influence of Diet

Rachel Pilla, DVM, PhD*, Jan S. Suchodolski, DrVetMed, PhD

KEYWORDS

• Healthy dog • Healthy cat • Protein • Fiber • Raw diet • Dysbiosis • Bile acids
• Short-chain fatty acids

KEY POINTS

- The gut microbiome is a functional organ, and dietary substrates are converted by different intestinal bacteria to metabolically active compounds that influence the host.
- Butyrate, for example, can be produced from either fiber or protein, suggesting that both increased fiber and increased protein in the diet may bring similar benefits and have the largest impact on the intestinal microbiome and metabolome composition.
- Although fiber and protein content appear to be main influencers of microbiome composition in both dogs and cats, the ideal fiber and protein intake to promote a healthy microbiome needs to be determined.
- Diet-induced changes in the microbiome of healthy dogs are less marked compared with microbiome changes associated with disease.

BACKGROUND

The gut microbiome is composed of bacteria, archaea, viruses, and eukaryotic organisms that reside in the gastrointestinal (GI) tract. The bacterial component is the largest and provides essential digestive functions, such as fermentation of fibers. The gut microbiome also contributes to host metabolism, protects against pathogens, and educates the immune system. Expanding knowledge of microbiome functions has revealed several remote connections leading to the coinage of terms such as the gut-brain axis, gut-skin axis, and others.

Many diseases, systemic or localized, are associated with dysbiosis. Gut dysbiosis is defined as changes in the composition of the gut microbiome that impact its function.[1] The increase in abundance of facultative anaerobic bacteria of the family Enterobacteriaceae is a hallmark of dysbiosis,[2] seen also in dogs.[3] The composition of the gut microbiota also has significant effects on immune function, and regulating the local

Gastrointestinal Laboratory, Department of Small Animal Clinical Sciences, Texas A&M University, Texas A&M College of Veterinary Medicine & Biomedical Sciences, 4474 TAMU, College Station, TX 77843-4474, USA
* Corresponding author.
E-mail address: rpilla@cvm.tamu.edu

Vet Clin Small Anim 51 (2021) 605–621
https://doi.org/10.1016/j.cvsm.2021.01.002 **vetsmall.theclinics.com**
0195-5616/21/

production of antibodies,[4] and the differentiation of intestinal helper T (Th) cell precursors. Intestinal inflammation also can be triggered by gut dysbiosis in different diseases through bile acid dysmetabolism,[5–7] or through the decreased production of anti-inflammatory molecules, such as short-chain fatty acids (SCFAs)[8–10] and indoles.[11,12] Although outside of the scope of this review, recent work has associated dysbiosis with obesity,[13,14] metabolic diseases,[15,16] cancer,[17] neurologic disfunctions,[18,19] and many others, both in dogs and in humans. However, caution should be taken when interpreting those findings, as a causation effect is yet to be proven, and the dysbiosis may be a symptom of the disease process rather than its cause.

The gut microbiome is responsive to nutrients. Changes in bacterial taxa often require large changes in dietary macronutrients; but alterations in bacterial-derived metabolites and, therefore, microbiota function may already occur due to the addition of micronutrients, and this is an emerging area of current microbiome research. Some bacterial species ferment different types of fiber and carbohydrates, and others are strongly proteolytic. Therefore, changes in the diet that affect the availability of such substrates in the gut will result in alterations of the microbiome and metabolome. Due to its resilience, dietary-induced changes in microbiome composition are maintained only by long-term maintenance of a specific diet. A good example is a study[20] in which healthy dogs were fed diets containing only purified amino acids and easily digestible starch for 32 weeks. At the end of the trial, dogs returned to the control diet, and microbiome composition quickly returned to baseline.[20]

Microbiome changes are individualized,[21] as the microbiome is an intrinsically redundant ecosystem, in which many unrelated species occupy the same niche.[22] This has a significant evolutionary advantage, because if only a single species performed an essential function, any aggression to the microbiome (such as antibiotic treatment) affecting that species would deprive the host of that function. Therefore, multiple species are necessary for microbiome resilience, and higher species richness is considered an indicator of a healthy microbiome.[22]

The GI tract regions are colonized with different bacterial populations. The composition varies according to luminal conditions, with a predominance of oxygen-tolerating bacteria in the small, and an abundance of strict anaerobes in the large intestine.[23,24] Because sampling from the proximal intestine is difficult, most clinical studies focus on fecal microbiota, and the abundance of most relevant bacterial species for gut health in dogs can be reliably measured in feces.[3] When analyzing the microbiome along the GI tract of cats, samples clustered by individual cat rather than by site of collection, indicating that fecal samples are also representative of the cat microbiome.[24]

METHODS FOR MICROBIAL ANALYSIS

Microbiological culture is useful for the subset of bacteria that are culturable, but molecular methods have largely replaced culture due to their ability to capture nonculturable bacteria.[25] Molecular methods, such as 16S ribosomal RNA (rRNA) gene sequencing and DNA shotgun sequencing, aim to measure the diversity of species present in the sample. That is accomplished by either amplifying and sequencing a fragment of a conserved region of the 16S rRNA gene, or by sequencing all available DNA in the sample (shotgun sequencing). Shotgun sequencing has the advantage of going beyond bacterial identification by also sequencing functional genes; however, it requires larger amounts of DNA from the sample, and is more expensive. Quantitative polymerase chain reaction (qPCR) is a quick, affordable, and reproducible method to quantify specific taxa that have been identified as clinically relevant.

Most studies focus on 16S rRNA gene sequencing, which generates phylogenetical data, and methods for sequencing and data analysis are in constant evolution.[26] Indeed, this is one disadvantage of these methods: different sequencing and/or data analysis methods may generate differences in the results, which prevents the development of reference intervals. When reviewing the literature, a wide variation in percentages of specific bacterial taxa can be seen, making comparisons between studies difficult.

Another limitation of most microbiome studies is that investigators typically compare the effects of environmental factors (eg, diet, storage, antibiotic treatment, breed influences, geography) with a control group or with its own baseline within the study, and often with a small sample size. Therefore, when changes (eg, due to diets) are observed, it is difficult to extrapolate the magnitude of these changes, and how they compare against a normal microbiota in a large reference population. Because of its high reproducibility, qPCR allows the development of reference intervals for specific taxa. One example is the canine fecal dysbiosis index (DI), a qPCR-based assay that quantifies 7 bacterial taxa, which are then combined into one single number.[27] Reference intervals for this assay have been established based on 120 healthy dogs from different countries and fed different commercial diets (https://tx.ag/DysbiosisGI). The DI can be used as a marker for normal microbiota, and is useful to track changes in microbiota over time in response to therapy in dogs.[26,28] The reference intervals for the 7 bacteria allow for comparison of effect sizes between studies, and whether changes in the microbiota fall within or outside the normal range (**Fig. 1**).

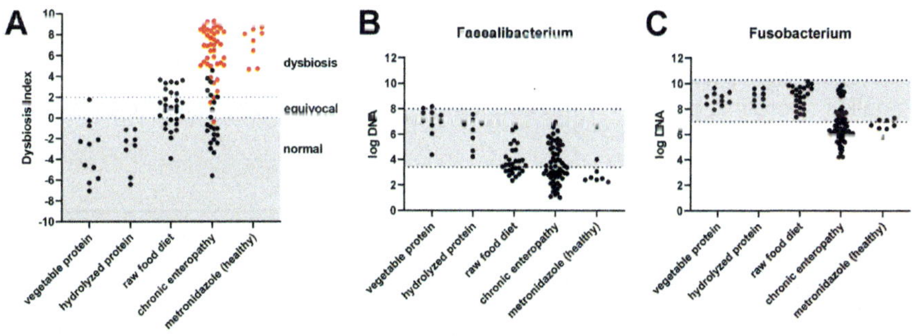

Fig. 1. The canine qPCR-based fecal DI (*A*) and key bacterial taxa *Faecalibacterium* (*B*) and *Fusobacterium* (*C*), both butyrate producers through different pathways (from carbohydrate and protein/amino acids, respectively), for different diet types, in comparison with chronic enteropathy[8] and metronidazole administration.[36] The gray areas indicate reference intervals, which allow comparison across studies and to a large reference population. Dots in red indicate dogs that also had a low abundance of *C hiranonis*, a beneficial bacterium that converts primary to secondary bile acids in the canine intestine. Dogs with chronic enteropathy and healthy dogs receiving metronidazole have a dysbiosis that is, associated with decreased *Faecalibacterium, Fusobacterium,* and *C hiranonis.* Lack of the latter results in abnormal bile acid metabolism. In contrast, dogs fed a raw food diet,[54] high in protein and fat, and low in fiber, have an increased fecal DI mostly driven due to low *Faecalibacterium* and increased *E coli* (not shown). The vegetable protein[44] and hydrolyzed protein diet[36] fed for 60 and 42 days, respectively, have similar macronutrient composition to commercial adult dog diets, despite the uniqueness of some ingredients. Accordingly, the fecal DI, and abundances of *Faecalibacterium* and *Fusobacterium* remained within normal reference intervals.

CORE MICROBIOTA

Key bacterial species are consistently present in fecal samples of healthy dogs, indicating the presence of a core fecal bacterial community. **Table 1** shows some of the most relevant bacterial taxa in fecal samples of dogs. The fecal microbiome of healthy dogs is co-dominated by 3 phyla: Firmicutes, Bacteroidetes, and Fusobacterium.[29,30] Within this core bacterial community, many major taxa belong to phylum Firmicutes, including Clostridia and Bacilli,[31,32] many of which are SCFA producers, such as *Faecalibacterium*. Bacteroidetes is another abundant phylum in fecal samples from dogs, including *Prevotella* and *Bacteroides*, which are highly variable in abundance between dogs.[3]

The genus *Fusobacterium* is typically associated with health in dogs. This is in contrast to people, in which *Fusobacterium nucleatum* is a pathogen associated with colorectal cancer.[33] In the GI tract of dogs, other *Fusobacterium* species, such as *Fusobacterium mortiferum* and *Fusobacterium perfoetens,* are typically observed,[34] and these seem to play a different role.[3] Fusobacteria are severely impacted by antibiotic treatment[35] and GI diseases,[26] and their recovery is slower than other phyla.[36] Therefore, in dogs Fusobacteria may be a therapeutic target for specific food ingredients that can increase their abundance.

Proteobacteria and Actinobacteria are also commonly identified and are typically colonizers of the small intestine, and in physiologic conditions will present in smaller numbers in fecal samples. For example, members of the family Enterobacteriaceae (eg, *Escherichia coli*) are facultative anaerobes, which allows them to take advantage of the oxygen available in the small intestine. Although part of the normal microbiome in small numbers, an increase of Enterobacteriaceae in fecal samples is a hallmark of dysbiosis[3] and is associated with many diseases, both within and outside of the GI tract.[8,37,38]

The literature on the fecal microbiome of healthy cats is less extensive. The fecal microbiome of cats is dominated in most studies by Firmicutes,[24,39–43] followed by smaller percentages of Proteobacteria, Actinobacteria, Bacteroidetes, and

Table 1
Relevant bacterial taxa in the fecal microbiome of dogs, organized according to the Greengenes database taxonomy[95]

Phylum	Class	Family	Genus/Species
Actinobacteria	Coriobacteriia	Coriobacteriaceae	*Collinsella*
Bacteroidetes	Bacteroidetes	Prevotellaceae	*Prevotella*
		Bacteroidaceae	*Bacteroides*
Firmicutes	Clostridia	Clostridiaceae	*Clostridium*
		Ruminococcaceae	*Faecalibacterium prausnitzii*
		Peptostreptococcaceae	*Peptostreptococcus*
		Lachnospiraceae	*Blautia*
		Veillonellaceae	*Megamonas*
	Bacilli	Streptococcaceae	*Streptococcus*
		Lactobacillaceae	*Lactobacillus*
		Turicibacteraceae	*Turicibacter*
Fusobacteria	Fusobacteriia	Fusobacteriaceae	*Fusobacterium*
Proteobacteria	Betaproteobacteria	Alcaligenaceae	*Sutterella*
	Gammaproteobacteria	Enterobacteriaceae	*E. coli*

Fusobacteria. One study compared the fecal microbiome of dogs and cats fed species-appropriate commercial diets, and found that cats had a larger number of species than dogs,[41] hinting at a higher diversity; however, more studies are needed to confirm that finding.

Although changes in microbiome composition can be important, they do not reflect changes in microbiome function. Recent studies are going beyond describing "Who is there?" and investigate the more pressing question of "What are they doing?" The study of bacterial metabolites through fecal metabolomics has revealed some major pathways regulated by bacteria, such as SCFA production, bile acid deconjugation and dehydroxylation, production of neurotransmitters such as serotonin and gamma-aminobutyric acid (GABA), and anti-inflammatory compounds such as indoles. Diet can influence bacterial metabolites, which can remotely affect organs such as the brain, skin, or muscle.

EFFECTS OF DIETS ON MICROBIOTA IN DOGS

Most microbiome studies in dogs have evaluated effects of extruded diets, which represent up to 95% of the dog food market. Extruded diets typically include a high carbohydrate load, but high-protein low-carbohydrate alternatives are available. Also increasingly popular are raw diets, frozen or freeze-dried, which are typically meat based and include low carbohydrate percentages. A small but increasing percentage of owners feed homemade diets, either raw or cooked.

Studies have shown that gut microbiome profiles in different species reflect their diet composition, especially when large macronutrient differences such as carnivore versus herbivore diets are considered.[44–46] In omnivore species, including humans, the short-term consumption of diets composed entirely of animal or plant products is enough to alter the microbial community structure and overwhelm interindividual differences in microbial gene expression.[46] In humans, the consumption of an animal-based diet increased the dietary intake of fat and protein, and decreased fiber intake to nearly zero. Such changes led to an increase in the abundance of bile-tolerant microorganisms and decreases the levels of Firmicutes, which includes species known to metabolize dietary plant polysaccharides.

For the canine gut microbiome, the ingredients seem to be less important than the overall macronutrient content. One study found that an extruded diet prepared exclusively with plant sources of protein did not significantly alter the microbiome of dogs when compared with a traditional (mixed animal and plant) extruded diet with similar macronutrient content.[44]

Major shifts in macronutrient composition were tested in a study in healthy dogs, which included 4 dry prescription diets formulated for weight loss, for renal disease, to be low-fat, or anallergenic.[47] The weight loss diet had the most drastic changes in macronutrients (higher protein and fiber) and resulted in the largest shift in microbiome composition. Increased protein content was associated with increased Fusobacteria. The abundance of SCFA producers *Bacteroides*, *Prevotella*, and *Faecalibacterium* was significantly increased in dogs fed the weight loss diet, and *Faecalibacterium* was increased in the low-fat diet. The weight-loss (28.1% fiber) and low-fat (8.6% fiber) diets both included soluble and insoluble fiber (beet pulp, fructooligosaccharide [FOS], and psyllium), and the increase in those genera is likely related to increased fiber content and different fiber types.

Different fibers have been studied for their prebiotic properties, and induce specific changes in the microbiome (**Table 2**). Most fibers act by enriching fiber-fermenting SCFA-producing Firmicutes.[29,48–52] Inulin-type fructans can increase SCFA,[48]

Table 2
Main effects of different types of fiber in the fecal microbiome and metabolome of dogs

Fiber Type	Main Findings	Method	References
Beet pulp	↓ Erysipelotrichi and Fusobacteria ↑ Firmicutes and Clostridia	16S rRNA seq.	Middelbos et al,[29] 2010
Inulin-type fructans	↑ Firmicutes, Erysipelotrichaceae, and Turicibacteraceae	16S rRNA seq.	Alexander et al,[50] 2018
Inulin	↓ Enterobacteriaceae ↑ *Megamonas* and *Lactobacillus*	16S rRNA seq.	Beloshapka et al,[52] 2013
Potato fiber	↓ *Prevotella* and *Fusobacterium* ↑ *Faecalibacterium, Lachnospira,* fecal acetate, propionate and butyrate	16S rRNA seq.	Panasevich et al,[48] 2013; Panasevich et al,[49] 2015
Soybean husk	↓ *Clostridium* cluster XI ↑ Total lactobacilli, *Faecalibacterium, Bacteroides-Prevotella-Porphyromonas*, and *Clostridium* cluster XIVa	qPCR	Myint et al,[51] 2017
Yeast cell wall	↑ *Bifidobacterium*	16S rRNA seq.	Beloshapka et al,[52] 2013

Abbreviations: qPCR, quantitative polymerase chain reaction; rRNA seq., ribosomal RNA sequencing.
↑ Up arrows indicate increased abundance
↓ Down arrows indicate decreased abundance

including acetate, butyrate and propionate, total fecal bile acids,[50] and decrease Enterobacteriaceae.[50,52]

A few studies[53–55] have evaluated the impact of meat-based raw diets on the gut microbiome of healthy dogs. Meat-based raw diets are typically very different in macronutrient content compared with control diets, with higher protein and lower carbohydrate and fiber. Dogs fed raw diets showed overall decreases in Firmicutes[54] and Bacteroidetes,[53] as shown in **Table 3**. Most decreased bacteria are associated with SCFA production from dietary carbohydrate,[56] indicating a decrease in carbohydrate fermentation due to decreased intake. Proteobacteria, Fusobacteria, and protein-associated genera increased in abundance.[53,54] One study with 6 dogs fed a raw diet for more than 1 year found increased microbiome diversity,[55] and an increased abundance of *Clostridium perfringens* and *Fusobacterium varium*, both known to produce butyrate from protein,[56] suggesting an adaptation to the diet.

Although Clostridiaceae can be associated with GI disease, it has been suggested that their increase when protein-rich diets are fed to dogs may not be detrimental to their health,[53] but are rather associated with protein digestion. In addition, Clostridiaceae were also found to positively correlate with protein digestibility and firmer fecal scores, and negatively correlate with fecal protein content (ie, more Clostridiaceae results in less undigested protein in feces) and less fecal output.[53]

Clostridium hiranonis is a bacterial species associated with normal bile acid (BA) metabolism,[6,57] and was found to increase in 2 studies with higher protein diets.[55,57] *C hiranonis* is often decreased in dogs with gastrointestinal disease, and after treatment with antibiotics (see **Fig. 1**). A study[54] reported normal BA metabolism in healthy dogs fed bones and raw foods (BARF) diets, with no significant difference from kibble-fed controls (see **Fig. 1**). BA metabolism is an important pathway not only for lipid

Table 3
Summary of findings from studies that evaluated the effect of high-protein diets on the fecal microbiome of dogs

Diet	Main Findings	Time on diet, n	Reference
Bones and raw foods (BARF)	↓ *Bifidobacterium* and *Faecalibacterium*; ↑ Fusobacteria, *Escherichia coli*, *Streptococcus*, and *Clostridium*	4 wk to 9 y, n = 27	Schmidt et al,[54] 2018
Red meat	↓ *Faecalibacterium*, *Peptostreptococcus*, *Bacteroides*, and *Prevotella* ↑ *Fusobacterium*, *Lactobacillus*, and *Clostridium*	9 wk, n = 7	Bermingham et al,[53] 2017
Raw diet	↑ Richness, evenness, *Clostridium perfringens*, *Clostridium hiranonis*, *Dorea*, and *Fusobacterium varium*	At least 1 y, n = 6	Kim et al,[55] 2017
Kibble with boiled beef	↓ *Faecalibacterium prausnitzii* ↑ *Clostridium hiranonis*, *Dorea*, *Slackia*, and unidentified Clostridiaceae	1 wk per combination, n = 11	Herstad et al,[57] 2017

digestion, but also for regulation of intestinal inflammation, and is commonly altered in chronic gastrointestinal diseases.[6,7]

Bifidobacterium, *Lactobacillus*, and *Faecalibacterium* are considered beneficial in omnivores, and the effect of diet on their abundances is often investigated.[58] Their benefit is due to their role in carbohydrate fermentation resulting in butyrate. The role of butyrate, an SCFA, in intestinal health is undisputed, as butyrate is the preferred energy source for colonocytes.[59]

However, butyrate can be found in fecal samples of all mammals regardless of their food sources. Therefore, in mammals that consume little to no carbohydrates, alternative pathways for butyrate production must be present. In a study comparing high-fat with high-starch diets in dogs, acetate, butyrate, and propionate levels were not different between dogs fed either diet, indicating that the production of SCFA in dogs is not exclusively dependent on carbohydrate content.[60] Supporting that hypothesis, another study[57] found that the addition of minced meat to a dry food diet actually led to a small increase in fecal butyrate and isovalerate.

A recent study has highlighted that in carnivores, Clostridiaceae, and in particular *C perfringens*, are associated with the butyrate kinase butyrate-synthesis pathway, which allows the production of butyrate from protein.[56] Another bacterium known to produce butyrate from protein sources is *F varium*,[61] which was more abundant in a group of dogs fed meat-based raw diets for more than 1 year, suggesting an adaptation of the microbiome to the long-term diet.[55] In addition, members of the Fusobacteriaceae family have been found to be more abundant in other carnivore species (cats,[62,63] wolves,[64,65] other carnivora[56,66]), and dogs fed high-protein raw diets.[53,54,67]

Those findings bring into question whether bacteria that specialize in carbohydrate fermentation bring the same benefits described in omnivores to the carnivore GI tract.[53] It is possible that in carnivores the butyrate production may be at least partially accomplished by other bacterial species such as members of the Clostridiaceae and Fusobacteriaceae families, which could be the reason for their increase in dogs fed raw diets.

Another bacteria-derived metabolite that can be affected by diet is GABA, a neurotransmitter, and its precursor gamma-hydroxybutyric acid (GHB).[54] BARF diets have also been found to increase fecal levels of GABA and GHB.[54] Ketogenic diets in mice have also led to microbiome-mediated increases in GABA,[68] and it is possible that the high fat and low carbohydrate content of BARF diets trigger similar changes. Both GABA and GHB are quickly absorbed from the GI tract when administered orally,[69,70] and fermented foods rich in GABA-producing bacteria (*Lactobacillus* and *Bifidobacterium*) are available in Japan for the treatment of hypertension.[71,72] The BARF diet also resulted in increased abundance of lactic acid bacteria such as Lactobacillales and *Steptococcus*,[54] which both of which can produce GABA.[73] The connection between the gut and the brain has been studied in many diseases, in dogs and other species, and ketogenic diets have been shown to be beneficial for dogs with neurologic diseases.[74,75] Recent studies[76,77] have shown that ketogenic diets impact microbiome composition, which may be one of the mechanisms by which they reduce seizure frequency.

EFFECTS OF DIETS ON MICROBIOTA IN CATS

High-protein/low-carbohydrate diets (HPLC), both extruded and raw, have been studied in cats compared with traditional moderate protein extruded diets. In cats, canned diets are an additional higher protein alternative, which is commonly fed alone or in combination with extruded diets. The use of moist foods in cats is supported by research indicating that their consumption leads to increased water intake,[78,79] decreased voluntary energy intake,[79] and decreased urine specific gravity,[79] which may be beneficial for certain health conditions.

Studies[80–82] have evaluated the microbiome of kittens weaned onto HPLC extruded diets compared with kittens weaned onto medium protein/medium carbohydrate (MP/MC) diets. There was some agreement between the studies, and their main findings are summarized in **Table 4**. Interestingly, species diversity was increased by HPLC,[82] and 5 genera that increased in HPLC-fed kittens[81] are known butyrate producers: *Clostridium* and *Eubacterium* may produce butyrate either from carbohydrate through the *but* pathway, or from protein through the *buk* pathway, whereas *Faecalibacterium*, *Ruminococcus,* and *Blautia* are producers through the *but* pathway.[56] Differences between kittens fed either diet affected 194 metabolic pathways, including pathways related to amino acid biosynthesis and metabolism, indicating that the protein:carbohydrate ratio has a significant effect on microbiome function.[82] However, the impact of such metabolite differences on overall health is still unknown.

The literature evaluating raw meat–based diets on the gut microbiome is less extensive in cats. Feeding raw 1-day-old to 3-day-old chicks,[83] or raw beef[84] to adult cats resulted in increases in genera known to be SCFA-producers[84,85] (see **Table 4**). Although the butyrate concentration was not increased in cats fed raw beef, the butyrate molar ratio was higher, indicating a shift in the proportions of different SCFAs. However, when plant fiber (2% as fed, inulin and cellulose) was added to raw beef, the microbiome became more similar to that of cats fed the control extruded diet, and fecal acetate:propionate:butyrate ratio was almost identical to that of controls.[84]

Similarly to raw diets, canned cat food has higher average protein and fat content, and lower carbohydrates content, compared with extruded dry foods. The microbiome of adult cats and kittens fed canned diets is more diverse[62,86] (see **Table 4**). As with other high-protein diets, many genera enriched by canned diets are associated with butyrate production, and may therefore be beneficial for intestinal health.[84]

Table 4
Summary of findings from studies that evaluated the effect of high-protein diets in the fecal microbiome of cats

Diet	Main Findings	Age	Time on Diet, n	Reference
High-protein low-carbohydrate dry food	↓ *Lactobacillus*, *Bifidobacterium*, and *Escherichia coli*	Kitten, weaning diet	8 wk, n = 7	Vester et al,[80] 2009
	↓ Actinobacteria, *Bifidobacterium*, *Dialister*, *Acidaminococcus*, *Megasphera*, and *Mitsuokella* ↑ Fusobacteria, *Clostridium*, *Faecalibacterium*, *Ruminococcus*, *Blautia*, and *Eubacterium*	Kitten, weaning diet	8 wk, n = 7	Hooda et al,[81] 2013
	↑ species diversity; Affected 194 metabolic pathways, including amino acid synthesis and metabolism	Kitten, weaning diet	8 wk, n = 6	Deusch et al,[82] 2014
to 3-day-old chicks	↑ *Peptococcus*, *Pseudobutyrivibrio*, and unidentified Lachnospiraceae	Adult	10 d, n = 5	Kerr et al,[83] 2014
Raw	↑ *Clostridium*, *Fusobacterium*, *Eubacterium*, and molar ratio of butyrate	Adult	3 wk, n = 12	Butowski et al,[84] 2019
Raw plus plant fiber	↓ *Clostridium*, *Fusobacterium*, and *Eubacterium* ↑ *Prevotella*	Adult	3 wk, n = 12	Butowski et al,[84] 2019
Canned	↓ Firmicutes, *Bacteroides*, *Lactobacillus*, and *Streptococcus* ↑ *Fusobacterium*, *Clostridium*, unidentified Peptostreptococcaceae and Prevotellaceae	Kitten, weaning diet	9 wk, n = 10	Bermingham et al,[86] 2013
	↓ *Lactobacillus*, *Megasphera*, and *Olsenella* ↑ richness, Fusobacteria, Proteobacteria, *Clostridium*, *Blautia*, *Bacteroides*, and unidentified Peptostreptococcaceae	Adult	5 wk, n = 16	Bermingham et al,[62] 2013
	↓ *Lactobacillus*, *Bifidobacterium*, and *Collinsella* ↑ *Bacteroides*, *Clostridium*, *Fusobacterium*, genes involved in vitamin biosynthesis, metabolism and transport	Kitten, weaning diet	9 wk, n = 10	Young et al,[88] 2016

Due to the strict carnivorous nature of cats, hindgut fermentation was considered unimportant.[87] However, several studies have evaluated the impact of dietary fiber on fecal microbiome composition in cats, and their results are summarized in **Table 5**. Similar to dogs, prebiotic fibers increase SCFA-producing bacterial

Table 5
Main effects of different types of fiber in the fecal microbiome and metabolome of cats

Fiber Type	Main Findings	Method	References
FOS	↑ *Bifidobacterium*	qPCR	Kanakupt et al.[89] 2011
	↑ Actinobacteria	16S rRNA seq.	Barry et al,[39] 2012
GOS	↑ *Bifidobacterium*	qPCR	Kanakupt et al,[89] 2011
FOS and GOS	↑ *Bifidobacterium,* total SCFA, butyrate and valerate	qPCR	Kanakupt et al,[89] 2011
FOS and inulin	↓ Gammaproteobacteria ↑ Veillonaceae	16S rRNA seq.	Garcia-Mazcorro et al,[42] 2017
Inulin	↓ *Faecalibacterium* and *Fusobacterium* ↑ *Bifidobacterium*	16S rRNA seq.	Young et al,[88] 2016
Cellulose	No changes	16S rRNA seq.	Barry et al,[39] 2012
Wool hydrolysate	No changes	16S rRNA seq.	Deb-Choudhury et al,[96] 2018
Pectin	↑ Firmicutes	16S rRNA seq.	Barry et al,[39] 2012
Mixed insoluble fibers	↓ isobutyric, 2-methylbutyric, and isovaleric acids ↑ *Blautia, Bacteroides, Turicibacter,* acetic and propionic acids	16S rRNA seq.	Wernimont et al,[97] 2019
Inulin and cellulose	↓ *Clostridium, Fusobacterium,* and *Eubacterium* ↑ *Prevotella, Bifidobacterium, Lactobacillus, Megamonas,* and unclassified Lachnospiraceae	16S rRNA seq.	Hooda et al,[81] 2013

Abbreviations: FOS, fructooligosaccharides; GOS, galactooligosaccharides; qPCR, quantitative polymerase chain reaction; rRNA seq., ribosomal RNA sequencing; SCFA, short-chain fatty acid.

genera,[39,81,87] but also *Bifidobacterium*.[81,86,88] The combination of FOS and galactooligosaccharides also led to increased concentrations of total SCFA, butyrate, and valerate.[89]

DIET VERSUS DISEASE EFFECTS ON THE MICROBIOME

Although diet can change microbiome composition significantly, and result in changes both in metabolic pathways and production of metabolites, those changes are typically much smaller than those that accompany disease.[26] In sick animals, and in particular those with gastrointestinal disease (eg, chronic enteropathies), microbiome diversity is quickly reduced, and many core species, such as *C hiranonis*, *Fusobacterium* spp, and *Faecalibacterium praunitzii*, are decreased[6,8,26,28] (see **Fig. 1**). Therefore, although dietary manipulations of microbiome composition can likely play a role in fostering a healthy and resilient microbe community, they are in most cases unlikely to generate changes comparable in magnitude to those observed in disease.

Diet modification, prebiotics, and probiotics are often used, alone or together with medications, to ameliorate clinical signs of diseases including diarrhea. The changes in microbiome composition associated with diarrhea are extensive and have been reviewed elsewhere,[26] and are accompanied by functional changes in digestion and motility that modify the luminal environment, further affecting microbiome composition. Hypoallergenic diets, formulated to reduce immunogenicity and facilitate digestion, do not significantly affect the microbiome of healthy dogs,[36,44] but have been associated with improved microbiome composition in dogs with food-responsive diarrhea.[44,90] Similarly, prebiotic fibers can aid recovery of beneficial bacterial populations and restore SCFA production. Probiotics, which are beneficial bacterial species, also can be fed to aid recovery. Although their colonization is typically transient,[31,91] probiotics can still be metabolically active during their transit, and produce beneficial metabolites that help improve clinical signs.[92] Probiotics have been reported to have a protective effect on acute diarrhea outbreaks, and to have beneficial effects on mucosal homeostasis,[93] speeding disease remission[94] in dogs with chronic diarrhea.

SUMMARY

The gut microbiome is a functional organ, and is responsive to the nutrient composition of diet. However, major shifts in microbiome composition are only observed with major changes in macronutrient composition, such as high-protein or high-fiber diets. More importantly, changes in bacterial composition may affect the production of metabolites in the gut. Indeed, fiber, starch, and protein content seem to be the key modulating players, and changes in those nutrient profiles cause rapid shifts in microbiome and metabolome composition, likely due to the changes in substrate availability. Because of the redundancy of the microbial communities, key metabolites can be produced by different bacteria. Butyrate, for example, can be produced from either fiber or protein, suggesting that both increased fiber or increased protein in the diet may bring similar benefits; however, the ideal levels of fiber and protein remain to be determined. The microbiome of healthy dogs and cats is resilient and adaptable, and it is capable of quickly restoring itself to baseline composition once the animal returns to its usual diet, indicating that sustained change requires long-term administration of a specific diet. Although diet affects the microbiome and metabolome of healthy dogs, changes associated with disease are of greater magnitude. In those cases, dietary change, prebiotic fibers, and probiotic bacteria can be beneficial to help improve microbial diversity and metabolite production.

DISCLOSURE

R. Pilla and J.S. Suchodolski are employed by the Gastrointestinal Laboratory at Texas A&M University, which provides assay for intestinal function and microbiota analysis on a fee-for-service basis.

REFERENCES

1. Zeng MY, Inohara N, Nunez G. Mechanisms of inflammation-driven bacterial dysbiosis in the gut. Mucosal Immunol 2017;10(1):18–26.
2. Rivera-Chavez F, Lopez CA, Baumler AJ. Oxygen as a driver of gut dysbiosis. Free Radic Biol Med 2017;105:93–101.
3. Vazquez-Baeza Y, Hyde ER, Suchodolski JS, et al. Dog and human inflammatory bowel disease rely on overlapping yet distinct dysbiosis networks. Nat Microbiol 2016;1:16177.

4. Tizard IR, Jones SW. The microbiota regulates immunity and immunologic diseases in dogs and cats. Vet Clin North Am Small Anim Pract 2018;48(2):307–22.
5. Duboc H, Rajca S, Rainteau D, et al. Connecting dysbiosis, bile-acid dysmetabolism and gut inflammation in inflammatory bowel diseases. Gut 2013;62(4): 531–9.
6. Guard BC, Honneffer JB, Jergens AE, et al. Longitudinal assessment of microbial dysbiosis, fecal unconjugated bile acid concentrations, and disease activity in dogs with steroid-responsive chronic inflammatory enteropathy. J Vet Intern Med 2019;33(3):1295–305.
7. Giaretta PR, Rech RR, Guard BC, et al. Comparison of intestinal expression of the apical sodium-dependent bile acid transporter between dogs with and without chronic inflammatory enteropathy. J Vet Intern Med 2018;32(6):1918–26.
8. Minamoto Y, Minamoto T, Isaiah A, et al. Fecal short-chain fatty acid concentrations and dysbiosis in dogs with chronic enteropathy. J Vet Intern Med 2019; 33(4):1608–18.
9. Duscha A, Gisevius B, Hirschberg S, et al. Propionic acid shapes the multiple sclerosis disease course by an immunomodulatory mechanism. Cell 2020; 180(6):1067–80.e16.
10. Park MJ, Pilla R, Panta A, et al. Reproductive senescence and ischemic stroke remodel the gut microbiome and modulate the effects of estrogen treatment in female rats. Transl Stroke Res 2020;11(4):812–30.
11. Bansal T, Alaniz RC, Wood TK, et al. The bacterial signal indole increases epithelial-cell tight-junction resistance and attenuates indicators of inflammation. Proc Natl Acad Sci U S A 2010;107(1):228–33.
12. Waclawikova B, El Aidy S. Role of microbiota and tryptophan metabolites in the remote effect of intestinal inflammation on brain and depression. Pharmaceuticals (Basel) 2018;11(3):63.
13. Kieler IN, Shamzir Kamal S, Vitger AD, et al. Gut microbiota composition may relate to weight loss rate in obese pet dogs. Vet Med Sci 2017;3(4):252–62.
14. Bermudez Sanchez S, Pilla R, Sarawichitr B, et al. Fecal microbiota in client-owned obese dogs changes after weight loss with a high-fiber-high-protein diet. PeerJ 2020;8:e9706.
15. Montoya-Alonso JA, Bautista-Castano I, Pena C, et al. Prevalence of canine obesity, obesity-related metabolic dysfunction, and relationship with owner obesity in an obesogenic region of Spain. Front Vet Sci 2017;4:59.
16. Jergens AE, Guard BC, Redfern A, et al. Microbiota-related changes in unconjugated fecal bile acids are associated with naturally occurring, insulin-dependent diabetes mellitus in dogs. Front Vet Sci 2019;6:199.
17. Zitvogel L, Daillere R, Roberti MP, et al. Anticancer effects of the microbiome and its products. Nat Rev Microbiol 2017;15(8):465–78.
18. Wu J, Zhang Y, Yang H, et al. Intestinal microbiota as an alternative therapeutic target for epilepsy. Can J Infect Dis Med Microbiol 2016;2016:9032809.
19. Jeffery ND, Barker AK, Alcott CJ, et al. The association of specific constituents of the fecal microbiota with immune-mediated brain disease in dogs. PLoS One 2017;12(1):e0170589.
20. Allaway D, Haydock R, Lonsdale ZN, et al. Rapid reconstitution of the faecal microbiome after extended diet-induced changes indicate a stable gut microbiome in healthy adult dogs. Appl Environ Microbiol 2020;86(13):e00562-20.
21. Johnson AJ, Vangay P, Al-Ghalith GA, et al. Daily sampling reveals personalized diet-microbiome associations in humans. Cell Host Microbe 2019;25(6): 789–802.e5.

22. Lozupone CA, Stombaugh JI, Gordon JI, et al. Diversity, stability and resilience of the human gut microbiota. Nature 2012;489(7415):220–30.
23. Honneffer JB, Steiner JM, Lidbury JA, et al. Variation of the microbiota and metabolome along the canine gastrointestinal tract. Metabolomics 2017;13(3):1–20.
24. Ritchie LE, Steiner JM, Suchodolski JS. Assessment of microbial diversity along the feline intestinal tract using 16S rRNA gene analysis. FEMS Microbiol Ecol 2008;66(3):590–8.
25. Blake AB, Suchodolski JS. Importance of gut microbiota for the health and disease of dogs and cats. Anim Front 2016;6(3):37–42.
26. Pilla R, Suchodolski JS. The role of the canine gut microbiome and metabolome in health and gastrointestinal disease. Front Vet Sci 2020;6:498.
27. AlShawaqfeh MK, Wajid B, Minamoto Y, et al. A dysbiosis index to assess microbial changes in fecal samples of dogs with chronic inflammatory enteropathy. FEMS Microbiol Ecol 2017;93(11):fix136.
28. Chaitman J, Ziese AL, Pilla R, et al. Fecal microbial and metabolic profiles in dogs with acute diarrhea receiving either fecal microbiota transplantation or oral metronidazole. Front Vet Sci 2020;7:192.
29. Middelbos IS, Vester Boler BM, Qu A, et al. Phylogenetic characterization of fecal microbial communities of dogs fed diets with or without supplemental dietary fiber using 454 pyrosequencing. PLoS One 2010;5(3):e9768.
30. Hand D, Wallis C, Colyer A, et al. Pyrosequencing the canine faecal microbiota: breadth and depth of biodiversity. PLoS One 2013;8(1):e53115.
31. Garcia-Mazcorro JF, Lanerie DJ, Dowd SE, et al. Effect of a multi-species synbiotic formulation on fecal bacterial microbiota of healthy cats and dogs as evaluated by pyrosequencing. FEMS Microbiol Ecol 2011;78(3):542–54.
32. Garcia-Mazcorro JF, Dowd SE, Poulson J, et al. Abundance and short-term temporal variability of fecal microbiota in healthy dogs. Microbiologyopen 2012;1(3):340–7.
33. Amitay EL, Werner S, Vital M, et al. Fusobacterium and colorectal cancer: causal factor or passenger? Results from a large colorectal cancer screening study. Carcinogenesis 2017;38(8):781–8.
34. Kim DH, Jeong D, Kang IB, et al. Modulation of the intestinal microbiota of dogs by kefir as a functional dairy product. J Dairy Sci 2019;102(5):3903–11.
35. Manchester AC, Webb CB, Blake AB, et al. Long-term impact of tylosin on fecal microbiota and fecal bile acids of healthy dogs. J Vet Intern Med 2019;33(6):2605–17.
36. Pilla R, Gaschen FP, Barr JW, et al. Effects of metronidazole on the fecal microbiome and metabolome in healthy dogs. J Vet Intern Med 2020;34(5):1853–66.
37. Xenoulis PG, Palculict B, Allenspach K, et al. Molecular-phylogenetic characterization of microbial communities imbalances in the small intestine of dogs with inflammatory bowel disease. FEMS Microbiol Ecol 2008;66(3):579–89.
38. Suchodolski JS, Xenoulis PG, Paddock CG, et al. Molecular analysis of the bacterial microbiota in duodenal biopsies from dogs with idiopathic inflammatory bowel disease. Vet Microbiol 2010;142(3):394–400.
39. Barry KA, Middelbos IS, Vester Boler BM, et al. Effects of dietary fiber on the feline gastrointestinal metagenome. J Proteome Res 2012;11(12):5924–33.
40. Eshar DL, Lee C, Weese JS. Comparative molecular analysis of fecal microbiota of bobcats (Lynx rufus) and domestic cats (Felis catus). Can J Vet Res 2018;83(1):42–9.

41. Handl S, Dowd SE, Garcia-Mazcorro JF, et al. Massive parallel 16S rRNA gene pyrosequencing reveals highly diverse fecal bacterial and fungal communities in healthy dogs and cats. FEMS Microbiol Ecol 2011;76(2):301–10.
42. Garcia-Mazcorro JF, Barcenas-Walls JR, Suchodolski JS, et al. Molecular assessment of the fecal microbiota in healthy cats and dogs before and during supplementation with fructo-oligosaccharides (FOS) and inulin using high-throughput 454-pyrosequencing. PeerJ 2017;5:e3184.
43. Marsilio S, Pilla R, Sarawichitr B, et al. Characterization of the fecal microbiome in cats with inflammatory bowel disease or alimentary small cell lymphoma. Sci Rep 2019;9(1):19208.
44. Bresciani F, Minamoto Y, Suchodolski JS, et al. Effect of an extruded animal protein-free diet on fecal microbiota of dogs with food-responsive enteropathy. J Vet Intern Med 2018;32(6):1903–10.
45. De Filippo C, Cavalieri D, Di Paola M, et al. Impact of diet in shaping gut microbiota revealed by a comparative study in children from Europe and rural Africa. Proc Natl Acad Sci U S A 2010;107(33):14691–6.
46. David LA, Maurice CF, Carmody RN, et al. Diet rapidly and reproducibly alters the human gut microbiome. Nature 2014;505(7484):559–63.
47. Mori A, Goto A, Kibe R, et al. Comparison of the effects of four commercially available prescription diet regimens on the fecal microbiome in healthy dogs. J Vet Med Sci 2019;81(12):1783–90.
48. Panasevich MR, Serao MCR, de Godoy MRC, et al. Potato fiber as a dietary fiber source in dog foods. J Anim Sci 2013;91(11):5344–52.
49. Panasevich MR, Kerr KR, Dilger RN, et al. Modulation of the faecal microbiome of healthy adult dogs by inclusion of potato fibre in the diet. Br J Nutr 2015;113(1):125–33.
50. Alexander C, Cross TL, Devendran S, et al. Effects of prebiotic inulin-type fructans on blood metabolite and hormone concentrations and faecal microbiota and metabolites in overweight dogs. Br J Nutr 2018;120(6):711–20.
51. Myint H, Iwahashi Y, Koike S, et al. Effect of soybean husk supplementation on the fecal fermentation metabolites and microbiota of dogs. Anim Sci J 2017;88(11):1730–6.
52. Beloshapka AN, Dowd SE, Suchodolski JS, et al. Fecal microbial communities of healthy adult dogs fed raw meat-based diets with or without inulin or yeast cell wall extracts as assessed by 454 pyrosequencing. FEMS Microbiol Ecol 2013;84(3):532–41.
53. Bermingham EN, Maclean P, Thomas DG, et al. Key bacterial families (Clostridiaceae, Erysipelotrichaceae and Bacteroidaceae) are related to the digestion of protein and energy in dogs. PeerJ 2017;5:e3019.
54. Schmidt M, Unterer S, Suchodolski JS, et al. The fecal microbiome and metabolome differs between dogs fed Bones and Raw Food (BARF) diets and dogs fed commercial diets. PLoS One 2018;13(8):e0201279.
55. Kim J, An JU, Kim W, et al. Differences in the gut microbiota of dogs (*Canis lupus familiaris*) fed a natural diet or a commercial feed revealed by the Illumina MiSeq platform. Gut Pathog 2017;9:68.
56. Vital M, Gao J, Rizzo M, et al. Diet is a major factor governing the fecal butyrate-producing community structure across Mammalia, Aves and Reptilia. Isme J 2015;9(4):832–43.
57. Herstad KMV, Gajardo K, Bakke AM, et al. A diet change from dry food to beef induces reversible changes on the faecal microbiota in healthy, adult client-owned dogs. BMC Vet Res 2017;13(1):147.

58. Turroni F, van Sinderen D, Ventura M. Genomics and ecological overview of the genus Bifidobacterium. Int J Food Microbiol 2011;149(1):37–44.
59. Rivera-Chavez F, Zhang LF, Faber F, et al. Depletion of butyrate-producing clostridia from the gut microbiota drives an aerobic luminal expansion of salmonella. Cell Host Microbe 2016;19(4):443–54.
60. Schauf S, de la Fuente G, Newbold CJ, et al. Effect of dietary fat to starch content on fecal microbiota composition and activity in dogs. J Anim Sci 2018;96(9):3684–98.
61. Potrykus J, White RL, Bearne SL. Proteomic investigation of amino acid catabolism in the indigenous gut anaerobe *Fusobacterium varium*. Proteomics 2008;8(13):2691–703.
62. Bermingham EN, Young W, Kittelmann S, et al. Dietary format alters fecal bacterial populations in the domestic cat (*Felis catus*). Microbiologyopen 2013;2(1):173–81.
63. Bermingham EN, Young W, Butowski CF, et al. The fecal microbiota in the domestic cat (*Felis catus*) is influenced by interactions between age and diet; a five year longitudinal study. Front Microbiol 2018;9:1231.
64. Wu X, Zhang H, Chen J, et al. Analysis and comparison of the wolf microbiome under different environmental factors using three different data of Next Generation Sequencing. Sci Rep 2017;7(1):11332.
65. Lyu T, Liu G, Zhang H, et al. Changes in feeding habits promoted the differentiation of the composition and function of gut microbiotas between domestic dogs (*Canis lupus familiaris*) and gray wolves (*Canis lupus*). AMB Express 2018;8(1):123.
66. Menke S, Meier M, Mfune JKE, et al. Effects of host traits and land-use changes on the gut microbiota of the Namibian black-backed jackal (*Canis mesomelas*). FEMS Microbiol Ecol 2017;93(11). https://doi.org/10.1093/femsec/fix123.
67. Sandri M, Dal Monego S, Conte G, et al. Raw meat based diet influences faecal microbiome and end products of fermentation in healthy dogs. BMC Vet Res 2017;13(1):65.
68. Olson CA, Vuong HE, Yano JM, et al. The gut microbiota mediates the anti-seizure effects of the ketogenic diet. Cell 2018;173(7):1728–41.e13.
69. Mason PE, Kerns WP 2nd. Gamma hydroxybutyric acid (GHB) intoxication. Acad Emerg Med 2002;9(7):730–9.
70. Thwaites DT, Basterfield L, McCleave PM, et al. Gamma-Aminobutyric acid (GABA) transport across human intestinal epithelial (Caco-2) cell monolayers. Br J Pharmacol 2000;129(3):457–64.
71. Barrett E, Ross RP, O'Toole PW, et al. gamma-Aminobutyric acid production by culturable bacteria from the human intestine. J Appl Microbiol 2012;113(2):411–7.
72. Iwatani S, Yamamoto N. Functional food products in Japan: a review. Food Sci Hum Wellness 2019;8(2):96–101.
73. Dhakal R, Bajpai VK, Baek KH. Production of gaba (gamma - Aminobutyric acid) by microorganisms: a review. Braz J Microbiol 2012;43(4):1230–41.
74. Molina J, Jean-Philippe C, Conboy L, et al. Efficacy of medium chain triglyceride oil dietary supplementation in reducing seizure frequency in dogs with idiopathic epilepsy without cluster seizures: a non-blinded, prospective clinical trial. Vet Rec 2020;187(9):356.
75. Law TH, Davies ES, Pan Y, et al. A randomised trial of a medium-chain TAG diet as treatment for dogs with idiopathic epilepsy. Br J Nutr 2015;114(9):1438–47.

76. Ma D, Wang AC, Parikh I, et al. Ketogenic diet enhances neurovascular function with altered gut microbiome in young healthy mice. Sci Rep 2018;8(1):6670.
77. Xie G, Zhou Q, Qiu CZ, et al. Ketogenic diet poses a significant effect on imbalanced gut microbiota in infants with refractory epilepsy. World J Gastroenterol 2017;23(33):6164–71.
78. Carciofi A, Bazolli R, Zanni A, et al. Influence of water content and the digestibility of pet foods on the water balance of cats. Braz J Vet Res Anim Sci 2005;42: 429–34.
79. Buckley CM, Hawthorne A, Colyer A, et al. Effect of dietary water intake on urinary output, specific gravity and relative supersaturation for calcium oxalate and struvite in the cat. Br J Nutr 2011;106(Suppl 1):S128–30.
80. Vester BM, Dalsing BL, Middelbos IS, et al. Faecal microbial populations of growing kittens fed high- or moderate-protein diets. Arch Anim Nutr 2009; 63(3):254–65.
81. Hooda S, Vester Boler BM, Kerr KR, et al. The gut microbiome of kittens is affected by dietary protein:carbohydrate ratio and associated with blood metabolite and hormone concentrations. Br J Nutr 2013;109(9):1637–46.
82. Deusch O, O'Flynn C, Colyer A, et al. Deep Illumina-based shotgun sequencing reveals dietary effects on the structure and function of the fecal microbiome of growing kittens. PLoS One 2014;9(7):e101021.
83. Kerr KR, Dowd SE, Swanson KS. Faecal microbiota of domestic cats fed raw whole chicks v. an extruded chicken-based diet. J Nutr Sci 2014;3:e22.
84. Butowski CF, Thomas DG, Young W, et al. Addition of plant dietary fibre to a raw red meat high protein, high fat diet, alters the faecal bacteriome and organic acid profiles of the domestic cat (Felis catus). PLoS One 2019;14(5):e0216072.
85. Liu B, Wang W, Zhu X, et al. Response of gut microbiota to dietary fiber and metabolic interaction with SCFAs in piglets. Front Microbiol 2018;9:2344.
86. Bermingham EN, Kittelmann S, Young W, et al. Post-weaning diet affects faecal microbial composition but not selected adipose gene expression in the cat (Felis catus). PLoS One 2013;8(11):e80992.
87. Rochus K, Janssens GP, Hesta M. Dietary fibre and the importance of the gut microbiota in feline nutrition: a review. Nutr Res Rev 2014;27(2):295–307.
88. Young W, Moon CD, Thomas DG, et al. Pre- and post-weaning diet alters the faecal metagenome in the cat with differences in vitamin and carbohydrate metabolism gene abundances. Sci Rep 2016;6:34668.
89. Kanakupt K, Vester Boler BM, Dunsford BR, et al. Effects of short-chain fructooligosaccharides and galactooligosaccharides, individually and in combination, on nutrient digestibility, fecal fermentative metabolite concentrations, and large bowel microbial ecology of healthy adults cats. J Anim Sci 2011;89(5):1376–84.
90. Kalenyak K, Isaiah A, Heilmann RM, et al. Comparison of the intestinal mucosal microbiota in dogs diagnosed with idiopathic inflammatory bowel disease and dogs with food-responsive diarrhea before and after treatment. FEMS Microbiol Ecol 2018;94(2). https://doi.org/10.1093/femsec/fix173.
91. Pilla R, Guard BC, Steiner JM, et al. Administration of a synbiotic containing enterococcus faecium does not significantly alter fecal microbiota richness or diversity in dogs with and without food-responsive chronic enteropathy. Front Vet Sci 2019;6:277.
92. Schmitz S, Suchodolski J. Understanding the canine intestinal microbiota and its modification by pro-, pre- and synbiotics - what is the evidence? Vet Med Sci 2016;2(2):71–94.

93. White R, Atherly T, Guard B, et al. Randomized, controlled trial evaluating the effect of multi-strain probiotic on the mucosal microbiota in canine idiopathic inflammatory bowel disease. Gut Microbes 2017;8(5):451–66.
94. Rossi G, Jergens A, Cerquetella M, et al. Effects of a probiotic (SLAB51) on clinical and histologic variables and microbiota of cats with chronic constipation/megacolon: a pilot study. Benef Microbes 2018;9(1):101–10.
95. DeSantis TZ, Hugenholtz P, Larsen N, et al. Greengenes, a chimera-checked 16S rRNA gene database and workbench compatible with ARB. Appl Environ Microbiol 2006;72(7):5069–72.
96. Deb-Choudhury S, Bermingham EN, Young W, et al. The effects of a wool hydrolysate on short-chain fatty acid production and fecal microbial composition in the domestic cat (Felis catus). Food Funct 2018;9(8):4107–21.
97. Wernimont S, Fritsch D, Jackson M, et al. Specialized dietary fibers alter microbiome composition & promote fermentative metabolism in the lower gastrointestinal tract of healthy adult cats (P20-045-19). Curr Dev Nutr 2019;3(Supplement_1):1807.

Calcium, Phosphorus, and Vitamin D in Dogs and Cats

Beyond the Bones

Jonathan Stockman, DVM[a], Cecilia Villaverde, BVSc, PhD[b], Ronald Jan Corbee, DVM, PhD[c,*]

KEYWORDS

• Metabolism • Renal • Urinary tract • Gastrointestinal • Cancer

KEY POINTS

- Calcium, phosphorus, and vitamin D have a key role in skeletal development and health as well as other important metabolic functions.
- Insufficient or unbalanced dietary provision of these nutrients can have multiple negative health impacts.
- Excess vitamin D intake may cause hypercalcemia and negative health effects in dogs and cats, and the health-related effects of high calcium and phosphorus intake are being studied.
- The dietary provision of calcium, phosphorus, and vitamin D and their interactions must be considered in patients with renal-urinary diseases.
- The rolo of vitamin D in chronic conditions, such as enteropathies and neoplasia, is receiving considerable attention, but research is still inconclusive, and no clinical recommendations can be made at this time.

INTRODUCTION

Calcium, phosphorus, and vitamin D are important essential nutrients in the dog and the cat. As such, these nutrients are required as a part of a complete and balanced diet. Most commercial diets for dogs and cats provide sufficient amounts of calcium, phosphorus, and vitamin D,[1–3] but homemade diets may be deficient or unbalanced in

---

J. Stockman is a consultant for Petco Animal Supplies, Inc. C. Villaverde has received honoraria for consulting and speaking engagements from pet food manufacturers. R.J. Corbee declares no conflict of interest regarding this article.

[a] Department of Clinical Veterinary Sciences, LIU College of Veterinary Medicine, Long Island University, 720 Northern Boulevard, Brookville, NY 11548, USA; [b] Expert Pet Nutrition, Fermoy, Cork P61KX38, Ireland; [c] Department of Clinical Sciences, Faculty of Veterinary Medicine, Utrecht University, Yalelaan 108, Utrecht 3584 CM, The Netherlands
* Corresponding author.
E-mail address: R.J.Corbee@uu.nl

Vet Clin Small Anim 51 (2021) 623–634
https://doi.org/10.1016/j.cvsm.2021.01.003 **vetsmall.theclinics.com**
0195-5616/21/

these nutrients, which may lead to negative outcomes.[4] Calcium and phosphorus are stored mostly in skeletal tissue, although they are present throughout the body. Bone metabolism and calcium and phosphorus absorption and retention are influenced by vitamin D as well as the relative dietary concentrations of these and other minerals. Although bone health is closely impacted by the nutrition and metabolism of these nutrients, these nutrients also impact animal physiology in many additional ways and have health impacts that transcend skeletal health alone. The following summary is aimed to explore and explain the various ways calcium, phosphorus, and vitamin D all play complex roles in canine and feline health.

The Nutritional Requirements for Calcium, Phosphorus, and Vitamin D in Dogs and Cats

Calcium and phosphorus are essential nutrients in dogs and cats, and therefore, they need to be provided in the diet in adequate amounts and in bioavailable forms. Calcium and phosphorus are the first and second most abundant minerals in the body, respectively, where they play both structural (such as of bone and teeth) and functional roles. For example, calcium is involved in blood coagulation and nerve impulse transmission, and phosphorus has a major role in energy metabolism as a component of adenosine triphosphate. The National Research Council gives a recommended allowance for calcium and phosphorus for different life stages (**Table 1**).[5] It also defines a safe upper limit for calcium of 4.5 g/1000 kcal of metabolizable energy for puppies, specifically those of large and giant breeds, where excess can result in skeletal abnormalities.[6,7] Adult dogs seem able to adequately handle high dietary calcium intakes.[8]

Vitamin D is also an essential nutrient in dogs and cats, because synthesis from sunlight exposure seems to be limited.[9,10] Therefore, it must be included in complete and balanced diets for dogs and cats in all life stages. Vitamin D plays an important role in calcium and phosphorus homeostasis and, consequently, its deficiency is associated with skeletal abnormalities. There is a lack of research on vitamin D requirements, especially in adult animals,[11] and the dietary recommendations[5,12,13] are educated estimates based on intakes that appear to support skeletal health. There is a growing body of research that supports the importance of vitamin D in other areas, as the vitamin D receptor is present in multiple tissues, which could result in changes in dietary recommendations in the future.[14–17]

Dietary Sources of Calcium, Phosphorus, and Vitamin D and Their Absorption and Bioavailability

Calcium and phosphorus in pet food can be provided by bony raw materials (from meat and fish). Phosphorus is also provided by meat and vegetable ingredients, such as cereals, although phosphorus in grains can be present as phytate, which has a reduced bioavailability compared with other forms in monogastric animals.[18]

Table 1
Recommended allowances (grams per 1000 kcal of metabolizable energy) for calcium and phosphorus for growth, maintenance, and reproduction in dogs and cats[5]

		Growth	Maintenance	Reproduction
Calcium	Dog	3	1	1.9
	Cat	2	0.72	2.7
Phosphorus	Dog	2.5	0.75	1.2
	Cat	1.8	0.64	1.9

Both minerals can also be provided as purified salts, together (as calcium phosphate salts) or separately.

Calcium and phosphorus availability is affected by several dietary factors, such as total amount and relative proportion to each other. Because of the close relationship of calcium and phosphorus, the Association of American Feed Control Officials (AAFCO) guidelines[12] recommend that commercial dog food not only meets the individual requirements but also provides a minimum calcium-to-phosphorus ratio of 1:1 and a maximum ratio of 2:1. Bioavailability is also affected by form and source. Data in cats have shown that highly soluble phosphate salts can result in increased absorption and postprandial serum levels compared with diets whereby it is provided by the bony raw materials,[19] which could affect phosphorus homeostasis negatively and contribute to renal damage.[20,21]

Dietary vitamin D is provided as cholecalciferol (vitamin D3) and ergocalciferol (vitamin D2), from animal and vegetable ingredients, respectively; it can also be added as a purified additive. Cats discriminate between vitamin D forms and use cholecalciferol more efficiently than ergocalciferol.[22] There is a lack of controlled, well-powered studies in dogs,[5,11] but vitamins D2 and D3 appear to have a similar potency in this species.[23]

Skeletal Development and Skeletal Health

Because the bone is the major reservoir of calcium and phosphorus, its metabolism is impacted by their relative homeostasis. During growth, imbalances of these nutrients have the most detrimental consequences, resulting in factures and limb deformities, such as valgus or varus stance, and incongruence of the elbow joint.[24–28] Vitamin D plays a key role in bone remodeling and bone growth by activating osteoblasts and osteoclasts. It is important for clinicians to distinguish between causes of limb deformities by nutritional evaluation, orthopedic examination, evaluation of radiographs, and determining plasma levels of calcium, phosphorus, parathyroid hormone (PTH), calcitonin (CT), and vitamin D metabolites.[29]

A common pitfall is to rule out insufficient calcium intake when plasma calcium levels are within the normal range. Even in cases of dietary calcium insufficiency, plasma calcium levels are usually kept within normal limits, unless the regulatory compensatory mechanisms fall short. Plasma calcium levels are strongly regulated because low calcium has immediate detrimental effects, such as cardiac arrhythmias, that can be fatal. Typically, with a low dietary calcium intake, radiographs will show decreased mineralization of bone, enlarged medullar areas, and thinner cortices that easily break (eg, green stick fractures). PTH levels will be increased as well as active vitamin D levels. Sometimes, deficient intake in both calcium and vitamin D occurs, which is often referred to as "all-meat syndrome." These cases may show signs of low vitamin D, such as enlarged growth plates and decreased mineralization of bone and cartilage. In adult animals, the bone will be gradually demineralized and replaced by connective tissue under the influence of fibroblast growth factor-23 (FGF-23).[30] Many times, these diets also lead to a high phosphorus intake, which exacerbates the pathologic condition by increasing PTH activity, resulting in more osteoclastic activity. In contrast, low phosphorus intake results in decreased levels of PTH.[31] In cases of adequate calcium and phosphorus but deficient vitamin D intake, enlarged growth plates can be seen radiographically as well as decreased mineralization of bone. PTH levels are expected to be high, and active vitamin D levels will be low. To prevent hypercalcemia, CT levels will be increased. In growing animals, this will result in decreased osteoclastic activity, as osteoclasts can no longer make contact to the matrix with their ruffled borders. Prolonged decrease of osteoclastic activity may result in enostosis, which can be visible on radiographs as an opaque cloud within the medullar area, and by painful reaction on deep palpation of the long bones during orthopedic examination. Treatment of these dietary imbalances is largely dependent on normalizing dietary intake, combined with pain medication and exercise instructions.[32]

The Importance of These Nutrients for Urinary Health

Urolithiasis is among the most common urinary diseases in companion animals. Uroliths and urinary crystals may occur as a result of multiple causes, including hereditary disease, infections, toxicity, and nutritional deficiency or excess. There are multiple uroliths and urinary crystals of varying compositions in dogs and cats, including organic and inorganic compounds. Some of the most common compounds are mineral salts, which include calcium and phosphorus. In fact, it is estimated that at least 90% of the uroliths in dogs and cats are composed of either calcium oxalate monohydrate or dehydrate compounds or struvite (magnesium-ammonium-phosphate hexahydrate).[33] Although crystalluria can be benign (with the exception of urethral plugs in male cats), crystal aggregation and nucleation may lead to the formation of uroliths.

The risk for urolith formation depends on the urinary saturation with minerals or organic compounds that precipitate into crystals[34]; however, this process also depends on the involvement of inhibitors of urolithiasis, including urinary proteins (nephrocalcin, uropontin, Tamm-Horsfall mucoprotein), urinary pH, and the presence and saturation of ions in the solution.[35,36]

Calcium oxalate urolithiasis

Hypercalcemia (of any cause) is a risk factor for the formation of calcium oxalate uroliths in both dogs and cats, as it may result in hypercalciuria.[37,38] Dietary phosphorus restriction below the established requirements may increase the risk for hypercalcemia, as a high calcium-to-phosphorus ratio may result in increased calcium absorption. When phosphorus intake is low, a decrease in FGF-23, which is a regulator of calcium and phosphorus excretion, results in increased activity of 1-alpha hydroxylase,[39] resulting in more active vitamin D, which increases intestinal calcium absorption and exacerbates hypercalciuria.

Normally, dogs and cats do not excrete much calcium in the urine even when the calcium intake is increased, as calcium homeostasis is regulated primarily via fecal excretion, presumably because dietary calcium absorption is reduced.[8,21] Increased dietary calcium was also found not to significantly change the urinary relative supersaturation for calcium oxalate.[8] However, in cases of hypercalcemia, the fractional excretion of calcium is increased, resulting in hypercalciuria.[33,40] Although hypercalciuria may not be a finding in all cases of canine and feline calcium oxalate urolithiasis,[41] it is a prominent risk factor.

Dogs with a medical history of calcium oxalate urolithiasis from highly predisposed breeds (miniature schnauzers, bichon frise, and shih tzu) were found to have greater urinary calcium excretion than control dogs of the same breed but not increased urinary oxalate excretion or overt hypercalcemia (although the ionized calcium was higher in case dogs).[42] The same researchers also found no increase in bone turnover markers in these dogs, possibly suggesting that the observed hypercalciuria is the result of increased intestinal calcium absorption or renal calcium leakage.[43]

Diets that are formulated to promote urine acidity may contain acidifiers, such as ammonium chloride, that have been shown to increase urinary calcium excretion.[44] Acidic urine may negatively impact urolith inhibitors, such as citrate or urinary mucoproteins, that prevent the formation of calcium oxalate crystals. It is thought that metabolic acidosis promotes osteoclast activity and inhibits osteoblasts for a net bone resorption and release of a strong calcium-containing alkaline buffer, hydroxyapatite.[45] The increase in bone turnover and the release of calcium increase the ionized calcium concentrations and can result in hypercalciuria and possibly increased risk for calcium oxalate urolithiasis.

Feeding a high-fiber diet has been suggested as a nutritional strategy for the management of hypercalcemia in both dogs and cats; however, conflicting evidence indicates that further research is needed as far as the clinical benefit of this approach, particularly because evidence suggests that soluble fiber may increase intestinal calcium absorption.[32,40,46–48] Because some fiber sources are high in oxalates, this should also be taken into account when formulating a diet plan.

Struvite urolithiasis

Urinary phosphorus excretion is influenced by its intake (amount and bioavailability) as well as the intake of sodium, calcium, and magnesium.[21,49] Increased dietary phosphorus is not sufficient to increase the relative supersaturation for struvite in cats or dogs to values that are considered supportive of crystallization.[8,21] As a result of hyperphosphatemia, increased PTH promotes urinary phosphorous excretion in the kidneys by reducing expression of sodium phosphate cotransporter on the apical membrane of the proximal tubule. The active form of vitamin D, calcitriol, increases urinary phosphorus excretion indirectly as it increases the sodium phosphorus transporters (NaPi-2b transporters) in the intestines.[50] There are no reports to the authors' knowledge of a higher incidence of struvite urolithiasis in dogs or cats with hyperphosphatemia, presumably because hyperphosphatemia most often occurs in cats who suffer from renal disease and may have other related metabolic complications, such as dilute urine and metabolic acidosis.

Sterile struvite urinary calculi in cats and dogs may be dissolved with a diet that is reduced in phosphorous, magnesium, and protein, which contribute the components of struvite urolithiasis, and with an acidic urinary pH (6.0 or lower).[51–53] Nonsterile struvite uroliths may be dissolved with use of targeted antimicrobial treatment primarily and complementary nutritional therapy.[52] Urine pH may be influenced by the dietary anion-to-cation balance. Therefore, a diet that is aiming to reduce urine pH may be lower in cations, such as calcium, sodium, or potassium, and higher in phosphate, sulfate, and chloride.[5] There are also acidifying compounds that may be added to the diet to achieve low urine pH, including phosphoric acid, methionine, and ammonium chloride. Base excess and urine pH appear to be more important than the relative mineral intake for struvite prevention.[54] Dietary prevention of recurrence of sterile struvite urolithiasis is possible with a diet that promotes urine dilution, targets an acidic pH, and provides reduced amounts of phosphorus and magnesium, although recurrence rates are unknown.[33] Addressing predisposing factors for infection, such as anatomic features and obesity, can help prevent the recurrence of nonsterile struvite.

Calcium phosphate and calcium carbonate urolithiasis

Calcium phosphate and calcium carbonate are often a small component of complex uroliths precipitated with struvite or calcium oxalate. Pure calcium phosphate or carbonate uroliths are uncommon in dogs and cats. Several calcium phosphate compounds include hydroxyapatite, brushite, whitlockite, and octacalcium phosphate, of which hydroxyapatite and calcium carbonate compounds are most common.[55] In dogs, many times these result from bacterial cystitis, as is struvite, and are formed under alkaline conditions.[33] Other conditions, such as hyperparathyroidism, that lead to hypercalciuria and hyperphosphaturia are also possible risk factors. Physical removal of these uroliths is usually necessary, although they may dissolve when the primary cause is addressed (for example, hyperparathyroidism).[56] Nutritionally, high dietary phosphorus in a bioavailable form may increase the relative supersaturation for brushite in cats.[21] Otherwise, there are no nutritional prevention strategies for these uroliths aside from addressing the primary cause (ie, bacterial cystitis) if possible.

In summary, calcium and phosphorus compounds are most common among those that are involved in precipitation in the canine and feline urinary system; however, the pathogenesis for these urinary calculi is complex, and simple dietary excess of these minerals is not the sole cause. As more data regarding the physiology and nutritional requirements and tolerance for calcium and phosphorus are accumulated, there will be a greater understanding of how best to nutritionally prevent and manage these in dogs and cats.

The Importance of These Nutrients for Renal Health

Calcium and phosphorus metabolism is commonly dysregulated in dogs and cats with chronic kidney disease (CKD), which has a major impact on the progression of disease and the associated clinical signs.

As discussed above, hypercalcemia may increase the risk of calcium oxalate urolithiasis as well as lead to soft tissue mineralization and possibly to kidney injury and impaired function. Hypercalcemia can be the result of dietary, metabolic, neoplastic, renal, and idiopathic causes in dogs and cats. The degree of hypercalcemia and its chronicity impacts prognosis. In cats, clinical signs of hypercalcemia are usually most severe when the increase in calcium is rapid.[40] Most often, clinical signs are noted when serum total calcium is higher than 14.0 mg/dL and ionized calcium is greater than 6.5 mg/dL (1.6 mmol/L). If serum total calcium increases to 16.0 mg/dL or if ionized calcium increases to above 7.5 mg/dL (1.9 mmol/L), clinical signs are severe and require hospitalization and immediate care.[40] A reduction in dietary vitamin D, which is one of the most important regulators of calcium absorption, is recommended when the cause of hypercalcemia is vitamin D toxicity. Some anecdotally recommend feeding a diet with moderately reduced calcium and vitamin D in addition to added insoluble fiber for all-cause hypercalcemia.[40] High dietary calcium on its own does not appear to be a cause of hypercalcemia or renal disease in dogs, such as Labrador retrievers and beagles.[8] It is unknown if dietary calcium reduction would benefit dogs with existing hypercalcemia.

Although regulatory mechanisms are aimed to maintain serum ionized calcium and inorganic phosphorus, shifts may occur and worsen with CKD progression and are associated with increased mortality.[57–59] A reduction of functioning nephrons, as occurs in advanced CKD, leads to lower glomerular filtration rate and a reduced phosphorus excretion, ultimately resulting in increased serum inorganic phosphorus. The result of this would be a compensatory increase in filtration, but with a gradual increase in the serum inorganic phosphorus set point, as compensation fails to keep up unless phosphorus intake is reduced. The retention of phosphorus can lead to soft tissue mineralization, which may further damage the renal tissue and lead to reduced renal function.[60]

The function of 1-α-hydroxylase enzyme is necessary to form calcitriol from calcidiol; this is reduced in CKD patients because of the decrease in renal mass and as a result of the activity of secreted FGF-23. Decreased calcitriol results in reduces calcium absorption from the intestines, decreased ionized calcium, and an increase in PTH.[39] PTH increase may lead to additional negative health implications, including osteodystrophy, pathologic fractures, and "rubber jaw."[60]

Serum phosphorus may remain in normal reference ranges thanks to compensatory mechanisms despite pathologic shifts in renal glomerular filtration, urine concentration, creatinine, PTH, and FGF-23.[39] Therefore, relying on increased serum phosphorus as a marker of CKD or as a primary indication to limit dietary phosphorus has important limitations. PTH and FGF-23 are not typically included in routine biochemistry panels; therefore, clinicians may not be aware of early dysregulation that occurs in CKD patients. Increases in FGF-23 and symmetric dimethylarginine, a biomarker for decreased glomerular filtration in early CKD, are intercorrelated in geriatric preazotemic cats.[61] The timing of these increases indicates that alterations in normal phosphorus metabolism occur in early CKD or even before CKD in cats.[62,63] Evidence regarding the potential benefits of early phosphorous intake reduction is lacking; however, the shifts in normal phosphorous metabolism may be nutritionally managed with dietary phosphorus restriction in advanced CKD (approximating or under the minimum accepted dietary requirements), as this may slow CKD progression and reduce related health complications.[60,64–67]

Recent data suggest that dietary phosphorus greater than 3.0 or 3.6 g/1000 kcal may lead to kidney damage and CKD in healthy cats when it is provided in a highly available form of soluble inorganic salts and when the ratio between calcium and phosphorus is low.[20,21] The relevance of this is highlighted by recent surveys that evaluated the total calcium and phosphorus in feline diets and found that approximately 33% of the tested products had a higher total phosphorus than 3.6 g/1000 kcal and highly variable calcium-to-phosphorus ratio (0.5–1.7).[2] Although the ratio between organic and inorganic phosphorus in those diets was not evaluated, several diets had a low calcium-to-phosphorus ratio in addition to high total phosphorus. However, there is no evidence that commercial cat foods indeed cause renal disease in healthy cats, as the aforementioned studies included experimental diets with a high proportion of soluble phosphorus salts possibly exceeding that of most commercial diets. There is no current maximum for dietary phosphorus for adult cats in the guidelines by AAFCO, nor is there a guidance regarding calcium-to-phosphorus ratio or the use of inorganic phosphorus salt additives.[12] Although more research is required to establish safety maximums, the authors believe that interim limits should be considered as well as a recommended calcium-to-phosphorous ratio greater than 1. In dogs, there is currently no evidence that high dietary phosphorus (up to 4.0 g/1000 kcal) in organic or inorganic form leads to renal injury when the calcium-to-phosphorus ratio is greater than 1[8]; however, further research to determine the tolerability of high dietary phosphorus in dogs is needed.

Vitamin D and Its Importance for Other Conditions Such as Gastrointestinal Disease and Cancer

The vitamin D receptor is present in multiple organs, such as the small intestine and colon. Apart from the traditional role of increasing calcium absorption by active transcellular transportation in the small intestine in the case of low plasma calcium levels,[68] calcitriol (active vitamin D) has additional important functions within the gastrointestinal tract. Calcitriol is needed to maintain the gastrointestinal barrier function by upregulation of tight junction protein expression,[69] the production of brush border enzymes,[70] as well as the formation of microvilli.[71] An intact gastrointestinal barrier prevents pathogen invasion and bacterial translocation; therefore, vitamin D is regarded as protective for chronic gastrointestinal diseases. Calcitriol further protects against damage to the gastrointestinal tract by suppressing tumor necrosis factor-alpha and nuclear factor kappa-beta pathways. These proinflammatory pathways play a key role in the first line of defense against pathogens; however, when overexpression occurs, this can contribute to chronic gastrointestinal diseases. The inhibition of these proinflammatory pathways makes calcitriol an interesting therapeutic option for multiple chronic inflammatory conditions (eg, osteoarthritis, atopic dermatitis), but so far, clinical studies in dogs and cats are lacking.

Vitamin D has several immune-modulating effects, demonstrated by in vitro studies, whereas the clinical effects are largely not yet elucidated.[72] Vitamin D–deficient mice are more prone to infection and support overgrowth by pathogenic bacteria because of inadequate response of the immune system.[71] Supplementation of vitamin D metabolites as a possible effective treatment or prevention of chronic gastrointestinal diseases in dogs and cats requires further investigation. Vitamin D also affects tissue fibrosis by suppressing the transforming growth factor-beta pathway, as was demonstrated in colon cell lines from people,[73] in gastrointestinal cells of mice,[74] and in the feline liver (hepatic stellate cells).[75] These studies suggest a possible preventative role for vitamin D in the progression of chronic inflammatory diseases to cancer (which has high relevance for prevention of colorectal cancer in people).

Together with the antifibrotic effects, vitamin D has antiproliferative effects. Calcitriol inhibits cyclins and enhances expression of inhibitors of cyclin-dependent kinases; however, clinical studies are scarce. Currently, the strongest clinical evidence is based on epidemiologic studies in people demonstrating lower odds ratios for colorectal cancer (0.88) and breast cancer (0.72) associated with increased vitamin D intake compared with a typical Western-type diet.[73] In people, deficient intake of vitamin D, combined with insufficient exposure to sunlight, is common, whereas most dogs and cats consume sufficient dietary vitamin D thanks to complete and balanced diets. Clinical studies in dogs and cats on the effects of vitamin D on different types of cancer have not been conducted thus far to the authors' knowledge.

CLINICS CARE POINTS

- Vitamin D might be protective for several inflammatory and proliferative diseases, like gastrointestinal disease and cancer, which are subjects for future research.

REFERENCES

1. Summers SC, Stockman J, Larsen JA, et al. Evaluation of nutrient content and caloric density in commercially available foods formulated for senior cats. J Vet Int Med 2020;34:2029–35.
2. Summers SC, Stockman J, Larsen JA, et al. Evaluation of phosphorus, calcium, and magnesium content in commercially available foods formulated for healthy cats. J Vet Int Med 2020;34(1):266–73.
3. Kritikos G, Weidner N, Atkinson JL, et al. Quantification of vitamin D3 in commercial dog foods and comparison with Association of American Feed Control Officials recommendations and manufacturer-reported concentrations. J Am Vet Med Assoc 2018;252:1521–6.
4. Hutchinson D, Freeman LM, McCarthy R, et al. Seizures and severe nutrient deficiencies in a puppy fed a homemade diet. J Am Vet Med Assoc 2012;241: 477–83.
5. NRC. Nutrient requirements of dogs and cats. Washington, DC: National Academies Press; 2006.
6. Nap RC, Hazewinkel HA. Growth and skeletal development in the dog in relation to nutrition; a review. Vet Q 1994;16:50–9.

7. Dobenecker B, Kasbeitzer N, Flinspach S, et al. Calcium-excess causes subclinical changes of bone growth in beagles but not in foxhound-crossbred dogs, as measured in X-rays. J Anim Physiol Anim Nutr (Berl) 2006;90:394–401.
8. Stockman J, Watson P, Gilham M, et al. Adult dogs are capable of regulating calcium balance, with no adverse effects on health, when fed a high-calcium diet. Br J Nutr 2017;117:1235–43, 31.
9. Morris JG. Ineffective vitamin D synthesis in cats is reversed by an inhibitor of 7-dehydrocholestrol-delta7-reductase. J Nutr 1999;129:903–8.
10. How KL, Hazewinkel HA, Mol JA. Photosynthesis of vitamin D in the skin of dogs cats and rats. Vet Q 1995;17(Suppl 1):S29.
11. Weidner N, Verbrugghe A. Current knowledge of vitamin D in dogs. Crit Rev Food Sci Nutr 2017;57:3850–9.
12. AAFCO. Official Publication. Atlanta (GA): Association of American Feed Control Officials; 2018.
13. FEDIAF. Nutritional guidelines for complete and complementary pet food for cats and dogs 2020. Available at: www.fediaf.org. Accessed October 8, 2020.
14. Allison LN, Jaffey JA, Bradley-Siemens N, et al. Immune function and serum vitamin D in shelter dogs: a case-control study. Vet J 2020;261:105477.
15. Osuga T, Nakamura K, Morita T, et al. Vitamin D status in different stages of disease severity in dogs with chronic valvular heart disease. J Vet Intern Med 2015; 29:1518–23.
16. Allenspach K, Rizzo J, Jergens AE, et al. Hypovitaminosis D is associated with negative outcome in dogs with protein losing enteropathy: a retrospective study of 43 cases. BMC Vet Res 2017;13:96.
17. Zafalon RVA, Risolia LW, Pedrinelli V, et al. Vitamin D metabolism in dogs and cats and its relation to diseases not associated with bone metabolism. J Anim Physiol Anim Nutr 2020;104:322–42.
18. Pallauf J, Rimbach G. Nutritional significance of phytic acid and phytase. Arch Tierernahr 1997;50:301–19.
19. Coltherd JC, Staunton R, Colyer A, et al. Not all forms of dietary phosphorus are equal: an evaluation of postprandial phosphorus concentrations in the plasma of the cat. Br J Nutr 2019;121:270–84.
20. Dobenecker B, Webel A, Reese S, et al. Effect of a high phosphorus diet on indicators of renal health in cats. J Feline Med Surg 2018;20:339–43.
21. Alexander J, Stockman J, Atwal J, et al. Effects of the long-term feeding of diets enriched with inorganic phosphorus on the adult feline kidney and phosphorus metabolism. Br J Nutr 2018;121:1–21.
22. Morris JG. Cats discriminate between cholecalciferol and ergocalciferol. J Anim Physiol Anim Nutr (Berl) 2002;86:229–38.
23. Delaney SJ. Serum ionized calcium, 25-hydroxyvitamin D, and parathyroid hormone in two dogs fed a homemade diet fortified with vitamin D2. In: 2015 Annual AAVN Symposium Order of Abstracts. J Anim Physiol Anim Nutr 2015;99:810–24.
24. Goedegebuure SA, Hazewinkel HA. Morphological findings in young dogs chronically fed a diet containing excess calcium. Vet Pathol 1986;23:594–605.
25. Hazewinkel HA, Van den Brom WE, Van 'T Klooster AT, et al. Calcium metabolism in great Dane dogs fed diets with various calcium and phosphorus levels. J Nutr 1991;121:S99–106.
26. Lauten SD, Cox NR, Brawner WR Jr, et al. Influence of dietary calcium and phosphorus content in a fixed ratio on growth and development in great Danes. Am J Vet Res 2002;63:1036–47.

27. Tryfonidou MA, Holl MS, Stevenhagen JJ, et al. Dietary 135-fold cholecalciferol supplementation severely disturbs the endochondral ossification in growing dogs. Domest Anim Endocrin 2003;24:265–85.
28. Hazewinkel HAW, Schoenmakers I. Hormonal and skeletal effects of excessive calcium intake during partial weaning and at prepubertal age in dogs. Compend Contin Educ Vet 2006;28(SUPPL):55.
29. Hazewinkel HAW, Tryfonidou MA. Vitamin D3 metabolism in dogs. Mol Cell Endocrinol 2002;197:23–33.
30. Verbrugghe A, Paepe D, Verhaert L, et al. Metabolic bone disease and hyperparathyroidism in an adult dog fed an unbalanced homemade diet. Vlaams Diergeneeskundig Tijdschrift 2011;80:61–8.
31. Kiefer-Hecker B, Bauer A, Dobenecker B. Effects of low phosphorus intake on serum calcium, phosphorus, alkaline phosphatase activity and parathyroid hormone in growing dogs. J Anim Physiol Anim Nutr 2018;102:1749–58.
32. Corbee RJ, Mars A. Enostosis, a diet induced disorder? In: ESVCN Congress Cirencester 2017 Proceedings, Royal Agricultural University Cirencester, September 20th-23rd 2017. p. 56.
33. Bartges J, Kirk C. Nutritional management of lower urinary tract disease. In: Fascetti AJ, Delaney SJ, editors. Applied veterinary clinical nutrition. New York: Wiley & Sons; 2012. p. 269–87.
34. Gupta M, Bhayana S, Sikka S. Role of urinary inhibitors and promoters in calcium oxalate crystallisation. Int J Res Pharm Chem 2011;1:793–8.
35. Mo L, Huang H-Y, Zhu X-H, et al. Tamm-Horsfall protein is a critical renal defense factor protecting against calcium oxalate crystal formation. Kidney Int 2004;66: 1159–66.
36. Hess B. The role of Tamm-Horsfall glycoprotein and nephrocalcin in calcium oxalate monohydrate crystallization processes. Scan Electron Microsc 1991;5:689.
37. Lulich JP, Osborne CA, Thumchai R, et al. Epidemiology of canine calcium oxalate uroliths: identifying risk factors. Vet Clin North Am Small Anim Pract 1999;29: 113–22.
38. Midkiff A, Chew D, Randolph J, et al. Idiopathic hypercalcemia in cats. J Vet Int Med 2000;14:619–26.
39. de Brito Galvao JF, Nagode LA, Schenck PA, et al. Calcitriol, calcidiol, parathyroid hormone, and fibroblast growth factor-23 interactions in chronic kidney disease. J Vet Emerg Crit Care (San Antonio) 2013;23:134–62.
40. de Brito Galvão JF, Parker V, Schenck PA, et al. Update on feline ionized hypercalcemia. Vet Clin North Am Small Anim Pract 2017;47:273–92.
41. Dijcker JC, Kummeling A, Hagen-Plantinga EA, et al. Urinary oxalate and calcium excretion by dogs and cats diagnosed with calcium oxalate urolithiasis. Vet Rec 2012;171:646.
42. Furrow E, Patterson E, Armstrong P, et al. Fasting urinary calcium-to-creatinine and oxalate-to-creatinine ratios in dogs with calcium oxalate urolithiasis and breed-matched controls. J Vet Int Med 2015;29:113–9.
43. Luskin AC, Lulich JP, Gresch SC, et al. Bone resorption in dogs with calcium oxalate urolithiasis and idiopathic hypercalciuria. Res Vet Sci 2019;123:129–34.
44. Ching SV, Fettman MJ, Hamar DW, et al. The effect of chronic dietary acidification using ammonium chloride on acid-base and mineral metabolism in the adult cat. J Nutr 1989;119:902–15.
45. Arnett TR. Acidosis, hypoxia and bone. Arch Biochem Biophys 2010;503:103–9.

46. Hiroshi H, Suzuki T, Kasai T, et al. Ingestion of guar gum hydrolysate, a soluble fiber, increases calcium absorption in totally gastrectomized rats. J Nutr 1999; 129:39–45.
47. Fantinati M, Priymenko N. Managing feline idiopathic hypercalcemia with chia seeds (Salvia hispanica L.): a case series. Front Vet Sci 2020;7:421.
48. McClain HM, Barsanti JA, Bartges JW. Hypercalcemia and calcium oxalate urolithiasis in cats: a report of five cases. J Am Anim Hosp Assoc 1999;35:297–301.
49. Pastoor F, Van't Klooster AT, Mathot J, et al. Increasing calcium intakes lower urinary concentrations of phosphorus and magnesium in adult ovariectomized cats. J Nutr 1994;124:299–304.
50. Rizzoli R, Fleisch H, Bonjour J-P. Role of 1,25-dihydroxyvitamin D3 on intestinal phosphate absorption in rats with a normal vitamin D supply. J Clin Invest 1977;60:639–47.
51. Calabrò S, Tudisco R, Bianchi S, et al. Management of struvite uroliths in dogs. Br J Nutr 2011;106:S191–3.
52. Dear JD, Larsen JA, Bannasch M, et al. Evaluation of a dry therapeutic urinary diet and concurrent administration of antimicrobials for struvite cystolith dissolution in dogs. BMC Vet Res 2019;15:273.
53. Torres-Henderson C, Bunkers J, Contreras ET, et al. Use of Purina Pro Plan Veterinary Diet UR Urinary St/Ox to dissolve struvite cystoliths. Top Companion Anim Med 2017;32:49–54.
54. Tarttelin MF. Feline struvite urolithiasis: factors affecting urine pH may be more important than magnesium levels in food. Vet Rec 1987;121:227–30.
55. Osborne C, Klausner J, Lulich J. Canine and feline calcium phosphate urolithiasis. In: Current veterinary therapy XII Kirk. Philadelphia: WB Saunders; 1995. p. 996–1001.
56. Adams L, Syme H. Canine ureteral and lower urinary tract diseases. In: Ettinger, Stephen J, Feldman, et al, editors. Textbook of veterinary internal medicine: diseases of the dog and the cat. 7th edition. St. Louis (MO): Elsevier Saunders; 2010. p. 2087.
57. Boyd L, Langston C, Thompson K, et al. Survival in cats with naturally occurring chronic kidney disease (2000–2002). J Vet Int Med 2008;22:1111–7.
58. Kuwahara Y, Ohba Y, Kitoh K, et al. Association of laboratory data and death within one month in cats with chronic renal failure. J Small Anim Pract 2006;47: 446–50.
59. Elliott J, Barber P. Feline chronic renal failure: clinical findings in 80 cases diagnosed between 1992 and 1995. J Small Anim Pract 1998;39:78–85.
60. Geddes RF, Finch NC, Syme HM, et al. The role of phosphorus in the pathophysiology of chronic kidney disease. J Vet Emerg Crit Care (San Antonio) 2013;23: 122–33.
61. Sargent HJ, Jepson RE, Chang Y-m, et al. Fibroblast growth factor 23 and symmetric dimethylarginine concentrations in geriatric cats. J Vet Intern Med 2019; 33:2657–64.
62. Finch N, Syme H, Elliott J. Risk factors for development of chronic kidney disease in cats. J Vet Intern Med 2016;30:602–10.
63. Finch NC, Syme HM, Elliott J. Parathyroid hormone concentration in geriatric cats with various degrees of renal function. J Am Vet Med Assoc 2012;241:1326–35.
64. Ross L, Finco D, Crowell WA. Effect of dietary phosphorus restriction on the kidneys of cats with reduced renal mass. Am J Vet Res 1982;43:1023–6.

65. Ross SJ, Osborne CA, Kirk CA, et al. Clinical evaluation of dietary modification for treatment of spontaneous chronic kidney disease in cats. J Am Vet Med Assoc 2006;229:949–57.
66. Brown SA, Rickertsen M, Sheldon S. Effects of an intestinal phosphorus binder on serum phosphorus and parathyroid hormone concentration in cats with reduced renal function. Int J Appl Res 2008;6:155–60.
67. Elliott J, Rawlings J, Markwell P, et al. Survival of cats with naturally occurring chronic renal failure: effect of dietary management. J Small Anim Pract 2000; 41:235–42.
68. Bikle DD Vitamin D. Biochemistry and physiology. In: Liao E, editor. Extraskeletal effects of vitamin D. contemporary endocrinology. Cham (Switzerland): Humana Press; 2018. p. 1–40.
69. Zhao H, Zhang H, Wu H, et al. Protective role of 1,25(OH)2vitamin D3 in the mucosal injury and epithelial barrier disruption in DSS-induced acute colitis in mice. BMC Gastroenterol 2012;12. Article number 57.
70. Chen A, Davis BH, Bissonnette M, et al. 1,25-Dihydroxyvitamin D3 stimulates activator protein-1-dependent Caco-2 cell differentiation. J Biol Chem 1999;274: 35505–13.
71. Barbáchano A, Fernández-Barral A, Ferrer-Mayorga G, et al. The endocrine vitamin D system in the gut. Mol Cell Endocrinol 2017;453:79–87.
72. Parravicini V, Caserta S. The immunomodulatory roles of vitamin D: new tricks for an old dog. Mol Interv 2010;10:204–8.
73. Ferrer-Mayorga G, Gómez-López G, Barbáchano A, et al. Vitamin D receptor expression and associated gene signature in tumour stromal fibroblasts predict clinical outcome in colorectal cancer. Gut 2017;66:1449–62.
74. Tao Q, Wang B, Zheng Y, et al. Vitamin D prevents the intestinal fibrosis via induction of vitamin D receptor and inhibition of transforming growth factor-beta1/ Smad3 pathway. Dig Dis Sci 2015;60:868–75.
75. Corbee RJ, Tryfonidou MA, Grinwis GCM, et al. Skeletal and hepatic changes induced by chronic vitamin A supplementation in cats. Vet J 2014;202:503–9.

Senior Pet Nutrition and Management

Julie A. Churchill, DVM, PhD[a,*], Laura Eirmann, DVM[b,c]

KEYWORDS

• Senior • Geriatric • Aging • Nutrition • Nutritional assessment

KEY POINTS

- Aging is a continuum with individual variation regarding the onset and degree of age-related physiologic and pathologic changes. This individual variation prevents a one-size-fits-all approach to senior nutrition.
- Physiologic changes associated with aging include changes in energy requirements, body composition, and certain nutrient requirements. In addition, senior pets are at risk of pathologic changes, risk of frailty and comorbidities that may require thoughtful nutrition planning.
- Every pet requires a nutritional assessment and specific recommendations. Frequent reassessment of the senior population is critical to ensure the nutrition plan continues to meet the needs of the elder pet who is at risk for various age-related health issues.
- There is no established Association of American Feed Control Officials nutrient profile for a senior life stage, so the nutrient composition of products marketed for senior pets varies widely.
- As end of life approaches, recognize the importance of feeding as part of the bond with the pet. Consider shifting the focus from eating the so-called right food to nurturing with foods to provide compassionate care.

INTRODUCTION

Senior pets represent approximately one-third of the pet population.[1] The point at which an individual progresses from the mature adult to senior life stage is variable. For this reason, age groupings are arbitrary demarcations that can help veterinary health care teams (VHCTs) focus attention on physiologic changes that occur at different stages. For cats, the American Association of Feline Practitioners (AAFP)–American Animal Hospital Association (AAHA) Feline Life Stage Guidelines group cats 11 to 14 years of age as seniors and cats more than 15 years of age as geriatric.[2] Dogs' life expectancies vary widely depending on breed and body size, and aging

[a] Veterinary Clinical Science Department, University of Minnesota College of Veterinary Medicine, 1352 Boyd Avenue, St Paul, MN 55108, USA; [b] Oradell Animal Hospital, 580 Winters Avenue, Oradell, NJ 07652, USA; [c] Nestle Purina PetCare, St Louis, MO, USA
* Corresponding author.
E-mail address: churc002@umn.edu

Vet Clin Small Anim 51 (2021) 635–651
https://doi.org/10.1016/j.cvsm.2021.01.004
0195-5616/21/Published by Elsevier Inc.

changes are also variable. Rather than characterize the senior life stage by specific age ranges, the 2019 AAHA Canine Life Stage Guidelines define the senior life stage as the last 25% of estimated lifespan through end of life.[3] Physiologic changes associated with aging may include loss of senses (hearing or vision), reduced energy requirements and lean body mass, as well as a decline in various organ functions.[4,5] Physiologic changes associated with aging may make a pet less tolerant of nutritional deficiencies or excesses.[6] Senior pets are more vulnerable or at risk for age-related health problems. Nutritional management can influence many of these chronic diseases. A vital component of preventive medical care should include a senior screen or health risk assessment for early detection of health problems and adjustments to care and prevent or slow the onset of age-related diseases. Every senior health screen should include a thorough nutritional assessment followed by an individualized nutritional recommendation.

NUTRITIONAL ASSESSMENT

Before recommending any diet changes, a nutritional evaluation should be performed. The goal of the nutritional assessment is to obtain the necessary information to provide a specific detailed nutrition recommendation. Nutritional assessment is an iterative process that includes evaluating the patient, all foods, and the feeding management (www.ACVN.org). Signalment, dietary and medical histories, and complete physical examination with appropriate diagnostic testing for the senior pet comprise the nutritional assessment. The AAHA and World Small Animal Veterinary Association (WSAVA) recommend a nutritional assessment and dietary recommendation every time a pet presents for veterinary consultation.[7,8] An accurate diet history is invaluable when assessing the nutritional health of the patient and is vital to formulating an individualized diet plan. Understanding the nutritional changes that occur with aging and identifying any changes in the individual patient can help the clinician better match the appropriate food with the patient's unique needs (**Table 1**). The patient, the food, and the pet owner's feeding practices are interrelated and require reassessment. Health and nutritional status are not static, especially in senior pets, but are a dynamic process worthy of continued reevaluation and treatment modifications to match the changing needs of the pet.

Patient Assessment

An initial assessment of the patient uses information collected as part of a health assessment: a complete medical and diet history, a thorough physical examination, and appropriate laboratory work (eg, complete blood count, serum biochemical profile, urinalysis, and thyroid function [feline]). Patient factors, including body weight and body condition score (BCS), are essential because food recommendations and feeding amounts are based on body condition and optimal body weight. Body weight and BCS should be recorded at each visit in a manner that allows the VHCT to observe trends. Several body scoring systems have been developed and evaluated in dogs and cats.[9–13]

Adopting a universal 9-point BCS, which has been more extensively validated than other BCS systems,[9,10,14–16] is preferable and is also the system that has been recommended by the WSAVA Global Nutrition Panel.[17] The 9-point BCS offers several advantages compared with other BCS and zoometric measures of adiposity,[12,13] most notably speed and simplicity to ensure consistent use in veterinary practices. A universal BCS would better enable VHCTs to interpret veterinary medical research, more consistently and accurately assess their patients' body conditions, and clearly

Table 1
Considerations to address nutritional/metabolic alterations of healthy aging pets

Key Nutrient/Metabolic Change	Feline and Canine	Rationale
Energy	Increase or decrease	Senior cats have a gradual decrease in MER through middle age (~11 y) and thereafter more commonly have an increase in MER associated with loss of body weight. Senior dogs commonly have decreased MER, but geriatric dogs are also more likely to be underweight
Water	No alteration or Increase	Reduced total body water, decreased sense of thirst, mobility conditions limiting access to water, and subclinical increases in water losses (urinary) increase risk of dehydration. Ensure easy access to water, offer higher-moisture foods, or add water/liquid to dogs' food Consider nutrient-enriched water supplement for cats
Protein	Increase (unless evidence of medical condition reducing protein tolerance)	Twenty percent of geriatric cats have decreased protein digestion Protein requirements of healthy senior cats and dogs increase with age because of compromised protein synthesis
Fat	Increase or decrease	An estimated 35% of geriatric cats have decreased fat digestion and may benefit from nutrient-dense highly digestible growth formula Dogs have no change in fat digestion with aging, and dietary fat intake should be adjusted to manage nutrient density of the diet and healthy BCS of the dog

(*continued on next page*)

Table 1
(*continued*)

Key Nutrient/Metabolic Change	Feline and Canine	Rationale
Long-chain omega-3 polyunsaturated fatty acids	No alteration or increase	Have shown promise in dogs with osteoarthritis, renal disease (*VCNA* Parker) heart disease (Freeman[79]) and some forms of cancer (*VCNA* Saker)
Antioxidants and medium-chain triglycerides	No alteration or increase	Valarie V. Tynes and Gary Landsberg's article, "Nutritional Management of Behavior and Brain Disorders in Dogs and Cats," in this issue

Abbreviations: BCS, body condition score; MER, maintenance energy requirement.

communicate with colleagues and clients. Using the 9-point system, each unit increase in the BCS greater than ideal is approximately equivalent to 10% to 15% more than ideal body weight.[18]

A muscle condition score (MCS) system, as recommended by the WSAVA, is also an essential component of the patient assessment. The MCS uses palpation of the skeletal musculature over the spine, skull, scapula, and pelvis, and is independent of body fat and BCS. An MCS has been developed and evaluated in both cats and dogs.[19,20] Senior dogs and cats experience sarcopenia, a loss of lean body mass (LBM) with age, unrelated to disease.[4,21] Sarcopenia is commonly accompanied by an increase in body fat, which may result in stable body weight. This loss of LBM may go unrecognized if the clinician relies on body weight trends and ignores MCS.[22,23] Evaluation of MCS in senior pets is an important first step in identifying age-related sarcopenia or cachexia (loss of muscle mass secondary to an underlying catabolic disease). Loss of LBM is important to recognize because it is associated with increased morbidity and mortality.[21,24]

The nutritional screening process (**Table 2**) can quickly identify patients with nutritional risks. Healthy seniors without identified risks, who are eating an appropriate nutritionally balanced diet, have a healthy body weight, healthy body and muscle conditions (BCS, MCS), and are free of significant physical or laboratory abnormalities need no further evaluation at this time, but a recommendation for the client is important. A pet-specific nutrition assessment and recommendation for healthy seniors can be done quickly. Nutritional recommendations should include the specific name of foods that match the pet's current nutritional needs, the amount and frequency for feeding, and a monitoring plan. In many of these healthy patients, the feeding recommendation involves little or no change, but it should include a verification and validation for the owner that the current food and feeding plan meets the pet's needs, and a documentation of the current feeding plan in the medical record. At a minimum, the monitoring should include body weight and BCS by the owner each month in order to detect changes early.

If nutritional risk factors or age-related problems are identified, an extended evaluation and management plan is indicated. This in-depth evaluation should address

Table 2
Initial screen: assessing for nutritional risk factors

Check When Any Risk Factors Present in the Patient	
Nutritional Screen for Risk Factors	**Require Extended Evaluation if (✓)**
History of:	
Treats/snacks/human foods >10% intake	
Inadequate information/inappropriate feeding/food	
Consuming unconventional diets	
Previous/ongoing medical problems	
Gastrointestinal signs	
Physical Examination:	
Any abnormal BCS ($\neq$5 out of 9)	
Any abnormal MCS	
Unintentional weight loss or gain	
New medical condition	
Poor skin hair coat	
Dental disease	

Adapted from the 2010 AAHA Nutritional Assessment Guidelines for Dogs and Cats. © American Animal Hospital Association, 2010.

changes that may indicate the onset of common age-related diseases that may be influenced by nutritional management (**Box 1**).

Diet Assessment

A comprehensive diet history is a critical component of the nutritional assessment of senior pets. To facilitate obtaining a comprehensive diet history, a form can be provided to the owner before the appointment (http://acvn.org/wp-content/uploads/2020/04/ACVN-Diet-History-Form-2020-FINAL_fillable.pdf). This form allows the caregivers an opportunity to look at pet food labels at home, measure the amount they are feeding, and perhaps keep a food diary before the visit. The diet history should identify all snacks, treats, and nutritional supplements by type and amount. The drug/supplement history should include questions about the use of food to administer medication, because it may comprise a significant portion of the pet's caloric intake. Diet history information combined with the patient assessment provides information about the patient's daily caloric requirements and specific nutrient intake. This nutrient intake should be compared with the patient's individual needs. For example, an overweight pet with a robust appetite should not be fed a calorie-dense product. Reducing the amount of a high-calorie product to limit calorie intake could lead to deficiencies of other essential nutrients[25,26] and increase hunger or undesirable food-seeking behaviors. Such pets would benefit from a diet specifically formulated to contain lower calories and a higher nutrient/calorie ratio.

Feeding management assessment

Feeding practices and preferences influence pets' intake. Multipet households may present competition, limiting the senior pet's access to food. A senior pet with mobility issues may have difficulty or pain associated with accessing food.

Box 1
Extended screening: assessing senior dogs for nutritionally relevant age-related factors

Extended evaluation: age-related diseases to evaluate in senior dogs

Abnormal body and muscle condition: change in weight and muscle mass?

Diet: is the pet eating appropriate amounts of balanced diet?
- Assess appetite and intake
- Assess ability to eat: prehension, mastication swallowing for those underweight and/or poor intake
- Perform oral examination: include periodontal, tonsils, or any oral abnormalities
- Assess sensory input: smell, vision, palatability of food; consider palatability enhancer if necessary

Mobility and access to food and water
- Is the pet able to walk, access food provided? Able to stand to eat and drink?
- Other pets or physical limitations impairing access?
- Mobility and exercise: is the pet's MCS normal (3 out of 3)?
- Presence of osteoarthritis, lameness, pain? Play a role in maintenance of comfort, fitness, and healthy BCS
- Activity minimizes sarcopenia
- Exercise and activity provide mental stimulation and environmental enrichment

Cognitive function
- Disorientation/confusion: becomes lost or confused, fails to recognize familiar people?
- Changed interactions with family members? Isolates or seeks attention less often?
- Change in sleep/activity cycles? Wander or pace, sleep more in day, less at night?
- Loss of house training (nonmedical reasons)

Change in clinical status to suggest disease onset
- Changes in energy, demeanor, and well-being
- Changes in urination or stool quality, frequency, or quantity

An extended evaluation is performed if more than 1 risk factor is identified in the nutritional screening process. This evaluation should include eating (both appetite and intake), oral examination, aspects of activity and mobility, sleep, cognitive function, and behavior.

Dental disease, common in senior pets, may limit intake because of pain or difficulty prehending. Age-related decline in sensory perception or cognition may require a different feeding strategy, such as warming food or hand feeding. Determine whether food is accurately measured, how much/how often food is offered, and how much is eaten. Ask whether there have been recent changes to the feeding plan and why, as well how the pet adapted to those changes. Senior pets becoming picky may be the first clue the owners notice of an underlying medical condition.

Reassessment and Modification of Treatment Plan

Nutritional assessment of geriatric pets is an ongoing process. Dogs and cats experience a variable and wide variety of metabolic changes as they age. It is important to communicate and engage pet owners to create the expectation of continued reassessment and treatment modifications that accommodate the specific changes observed in each individual pet, rather than adopting a general senior protocol. A vigilant monitoring plan allows early detection of problems if they arise and a better opportunity to intervene or modify the pet's individualized nutritional plan to improve its health. Partner with clients to help ensure success and maintain adherence to the feeding and monitoring goals.

EFFECTS OF AGING ON NUTRITIONAL NEEDS

Energy

Aging can result in both structural and functional changes of the gastrointestinal tract. However, clinically relevant differences in nutrient absorption between young adult and geriatric dogs have not been reported.[27,28] In contrast, approximately one-third of cats greater than 12 years of age have decreased fat digestibility and approximately 20% of cats greater than 14 years of age have reduced protein digestibility.[22] Maintenance energy requirement (MER) is defined as the energy required to keep an animal at a state of energy equilibrium such that caloric intake matches energy expedition resulting in stable body weight. MER varies depending on factors such as breed, activity level, health, neuter status, and age. As dogs age, MER decreases ~25%, with the greatest decline at middle age,[29] although some studies report an even greater decline in MER with age.[30] In cats, MER seems to decrease by approximately 3% per year for the first 11 years of life, but, after ~12 years of age, MER tends to increase, and weight loss and decreases in LBM are common.[31–33]

Because of the wide range of individual energy requirements across the senior pet population, each senior needs frequent monitoring to adjust energy intake to match that individual's needs. Aging pets may be less active than young adults, which contributes to reduced MER. If no adjustments are made to energy intake to account for the reduced caloric requirement, the senior pet may gain unhealthy weight. A less calorie-dense diet with a higher nutrient to calorie ratio would be beneficial to promote ideal weight while delivering sufficient intake of essential nutrients. Results from a lifelong study performed in dogs revealed lower disease incidence, later onset of disease, and increased life span in calorically restricted animals. Dogs fed to maintain a lean body condition lived an average of 13.0 years compared with 11.2 years in the heavier control group.[34] Thus, maintaining energy balance to maintain optimal body condition should be one of the most important health goals for senior pets. In 1 study following a colony of aging cats, body weight decreased starting about 2.5 years before end of life, before clinical evidence of underlying disease.[22] For this reason, clinicians should take note of subtle declines in body weight and recommend appropriate diagnostics with the goal of earlier diagnosis of an underlying medical condition. Evaluating changes in body weight and body condition in conjunction with food intake also allows veterinarians to investigate possible underlying disorders. Weight loss despite increased food intake in a senior cat increases the index of suspicion for diseases such as hyperthyroidism. Weight gain with stable caloric intake may occur in a senior dog with decreased mobility because of osteoarthritis (OA) or certain endocrinopathies, such as hypothyroidism. Unhealthy weight gain exacerbates several age-related conditions, including OA, so caloric intake must be adjusted. Maintaining energy balance to maintain optimal body condition should be one of the most important health goals for senior pets.

Water

The prevalence of dehydration in elderly humans is 20% to 30%. It is mainly secondary to reduced thirst sensation and reduced ability to concentrate urine. Hypohydration or chronic mild hydration in human elders is associated with frailty, morbidity, and mortality.[35] Mild dehydration has also been associated with impaired cognition, mood, and pain sensation in humans.[36–38] Although optimal water recommendations for senior dogs and cats remain unknown, it is prudent to closely monitor water intake in this population. Older pets with decreased mobility may need management modifications, including an increased number of water bowls in multiple locations to facilitate access to clean fresh water at all times. Water intake should be monitored or ensured when older dogs are exercising or exposed to hot environments. Senior pets may also be at risk of dehydration if they have subclinical renal insufficiency. When a senior pet has a good appetite but water intake is suspect, changing to a moist food, adding water to the food as the pet tolerates it, or considering a nutrient-enriched water supplement to improve hydration should be considered.

Protein

Protein requirements increase with age because of increased protein turnover and reduced protein synthesis.[39,40] Healthy senior pets do not benefit from protein restriction[41] and may be harmed by limiting dietary protein.[42,43] Insufficient or marginal protein intake contributes to sarcopenia. Thus, protein restriction of seniors could be more detrimental than protein deficiency in younger animals.[44] Although nutrition alone does not prevent loss of LBM, providing adequate dietary protein is an essential component to limit this loss. As a general guideline for estimating adult daily protein needs, provide at minimum 2.55 g protein per kilogram body weight (or ~ 1 g protein per pound body weight) for dogs,[8,20,21] and ~5 g protein per kilogram body weight (~2 g per pound body weight) for cats.[45–48] There is growing support that, like healthy senior people, senior pets may require approximately 50% more dietary protein than adults.[49] This level of protein intake should minimize risk of protein deficiency, help minimize loss of LBM, and should only be restricted when medically indicated.

Because of the wide variation in energy needs as pets age, protein intake should be assessed in the context of the individual's energy needs. For example, older dogs generally require fewer calories, or less food, than younger dogs, whereas senior cats may or may not need calorie adjustments to maintain healthy body weight. In general, diets for older dogs should contain not only lower calories but a higher percentage of protein or a higher protein/calorie ratio in order to meet the dog's age-related nutritional needs. Based on the diet history, ensure that the pet is meeting daily protein needs. Regular reassessment of MCS to monitor LBM is important in managing the nutritional health of seniors.

WHAT IS A SENIOR PET FOOD?

Pet owners perceive that most pets, including senior dogs, are healthy and do not require a therapeutic food,[50] but they are still left with hundreds of pet foods options. Advice and information recommending the best food is available almost anywhere, from trainers to pet food retailers, from magazines, Internet sources, and social media. In a survey of pet owners' opinions about nutritional requirements of senior dogs, most responded that senior dogs have different nutritional needs than adults, with seniors needing fewer calories and less fat, sodium, protein, and carbohydrates.[51] However, the Association of American Feed Control Officials (AAFCO) has established nutrition guidelines for growth, reproduction, and adult maintenance, but there is no established nutrient profile to meet the geriatric life stage needs.[52] The nutrient and caloric content of products marketed for both senior dogs and cats is widely variable.[51,53] There is a wide discrepancy between perceived needs of senior pets and actual diet composition of products marketed for senior pets. This discrepancy makes it even more critical for the VHCT to play an active role in providing credible nutritional advice, especially for senior dogs and cats that have unique nutritional concerns.

NUTRITIONAL INTERVENTION OF SELECTED AGE-RELATED DISEASES

Although the most common age-related conditions in pets are best managed with a multimodal approach combining nutritional strategies, exercise or environmental enrichment, and medical management, the following discussion focuses on nutritional management. This issue of *VCNA* has several chapters devoted to the nutritional management of specific disease conditions. Therefore, this article highlights nutritional concerns of generally healthy senior pets. The following discussion focuses on comorbid conditions that occur commonly in aging pets and are often overlooked or dismissed as simply aging changes, when nutritional intervention for these conditions can play an important role in optimizing health.

ABNORMAL BODY WEIGHT

Overweight/Obese

Hyperadiposity, the most prevalent form of malnutrition, contributes to many of the diseases linked to obesity.[54–56] However, pets that are overweight often go unrecognized or may not have this health concern addressed. The canine lifespan study[34] showed the benefits of maintaining a lean body condition and many negative health consequences with as little as 25% weight gain above healthy ideal BCS (4.5–5 out of 9). For information regarding maintaining or achieving healthy body weight, see Megan Shepherd's article, "Canine and Feline Obesity Management," in this issue. In contrast with dogs, evidence suggests cats with BCS up to 6 out of 9 may be associated with longevity.[57]

Underweight

Cats greater than 12 years old more commonly experience weight loss with advancing age and have a greater likelihood of being underweight than young adult cats.[58,59] Identifying weight loss or underweight senior cats is important because underweight cats are more likely to have a greater morbidity and mortality.[57] Weight loss has been shown to precede diagnoses of disease in cats,[60,61] and early detection may provide an opportunity for early diagnosis and nutritional or medical intervention. To address unintentional weight loss, either increase the amount of the current food or transition to a more calorie-dense diet.

DEGENERATIVE JOINT DISEASE

OA is common in senior cats[62] and is the most prevalent joint disorder in dogs, affecting as many 1 in 5 dogs, with OA increasing in incidence and severity with advancing age.[63] Being overweight or obese is recognized as a primary risk factor.[64] Poor mobility and decreased activity are each components of a frailty score in dogs. Increased frailty is associated with shorter time to death.[65] Nutritional strategies for improving geriatric health span and minimizing OA include weight and muscle management, and provision of omega-3 fatty acids.

Weight and Muscle Management

Correction of hyperadiposity can improve clinical signs of lameness in arthritic dogs.[66] Scientific data are limited regarding cats with OA; however it is assumed, as in other species, that obesity management is important in reducing inflammatory mediators and pain associated with OA. Strategies to maintain healthy body weight, BCS, and LBM and prevent sarcopenia should be prioritized for senior pets. This management can be achieved by selecting a complete and balanced diet that supplies protein and other nutrients while providing the number of calories to prevent excess body fat gain. The nutritional goal is to delay onset and prevent progression of OA, maintain LBM, and delay frailty.

Long-Chain Omega-3 Polyunsaturated Fatty Acids

Intake of omega-3 polyunsaturated fatty acids (n-3-PUFAs) shows the greatest evidence for synovial antiinflammatory effects in dogs[67–69] and cats[62,70] compared with other nutraceuticals. The n-3-PUFAs eicosapentaenoic acid (EPA) and docosahexaenoic acid (DHA) compete with arachidonic acid in cell membranes to yield fewer inflammatory leukotrienes, prostaglandins, and thromboxanes, which reduce the pain of OA. Marine oils (EPA>DHA)[71] are more effective compared with shorter-chain plant-source n-3 oils. Studies have shown the beneficial effects of supplementing n-3-PUFAs in dogs with lameness secondary to OA.[68,69,72] There is currently no standard accepted dose of omega-3 fatty acids for dogs or cats. In dogs, a general recommended range of doses for OA is a combination of EPA and DHA of 230 to 310 mg/kg of metabolic body weight, whereas doses of 90 to 110 mg/kg body weight were also effective.[68,69,73] In cats with OA, a diet containing 188 mg of omega-3 fatty acids/100 kcal or a similar amount of added supplement alone improved owners' perception of their cats' activity.[62,70] Veterinary diets formulated to help pets with OA have enriched concentrations of n-3-PUFA with EPA and DHA. The therapeutic joint diets also include some combination of proteoglycan precursors (glucosamine and chondroitin sulfate) and antioxidants. Consumption of therapeutic diets may allow reduction in nonsteroidal antiinflammatory drug use. Note that these diets are better suited for pets that are not significantly overweight, because the therapeutic joint diets are not intended for weight reduction, and limiting food to achieve weight loss may not only lead to nutrient deficiencies but may also not deliver the therapeutic level of supplements. For this reason, a new generation of combination therapeutic diets formulated as combination weight loss and mobility supplements are entering the market.

COGNITIVE DYSFUNCTION

As many as 20% to 68% of middle-aged to elderly dogs are thought to experience cognitive dysfunction or behavioral changes, which can manifest in varying degrees of mental decline[74] (see **Table 2**). Nutraceuticals may have potential use both in prevention and treatment but are best when combined with environmental enrichment.[75–77] Antioxidants and medium-chain triglycerides have shown promise in helping dogs with cognitive dysfunction, as addressed in the Valarie V. Tynes and Gary Landsberg's article, "Nutritional Management of Behavior and Brain Disorders in Dogs and Cats," in this issue.

SUPPLEMENTS VERSUS ENRICHED DIETS

One caveat for the use of nutraceutical supplementation is that they have not been adequately assessed for efficacy, optimal doses, or nutrient interactions. When considering whether to select a diet containing the supplement or to prescribe a supplement, consider the nutrient composition of the base diet. Ensure that the base diet meets the macronutrient needs of the patient and determine whether it will provide an adequate dose of the intended supplement when fed to meet the energy needs of the individual pet. If not, it is prudent to select a more appropriate diet and give the intended dose of supplement (**Box 2** Provides an example of supplement dosing).

THE CONUNDRUM OF COMORBIDITIES

Making a nutritional recommendation seems straightforward when the senior pet is healthy or has only a single problem. Challenges arise when patients present with multiple seemingly competing or conflicting comorbidities, such as overweight patients

Box 2
Examples of supplement dosing with enriched food versus supplement administration

Two senior 10-kg mixed-breed dogs with OA

Both dogs are at their healthy weight with a body condition of 5 out of 9

A hypothetical joint supplement (Y) has been recommended for both dogs at a standard dose of 40 mg/kg body weight

The daily dose for each dog: 10 kg $\times$ 40 mg/kg = 400 mg of supplement Y per day

One pet food company just released a new therapeutic food formula BegoneOA. This therapeutic dog food has a caloric density of 370 kcal/cup, which contains 75 mg supplement Y/100 kcal.

Is it better to give each dog the Y supplement or feed a food with the Y supplement incorporated into the formulation?

Dog A: current daily intake of 1.5 cups/d of an adult maintenance food (380 kcal/cup) for a total of 570 kcal/d to maintain his healthy weight
The BegoneOA food fed at 570 kcal/d would provide:
75 mg/100 kcal $\times$ 5.7[100 kcal] = 427.5 mg of supplement Y
The food **would provide** an appropriate daily supplement dose for dog A.

Dog B: current daily intake is 1.5 cups/d of a healthy weight product (300 kcal/cup) for a total of 450 kcal/d
The BegoneOA food fed at 450 kcal/d would provide:
75 mg/100 kcal $\times$ 4.5[100 kcal] = 337.5 mg of supplement Y
The food would **not** provide the 400 mg recommended daily supplement dose for dog B. The dog should continue eating his current food and receive 400 mg of supplement Y per day or change to the therapeutic food and supplement an **additional** 63 mg of supplement Y per day to achieve the recommended dose.

with renal disease or cancer and pancreatitis. Except for obesity and OA, there is little research in how to manage multiple problems. However, in the absence of evidence, patients must eat. A general approach to prioritizing comorbidities is described in **Box 3**. **Table 3** lists typical ranges of nutrient modification to consider when managing multiple medical conditions. For example, an overweight senior cat or dog with early kidney disease may benefit from a modestly high-protein, lower-phosphorus diet.[41] Once a diet plan is implemented, the patient is monitored to see whether the desired effect is achieved with a repeated nutritional assessment and modifications to the plan as necessary in an iterative process.

END-OF-LIFE CONSIDERATIONS

Nutrition and nurturing are intimately linked, and food is a primary way of caring for pets. When the pet approaches end of life and is facing advanced stages of a progressive life-limiting illness or disability, realigning nutrition goals is usually indicated. Nutrition is a component of the integrated end-of-life treatment plan outlined in the 2016 AAHA/International Association for Animal Hospice and Palliative Care (IAAHPC) End-of-Life Care Guidelines.[78] Provide empathetic nonjudgmental communication regarding nutrition with the goal of maximizing patient comfort and minimizing suffering while supporting the caregiver. The veterinarian should assess and monitor the patient's hydration status, food intake, and feeding behaviors. Address underlying causes of hyporexia or dysrexia such as nausea or discomfort when possible. Help set expectations with the caregiver that will reduce stress for both the patient and family during this critical time. Consider giving the pet and caregiver permission to skip a meal or resume favorite foods that might have been discouraged in the past because

Box 3
Nutritional prioritization process for comorbidities

There is little evidence for best practices for managing senior pets with multiple conditions or comorbidities, but patients must eat to support their needs and support their quality of life. One approach is to perform a nutritional triage or prioritization, considering the following elements of the patient's status:

- Consider nutrients of concern or nutritional evidence to:
  - Try to meet needs for species and senior life stage
- Consider medical condition's onset: is it acute or chronic?
- Prioritize conditions affecting clinical signs and the patient's quality of life, and the degree or severity.
- Prioritize medical problems next based on the prognosis and/or progressive nature of each.
  - Build a key nutrient profile wish list
    - Nutrient profile for management of each disease
    - Consider contraindications or intolerance
  - Find a balance or prioritize management of diseases
  - Check **Table 3** to consider key nutrient ranges desired to manage the patient's individual needs
  - Select a therapeutic diet or seek board-certified veterinary nutritionist assistance for homemade formulation
- Make a nutritional recommendation
  - Exact product name, form, and flavor
  - Specific amount to feed
  - Frequency to feed
  - Monitoring or follow-up plan

Table 3
Information[b] for assessing products with nutrient modifications

Nutrient Modification	AAFCO[a] Minimum	Low	Moderate	High
Protein: Dog (g/100 kcal)	4.5	<5	6–7	>9
Protein: Cat (g/100 kcal)	6.5	<7	7–8	>10
Fat: Dog (g/100 kcal)	1.4	<2 (ultralow)	2.5–3.5 (low)	>5
Fat: Cat (g/100 kcal)	2.3	<3	4–4.5	>5
Phosphorus: Dog (mg/100 kcal)	100	<100	<150	>200
Phosphorus: Cat (mg/100 kcal)	125	<125 (ultralow)	<160 (low)	>200
Sodium: Dog (mg/100 kcal)	20	<70 (ultralow)	<100 (low)	>250
Sodium: Cat (mg/100 kcal)	50	<70 (ultralow)	<100 (low)	>250
Combined EPA and DHA: Dog (mg/100 kcal)	NA	NA	~10–15	>15 (wide variation)
Combined EPA and DHA: Cat (mg/100 kcal)	NA	NA	—	15 (wide variation)

Typical nutrient ranges and AAFCO minimum levels for adult canine and feline maintenance to use as reference when selecting products with nutrient modifications to either enrich or restrict a particular nutrient.

[a] AAFCO 2020 Official Publication adult maintenance minimums.

[b] There are no currently established values for low, moderate, and high nutrient ranges. The specific ranges provided in this table are based on the authors' opinions and clinical experience with commercially available foods.

of the underlying medical condition. Veterinary professionals are aware that decreased water and food intake are often part of the normal end-of-life process. However, caregivers may be under the impression that they just have not found the right food the pet will eat. This false assumption can be highly stressful to both the pet and the caregiver. Discourage force-feeding, which may lead to food aversion and is stressful to both the pet and caregiver. Instead, reframe realistic expectations of food intake and encourage coaxing and reassurance to both the pet and caregiver.

SUMMARY

Senior pets are increasingly becoming a sizable proportion of patients seen in primary care. Therefore, an iterative, proactive approach to making nutrition assessments and patient-specific recommendations to support optimal health and body condition contributes to their health spans. More frequent health and nutritional screens beginning when pets are middle aged improve disease surveillance and early detection, allowing medical and nutritional intervention.

DISCLOSURE

Funding sources: none.

Conflicts of interest: J.A. Churchill: none. L. Eirmann: Veterinary Communications Manager, Nestle Purina Petcare.

REFERENCES

1. AVMA pet ownership and demographics sourcebook, 2017-2018 Edition. Schamburg (IL): American Veterinary Medical Association; 2018.
2. Vogt AH, Rodan I, Brown M, et al. AAFP-AAHA: Feline life stage guidelines. J Am Anim Hosp Assoc 2010;46:70–85.
3. Creevy KE, Grady J, Little SE, et al. 2019 AAHA Canine Life Stage Guidelines. J Am Anim Hosp Assoc 2019;55:267–90.
4. Kealy RD. Factors influencing lean body mass in ageing dogs. Compend Contin Educ Pract Vet 1999;21:34–7.
5. Lawler DF, Larson BT, Ballam JM, et al. Diet restriction and ageing in the dog: major observations over two decades. Br J Nutr 2008;99:793–805.
6. Fahey GC Jr, Barry KA, Swanson KS. Age-related changes in nutrient utilization by companion animals. Annu Rev Nutr 2008;28:425–45.
7. Baldwin K, Bartges J, Buffington T, et al. AAHA nutritional assessment guidelines for dogs and cats. J Am Anim Hosp Assoc 2010;46:285–96.
8. Freeman L, Becvarova I, Cave N, et al. WSAVA nutritional assessment guidelines. J Small Anim Pract 2011;52:385–96.
9. Laflamme D. Development and validation of a body condition score system for dogs. Canine Pract 1997;22:10–5.
10. Laflamme D. Development and validation of a body condition score system for cats: a clinical tool. Feline Pract 1997;25:13–8.
11. German AJ, Holden SL, Moxham GL, et al. A simple, reliable tool for owners to assess the body condition of their dog or cat. J Nutr 2006;136:2031S–3S.
12. Witzel AL, Kirk CA, Henry GA, et al. Use of a novel morphometric method and body fat index system for estimation of body composition in overweight and obese dogs. J Am Vet Med Assoc 2014;244:1279–84.

13. Witzel A, Kirk C, Henry G, et al. Use of a morphometric method and body fat index system for estimation of body composition in overweight and obese cats. J Am Vet Med Assoc 2014;224:1285–90.
14. German AJ, Holden SL, Bissot T, et al. Use of starting condition score to estimate changes in body weight and composition during weight loss in obese dogs. Res Vet Sci 2009;87:249–54.
15. Bjornvad C, Nielsen D, Armstrong P, et al. Evaluation of a nine-point body condition scoring system in physically inactive. Am J Vet Res 2011;72:433–7.
16. Flanagan J, Bissot T, Hours MA, et al. Success of a weight loss plan for overweight dogs: The results of an international weight loss study. PLoS One 2017; 12:e0184199.
17. WSAVA Global Nutrition Committee Nutrition Toolkit. Available at: https://wsava.org/wp-content/uploads/2020/05/WSAVA-Global-Nutrition-Toolkit-English.pdf. Accessed July 15, 2020.
18. Laflamme DP. Companion animals symposium: obesity in dogs and cats: what is wrong with being fat? J Anim Sci 2012;90:1653–62.
19. Michel KE, Anderson W, Cupp C, et al. Correlation of a feline muscle mass score with body composition determined by dual-energy X-ray absorptiometry. Br J Nutr 2011;106(Suppl 1):S57–9.
20. Freeman LM, Michel KE, Zanghi BM, et al. Evaluation of the use of muscle condition score and ultrasonographic measurements for assessment of muscle mass in dogs. Am J Vet Res 2019;80:595–600.
21. Cupp C, Kerr WW. Effect of diet and body composition on life span in aging cats. Proceedings of the Nestle Purina Companion Animal Nutrition Summit: focus on gerontology. March 26–27, 2010. Clearwater Beach, FL.
22. Perez-Camargo G. Cat nutrition: What is new in the old? Compend Contin Educ Pract Vet 2004;(Suppl 26):5–10.
23. Koopman R, van Loon LJ. Aging, exercise, and muscle protein metabolism. J Appl Physiol 2009;106:2040–8.
24. Evans WJ. Skeletal muscle loss: cachexia, sarcopenia, and inactivity. Am J Clin Nutr 2010;91:1123s–7s.
25. Linder DE, Freeman LM, Morris P, et al. Theoretical evaluation of risk for nutritional deficiency with caloric restriction in dogs. Vet Q 2012;32:123–9.
26. Gaylord L, Remillard R, Saker K. Risk of nutritional deficiencies for dogs on a weight loss plan. J Small Anim Pract 2018;59(11):695–703.
27. Larsen JA, Farcas A. Nutrition of aging dogs. Vet Clin North Am Small Anim Pract 2014;44:741–59.
28. Swanson KS, Kuzmuk KN, Schook LB, et al. Diet affects nutrient digestibility, hematology, and serum chemistry of senior and weanling dogs. J Anim Sci 2004;82: 1713–24.
29. Laflamme D, Martineau B, Jones W, et al. Effect of age on maintenance energy requirements and apparent digestibility on canine diets. Comp Contin Educ Pract Vet 2000;22:113.
30. Speakman JR, van Acker A, Harper EJ. Age-related changes in the metabolism and body composition of three dog breeds and their relationship to life expectancy. Aging cell 2003;2:265–75.
31. Laflamme D, Ballum JM. Effect of age on maintenance energy requirements of adult cats. Compend Contin Educ Pract Vet 2002;24:82.
32. Cupp C, Perez-Camargo G, Patil A. Long-term food consumption and body weight changes in a controlled population of geriatric cats. Compend Contin Educ Pract Vet 2004;26:60.

33. Laflamme D, Gunn-Moore D. Nutrition of aging cats. Vet Clin North Am Small Anim Pract 2014;44:761–74, vi.
34. Kealy RD, Lawler DF, Ballam JM, et al. Effects of diet restriction on life span and age-related changes in dogs. J Am Vet Med Assoc 2002;220:1315–20.
35. Lorenzo I, Serra-Prat M, Yébenes JC. The role of water homeostasis in muscle function and frailty: a review. Nutrients 2019;11:1857.
36. Armstrong LE, Ganio MS, Casa DJ, et al. Mild dehydration affects mood in healthy young women. J Nutr 2012;142:382–8.
37. Ganio MS, Armstrong LE, Casa DJ, et al. Mild dehydration impairs cognitive performance and mood of men. Br J Nutr 2011;106:1535–43.
38. Benton D, Young HA. Do small differences in hydration status affect mood and mental performance? Nutr Rev 2015;73(Suppl 2):83–96.
39. Wannemacher RW Jr, McCoy JR. Determination of optimal dietary protein requirements of young and old dogs. J Nutr 1966;88:66–74.
40. Richardson A, Birchenall-Sparks MC. Age-related changes in protein synthesis. Rev Biol Res Aging 1983;1:255–73.
41. Churchill J, Polzin D, Osborne C. The influence of dietary protein, lipid, phosphorus and sodium on renal structure and function in geriatric dogs. PhD thesis. St Paul (MN): Department of Clinical Sciences: University of Minnesota, College of Veterinary Medicine; 2001.
42. McMurray DN. Effect of moderate protein deficiency on immune function. Compend Contin Educ Pract Vet 1999;21:21–4.
43. Wolfe RR. The underappreciated role of muscle in health and disease. Am J Clin Nutr 2006;84:475–82.
44. Laflamme DP. Nutrition for aging cats and dogs and the importance of body condition. Vet Clin North Am Small Anim Pract 2005;35:713–42.
45. Protein and Amino acids. Nutrient requirements of the dog and cat. National research Council. Washington, DC: The National Academies Press; 2006. p. 111–38.
46. Hewson-Hughes AK, Hewson-Hughes VL, Miller AT, et al. Geometric analysis of macronutrient selection in the adult domestic cat, Felis catus. J Exp Biol 2011; 214:1039–51.
47. Zoran DL, Buffington CA. Effects of nutrition choices and lifestyle changes on the well-being of cats, a carnivore that has moved indoors. J Am Vet Med Assoc 2011;239:596–606.
48. Laflamme DP, Hannah SS. Discrepancy between use of lean body mass or nitrogen balance to determine protein requirements for adult cats. J Feline Med Surg 2013;15:691–7.
49. Laflamme DP. Understanding the nutritional needs of healthy cats and those with diet-sensitive conditions. Vet Clin North Am Small Anim Pract 2020;50(5):905–24.
50. Laflamme DP, Abood SK, Fascetti AJ, et al. Pet feeding practices of dog and cat owners in the United States and Australia. J Am Vet Med Assoc 2008;232:687–94.
51. Hutchinson D, Freeman L, Schreiner M, et al. Survey of opinions about nutritional requirements of senior dogs and analysis of nutrient profiles of commercially available diets for senior dogs. Intern J Appl Res Vet Med 2011;9:68–79.
52. Association of animal feed control Officials 2020 Official Publication. Champaign, IL: Association of American Feed Control Officials; 2020.
53. Summers SC, Stockman J, Larsen JA, et al. Evaluation of nutrient content and caloric density in commercially available foods formulated for senior cats. J Vet Intern Med 2020;34:2029–35.

54. Gayet C, Leray V, Saito M, et al. The effects of obesity-associated insulin resistance on mRNA expression of peroxisome proliferator-activated receptor-gamma target genes, in dogs. Br J Nutr 2007;98:497–503.
55. Eirmann L, Freeman LM, Laflamme D. Comparison of adipokine concentration and markers of inflammation in obese versus lean dogs. Int J Appl Res Vet Med 2009;196–205.
56. German AJ, Hervera M, Hunter L, et al. Improvement in insulin resistance and reduction in plasma inflammatory adipokines after weight loss in obese dogs. Domest Anim Endocrinol 2009;37:214–26.
57. Teng KT, McGreevy PD, Toribio JL, et al. Strong associations of 9-point body condition scoring with survival and lifespan in cats. J Feline Med Surg 2018;20(12): 1110–8.
58. Armstrong PJ, Lund EM. Changes in body composition and energy balance with aging. Vet Clin Nutr 1996;3:83–7.
59. Courcier EA, Mellor D, Thomson RM, et al. A cross sectional study of the prevalence and risk factors for owner misperception of canine body shape in first opinion practice in Glasgow. Prev Vet Med 2011;102:66–74.
60. Freeman LM, Lachaud MP, Matthews S, et al. Evaluation of weight loss over time in cats with chronic kidney disease. J Vet Intern Med 2016;30:1661–6.
61. Baez JL, Michel KE, Sorenmo K, et al. A prospective investigation of the prevalence and prognostic significance of weight loss and changes in body condition in feline cancer patients. J Feline Med Surg 2007;9:411–7.
62. Corbee RJ, Barnier MM, van de Lest CH, et al. The effect of dietary long-chain omega-3 fatty acid supplementation on owner's perception of behaviour and locomotion in cats with naturally occurring osteoarthritis. J Anim Physiol Anim Nutr 2013;97(5):846–53.
63. Roush JK, McLaughlin R, Radlinsky M. Understanding the pathophysiology of osteoarthritis. Vet Med 2002;97:108–12.
64. Foye P, Stitik T, Chen B, et al. Osteoarthritis and body weight. Nutr Res 2000;20: 899–903.
65. Hua J, Hoummady S, Muller C, et al. Assessment of frailty in aged dogs. Am J Vet Res 2016;77:1357–65.
66. Impellizeri J, Tetrick M, Muir P. Effect of weight reduction on clinical signs of lameness in dogs with hip osteoarthritis. J Am Vet Med Assoc 2000;216:1089–91.
67. Bartges J, Budsberg S, Pazak H. Effects of different n6:n3 fatty acid ratio diets on canine stifle osteoarthritis. Orthopedic Research Society 47th Annual Meeting San Francisco, CA, February 25-28, 2001.
68. Roush JK, Dodd CE, Fritsch DA, et al. Multicenter veterinary practice assessment of the effects of omega-3 fatty acids on osteoarthritis in dogs. J Am Vet Med Assoc 2010;236:59–66.
69. Moreau M, Troncy E, Del Castillo JR, et al. Effects of feeding a high omega-3 fatty acids diet in dogs with naturally occurring osteoarthritis. J Anim Physiol Anim Nutr 2013;97(5):830–7.
70. Lascelles BD, DePuy V, Thomson A, et al. Evaluation of a therapeutic diet for feline degenerative joint disease. J Vet Intern Med 2010;24:487–95.
71. Sierra S, Lara-Villoslada F, Comalada M, et al. Dietary eicosapentaenoic acid and docosahexaenoic acid equally incorporate as decosahexaenoic acid but differ in inflammatory effects. Nutrition 2008;24:245–54.
72. Roush JK, Cross AR, Renberg WC, et al. Evaluation of the effects of dietary supplementation with fish oil omega-3 fatty acids on weight bearing in dogs with osteoarthritis. J Am Vet Med Assoc 2010;236:67–73.

73. Bauer J. Timely topics in nutrition: therapeutic use of fish oils in companion animals. J Am Vet Med Assoc 2011;293:1441–51.
74. Azkona G, García-Belenguer S, Chacón G, et al. Prevalence and risk factors of behavioural changes associated with age-related cognitive impairment in geriatric dogs. J Small Anim Pract 2009;50:87–91.
75. Pan Y, Landsberg G, Mougeot I, et al. Efficacy of a therapeutic diet on dogs with signs of cognitive dysfunction syndrome (CDS): A prospective double blinded placebo controlled clinical study. Front Nutr 2018;5:127.
76. Pop V, Head E, Hill MA, et al. Synergistic effects of long-term antioxidant diet and behavioral enrichment on beta-amyloid load and non-amyloidogenic processing in aged canines. J Neurosci 2010;30:9831–9.
77. Fahnestock M, Marchese M, Head E, et al. BDNF increases with behavioral enrichment and an antioxidant diet in the aged dog. Neurobiol Aging 2012;33:546–54.
78. Bishop G, Cooney K, Cox S, et al. 2016 AAHA/IAAHPC End-of-Life Care Guidelines. J Am Anim Hosp Assoc 2016;52:341–56.
79. Freeman LM. Beneficial effects of omega-3 fatty acids in cardiovascular disease. J Small Anim Pract 2010;10:462–70.

Canine and Feline Obesity Management

Megan Shepherd, DVM, PhD

KEYWORDS

- Overweight • Weight loss • Body weight • Body condition score (BCS) • Nutrition
- Communication • Prevention • Risk factors

KEY POINTS

- Be a guide for the pet parent; an authoritarian approach may not be successful; offer options when possible. Work with the pet parent to identify potential barriers to weight loss success (eg, financial resources, other pets in the household, and multiple people feeding the pet).
- Formulate an initial weight loss plan with an intent to restrict energy/calories.
- The recommended diet should meet all essential nutrient requirements (protein, vitamins, and minerals) when fed to restrict calorie intake. Be specific about diet options and how much per day.
- Treats must be accounted for; if fed, include treats in the pet's daily calorie goal, be specific about which treat(s) and how much per day.
- Monitor body weight every 2 weeks to 4 weeks to determine if the initial plan is working. If not and the plan was not implemented, find out why not. If not and the plan was implemented, restrict calories further.

INTRODUCTION/BACKGROUND

In 2018%, 60% of cats and 56% of dogs in the United States were reported by veterinarians as overweight or obese.[1] From 2008 to 2018, the reported incidence of overweight or obese rose 3% in cats and 12% in dogs.[2] Overweight and obese body conditions (herein referred to as overweight) reduce quality of life[3] and longevity.[4–7] Overweight increases the risk of some cancers,[8] insulin/glucose dysregulation (including diabetes mellitus in cats),[9–12] and joint/mobility issues.[13–15] Overweight pets are less active[16–18] and less social.[19] Additionally, overweight is associated with other comorbidities, such as urinary tract infection,[20] hypertriglyceridemia,[12] altered cardiorespiratory function,[21–23] and potentially liver dysfunction.[24] Pet obesity and related health disparities are monetary and emotional burdens for pet parents.[25,26] Furthermore, challenges to effective overweight management include

Department of Large Animal Clinical Sciences, Virginia-Maryland College of Veterinary Medicine, Phase II Duck Pond Drive, Virginia Tech Mail Code 0442, Blacksburg, VA 24061, USA
E-mail address: meshephe@vt.edu

Vet Clin Small Anim 51 (2021) 653–667
https://doi.org/10.1016/j.cvsm.2021.01.005 vetsmall.theclinics.com

awareness ("My pet is overweight?"), education ("So what if my pets overweight?"), emotions ("Food is how I show my pet I love them."), and behavior ("My pet begs for food.").[27] Therefore, prescribed weight loss plans should be instituted for the overweight pet to manage/reduce the risk of overweight comorbidities, preserve quality of life, and reduce pet parent distress. Exercise alone may not be adequate for successful weight loss.[28] Controlled exercise and physical rehabilitation, however, can greatly complement calorie restriction[29] and help preserve lean muscle.[30]

ASSESS THE PATIENT

Diagnosis of pet overweight is described elsewhere[18,31,32] and is performed most commonly using a subjective body condition score (BCS) system. The author uses a 9-point BCS system, along with a subjective assessment of muscle condition score (MCS).[33] Furthermore, the author estimates target body weight (BW)[34] assuming each BCS point (9-point scale) above ideal/target represents 10% of current overweight BW. For example, if a 9.1-kg (20-lb) pet has a BCS of 8/9 and the target BCS is 5/9, then the pet is 30% over target (or 130% of target); thus, target weight is estimated at 7 kg (15.4 lb) (9.1 kg/1.3 = 7 kg). Alternately, a practical online calculator[35] may be used to estimate target weight using a different approach. The focus of this article is on managing the overweight pet without a conflicting comorbidity. Effective weight loss, however, helps manage conditions secondary to or worsened by obesity.

ASSESSING THE CURRENT/PAST DIET

Evaluating a current diet and/or diet history can help refine the energy and nutrient goals for the prescribed weight loss plan. The author recognizes that evaluating a current/past diet is time-consuming, at least for pets with complicated or dynamic diets.[36] Therefore, as discussed later, the author provides general guidance on starting a weight loss plan in absence of a detailed analysis of the current diet. Regardless, diet history taking is a key point of a pet's medical record and especially important in managing nutrition-sensitive conditions like overweight. The style of nutrition inquiry (phrasing of question) influences the depth of information retrieved.[37,38] Furthermore, although effective history taking may add a little more time to an appointment, spending a little extra time up-front can save time in the long run.[39] Both a diet history form and a more detailed nutritional assessment checklist are available for use as part of the World Small Animal Veterinary Association Global Nutrition Guidelines (https://wsava.org/global-guidelines/global-nutrition-guidelines/).[33]

GETTING CLIENTS ON BOARD

Nutrition communication is key to successful implementation of a prescribed weight loss plan. Effective veterinarian–pet parent communication has a positive impact on pet health,[40–43] and pet parents report veterinarians to be the most trusted sources of nutrition information.[44] Pet parent compliance is positively associated with weight loss sucess.[28] The incidence of veterinarian–pet parent nutrition communication, however, appears to be low.[37,44] Furthermore, veterinary judgment and pet parent guilt can be barriers to effective communication and patient care. Therefore, veterinarians should avoid blaming the pet parent and use of fat-shaming terminology (eg, chunky or fat).[45]

Veterinarians should consider pet parent goals and serve as a guide, rather than an authoritarian, and provide options when possible.[37,46–48] Pet parent goals may be influenced by readily available so-called expert nutrition information online,[49–54] which may complicate nutrition communication. See Chapter 1 for more information on communicating with clients about nutrition issues.

Veterinarians should explore potential barriers to success that the pet parent is concerned about. Is there a person in the household who may be unable to adhere to the plan (eg, a person with dementia)? If so, adjust for it. For example, if there is a person who always shares a bit of food and that is unavoidable, then consider that food in total daily calories as a treat. Multipet households can be another barrier, especially for feline households. The overweight cat may be kept away from the lean cats' food by feeding the lean cat(s) in a space inaccessible to the overweight cat (eg, box or space with a small opening or high up). Note that as an overweight cat loses weight, size decreases and activity hopefully improves, so some strategies do not work in the long run. Several commercial feeders exist that allow only lean cat(s) to access food if their collar or microchip is programmed to the feeder. Furthermore, collar or microchip-based pet doors may be used to feed only the lean cat(s) in a room or closet.

FORMULATING A PLAN

Chronic positive energy imbalance is the primary risk factor for obesity; thus, prescribed weight loss plans need to include strategic energy restriction. The level of energy restriction needed varies by individual. For patients that are simply overfed, a strict weight loss plan may not be needed. For example, for the adult dog whose BCS has crept up to 6/9, but whose overall energy requirements are about average for adult maintenance, treats may be cut back and/or a lower-calorie over-the-counter food may be selected. This section focuses, however, on formulating a plan for patients in need of a strict weight loss plan.

Body condition negatively correlates with energy requirement.[55] Therefore, strict weight loss plans must promote negative energy balance to metabolize excess adipose/fat tissue. The author calculates the initial daily energy goal (kilocalories per day) as 100% of resting energy requirements (RERs) (70 kcal/kg$^{0.75}$) at target weight for dogs and 80% of RERs at target weight for cats (**Box 1**).[34] Some pets require severe energy restriction (eg, 50% of RERs) to achieve weight loss. The author suggests working with a veterinary nutritionist in such cases.

The recommended diet should meet all essential nutrient requirements (protein, fatty acids, vitamins, and minerals)[56] when fed to meet the prescribed restricted energy/calorie goal.[57] Meeting protein requirements (at least 3.28 g/kg$^{0.75}$ for the dog and 4.96 g/kg$^{0.67}$ for the cat)[57] is important in maintaining lean muscle mass, which has a positive influence on basal metabolic rate and promotes satiety. Furthermore, feeding a high-protein diet (exceeding protein requirements) may help preserve lean muscle during weight loss.[58] Although resting energy expenditure in dogs did not differ whether fed a high-fat/low-carbohydrate or low-fat/high-carbohydrate diet,[59] dietary fat should be limited,[10] because it is twice as energy dense compared with protein and nonfiber carbohydrates. Exceeding omega-3 fatty acid requirements (eicosapentaenoic acid and docosahexaenoic acid) may be helpful because obesity promotes a chronic state of inflammation, and it may be especially helpful if concurrent joint disease is present. Increasing insoluble fiber (eg, cellulose powder or soybean hulls), in addition to limiting fat, helps promote satiety. Calorie restriction leads to food volume reduction, which may cause or perpetuate food seeking behavior and thus cause pet parent stress. Cats seem skilled at disruptive food-seeking behavior (ie, waking the owner at night or destroying carpet). Therefore, promoting satiety or attempts to disrupt food-seeking behavior are important for effective implementation of a weight loss plan (**Box 2**). Carnitine is not considered an essential nutrient but may be

Box 1
Case example 1—successful and uncomplicated overweight management in a cat

An 8-year-old female, spayed, domestic shorthair cat enrolled in a weight loss study

Initial BW: 6.7 kg (14.8 lb)

Initial BCS: 8/9

Initial MCS: normal

History: unremarkable

Initial diet: commercial feline kibble

Target BCS: 5/9

Target BW: 5.2 kg (11.4 lb)

Prescribed daily calories: calculated target 192 kcal (RERi*0.8), with 100% met with a dry commercial veterinary weight loss diet; due to volume rounding, actual initial calories were 214 kcal (RERi*0.9)

Updates (number of months since initial work-up)

- 1 mo—6.6 kg (14.4 lb), no change
- 2 mo—6.6 kg (14.4 lb), reduce to 192 kcal
- 3 mo—6.4 kg (14.0 lb), reduce to 161 kcal
- 4 mo—6.3 kg (13.8 lb), reduced to 120 kcal (RERi*0.5)
- 5 mo—5.8 kg (12.8 lb), recommended 1/4-C chopped fresh zucchini to manage food-seeking behavior
- 6 mo—5.5 kg (12.1 lb), no change, does not like vegetables, food-seeking behavior subsided
- 7 mo—5.4 kg (11.8 lb), no change
- 8 mo—5.1 kg (11.3 lb), no change
- 9 mo—4.8 kg (10.6 lb), BCS 5/9, MCS normal, increased to 166 kcal to maintain
- 10 mo—4.6 kg (10.2 lb), BCS 5/9, MCS normal

beneficial during calorie restriction. Carnitine facilitates fat metabolism and may help preserve muscle mass during weight loss.[60]

UTILIZING COMMERCIAL PET FOOD

A large majority of pets are fed commercial pet food, especially dry/kibble.[49,61–63] Although dry food is a risk factor for obesity in young cats, living indoors and physical

Box 2
Managing food-seeking behavior

High-protein, high-fiber commercial diet or homemade recipe

Using food toys or puzzles to extend meal time and possibly increase activity

Feeding small frequent meals to reduce time between meals and spreading meals evenly throughout the day (eg, feeding right before bedtime to prevent being woke early by a hungry pet)

Using automatic feeders to disassociate the pet parent from the food and to deliver food during times when food-seeking behavior is most disruptive (eg, when the pet parent is sleeping or studying)

Feeding high-fiber foods fed between meals or to add bulk to a meal (eg, vegetables [see **Table 2**])

Responding to food-seeking behavior with a quality-time distraction: play, walk, groom, pet/rubs

inactivity pose a greater risk for feline obesity (discussed later).[64] Commercial diets not formulated for obesity management, including over-the-counter weight management/light varieties, typically are not nutrient fortified enough to be fed during a weight loss plan (**Table 1**). Commercial veterinary weight loss diets are lower in calories and more nutrient fortified on an energy basis (eg, grams of nutrient per 1000 kcal [Mcal]), which helps prevent nutrient deficiencies, prevent muscle loss, and improve fat metabolism during a prescribed weight loss plan.[56,58,65] These diet characteristics also help previously overweight pets maintain healthy weight post–weight loss.[56,58,65]

Lower pet parent income and increasing pet parent age are risk factors for canine obesity.[61] The cost of a veterinary weight loss diet may be a concern for some clients. Commercial dry food is more economical than commercial wet/canned food.[66,67] Furthermore, German and colleagues[68] reported that veterinary weight loss diets are cost-neutral, once all aspects of the diet (food and treats) are controlled for. However, the up-front cost of a veterinary weight loss diet may be offset by cost-savings in disease prevention (eg, prevent or reduced cost of managing joint disease or diabetes mellitus). Veterinarians, however, should help clients navigate options to find the most practical and nutritionally appropriate approach.

UTILIZING A HOMEMADE DIET

Properly formulated homemade diets may cost more than commercial dry diets but are more economical than commercial wet/canned food.[66,67] Furthermore, the cost of homemade diets may be minimized, depending on how ingredients are sourced (eg, purchasing in bulk). Pedrinelli and colleagues[55] reported that dogs fed a homemade recipe had a higher daily energy requirement and were less likely to be

Table 1
Macronutrient comparison of select commercial dog foods[a]

Diet Categories[b]	Veterinary/ Prescription Weight Loss Diets[c]	Over-the-Counter Weight Management/ Light Diets[d]	Over-the-Counter Adult Maintenance Dog Foods[e]
Crude protein (g/Mcal)	82–115	77–85	62–70
Crude fat (g/Mcal)	22–37	28–33	36–44
Crude fiber (g/Mcal)	36–65	6–38	3–5
Calcium (g/Mcal)	2.8–3.6	2.4–3.6	2.5–3.3
Phosphorus (g/Mcal)	2.2–2.8	1.8–2.8	1.9–2.4
Metabolizable energy (kcal/g as fed)	3.0–3.2	3.0–3.5	3.6–4.0
Metabolizable energy (kcal/cup[f])	214–291	271–274	340–387

[a] Products were selected from manufacturers that produced dry/extruded diets across all 3 diet categories.
[b] Nutrient concentrations are listed per megacalorie, as provided per manufacturer's typical analysis.
[c] Hill's Prescription Diet, Metabolic, Chicken Flavor; Purina ProPan Veterinary Diets OM Overweight Management; and Royal Canin Veterinary Diet Satiety Support.
[d] Hill's Science Diet Light, Adult 1-6, Chicken & Barley; Purina ProPlan Adult Weight Management; and Royal Canin Weight Control.
[e] Hill's Science Diet, Adult 1-6; Purina ProPlan Adult Complete Essentials Shredded Blend Chicken & Rice; and Royal Canin Adult Medium.
[f] 1 cup = 8 fl oz volume.

overweight compared with dogs fed commercial food. Furthermore, Wall and colleagues[63] reported that cats fed a homemade recipe had a lower risk of obesity. Not all studies have found homemade pet food superior to commercial pet food, however, in the context of overweight condition.[69] Homemade diets allow for accommodation of specific pet parent preferences,[49,50,62,70–72] such as specific diet or ingredient characteristics (eg, natural,[73,74] holistic, gourmet,[75] grain-free, or meat as first ingredient) or avoidance of commercial pet food,[76,77] while meeting the nutrient needs of the pet. For pets with extremely low energy needs (eg, 50% of RERs for estimated target weight), then a homemade diet may be ideal because it can be tailor-made to the individual pet. Whether a homemade diet is right for an overweight pet largely is dependent on owner factors, especially owner compliance.[78] Feeding a properly formulated homemade diet is a larger time commitment. Swapping out ingredients, without reformulation, likely renders a recipe incomplete or unbalanced. Furthermore, the author cautions against feeding a raw meat–based homemade or commercial diet due to risks to both the pets and humans.[79–82] The author encourages veterinarians and pet parents to work with a veterinary nutritionist in formulating a homemade diet because there are many published recipes that are not formulated properly, which can lead to serious health disparities.[83–85] Pets previously on a homemade diet may be transitioned to a commercial veterinary weight loss diet, although slow transition may be needed for pets with strong opinions about their food.

TREATS

Treats are fed commonly and should be accounted for.[86] Pet parents have a variety of ways of expressing love/care to their pet, such as play and petting; however, food commonly is used to show affection and in training.[87,88] Treats vary and may include commercial pet treats (biscuits and chews), table scraps, and other human food (eg, cheese).[86] Treats, when fed, should be limited to 10% of total daily calories because they contribute to daily calories and dilute the essential nutrients provided by a complete and balanced commercial dog food or homemade recipe. Examples of treats and calorie content are found in **Table 2**. Vegetables are a great treat option for the food-motivated pet, even cats, although cats likely need a low-calorie flavor enhancer.[89] The need for food for medication delivery should be considered, as needed, and factored into total daily calories. For example, the 10% of daily calories from treats goal may be divided into 5% for medication administration and 5% for treats.

FEEDING MANAGEMENT

Feeding management can make or break a weight loss plan. For example, feeding a commercial veterinary weight loss food to an obese pet ad libitum likely will not lead to success. When using a bowl or plate to offer food, consider the size, because the perception of a mostly empty bowl/plate may cause a pet parent stress. Small bowls and measuring scoops reduce the likelihood of a pet parent overfeeding.[90] Feeding frequency may have a positive influence on voluntary activity in cats.[91] Food-dispensing toys slow food consumption, reduce time between meals, and can encourage activity.[92,93] Reducing time between meals may reduce begging and improve owner-perceived quality of life.[94] Furthermore, food toys, as an environmental enrichment tool, can offset the higher risk of obesity in indoor cats.[64] Ensure the pet parent understands the purpose of the recommendations and monitoring plan.[37]

Table 2
Energy/calorie content of some treat options, excluding commercial pet treats

Options	kcal/unit[a,62]
Green beans: fresh/raw[b]	31 kcal/C, 1/2″ pieces
Green beans: canned, no sodium/salt added, drained	34 kcal/C; 153 g/C
Zucchini: fresh/raw[b]	21 kcal/C, chopped
Broccoli: fresh/raw[b]	31 kcal/C, chopped
Carrot: baby, fresh/raw[b]	4 kcal/medium; 10 g/medium
Carrot: fresh/raw[b]	52 kcal/C, chopped
Cauliflower: fresh/raw[b]	27 kcal/C, chopped
Lettuce: fresh/raw	10 kcal/C, shredded; 75 kcal/medium head; 6″ diameter
Apples: fresh/raw	65 kcal/C, chopped; 95 kcal/medium; 3″ diameter
Strawberries: fresh/raw	4 kcal/medium strawberry; 1–1.25″ diameter
Raspberries: fresh/raw	1 kcal/raspberry
Watermelon: fresh/raw and diced	46 kcal/C; 154 g/C
Mozzarella cheese	80 kcal/oz; 1 oz = 1/4 C, shredded
Cheddar cheese	110 kcal/oz; 1 oz = 1/4 C, shredded
Chicken breast: boneless and skinless, cooked	231 kcal/C
Egg: whole, cooked	60 kcal/large egg
Ground beef: 90% lean, cooked, juices retained	65 kcal/oz
Peanut butter: creamy	95 kcal/tbsp

[a] 1 C = 8 fl oz volume.
[b] Vegetables may be cooked, after measuring, without added ingredients (salt, sauce, and butter).

MONITORING

Monitoring is critical to determine if the initial plan is appropriate, regardless of how a weight loss plan is established.[35,95] BW should be assessed every 2 weeks to 4 weeks. Ideally, BCS and MCS also are re-evaluated every 2 weeks to 4 weeks and it is essential to monitor when a pet is close to achieving target BW. If a pet has achieved the estimated target weight but still has a BCS greater than 5/9, then weight loss should continue. Target weight loss is 1% to 2% per week for dogs and 0.5% to 2% per week for cats (see **Box 1**).[34] If losing too fast, add 20% calories (120% of original daily energy/calorie recommendation); the author rarely observes pets losing too fast on a prescribed weight loss plan. Rapid weight loss may be associated with lean tissue loss (eg, muscle), which may have a negative impact on long-term healthy weight maintenance. Even at a target weight loss rate, weight loss takes months and veterinarians can help pet parents stay motivated through regular rechecks.[89] If a pet is losing too slowly (<1% BW per week for dogs; <0.5% BW per week for cats) or weight loss has plateaued, check in with the pet parent. If a pet parent has implemented the prescribed weight loss plan, then reduce daily calories by 10% to 20% (80%–90% of original daily energy recommendation).

It is the author's observation that weight loss plans are effective when implemented, but there are challenges to implementation. If a pet parent has not been able to implement a prescribed weight loss plan, then explore what barriers have developed.

Barriers vary by household and may include disruptive food-seeking behavior (see **Box 2**), family/friends/neighbors not adhering to the weight loss plan, and/or continued access to another pet's food. See Case example 2 (**Box 3**), which highlights real-life barriers to implementation.

Once a pet has achieved a BCS of 5/9, calories may need to be increased (10%–20%) to cease further weight loss. The pet likely always will have lower-than-average energy requirements, even once the target BCS has been achieved. Therefore, weight loss is the initial goal and maintenance of healthy BCS is the secondary/long-term goal.

Box 3
Case example 2—unsuccessful and complicated overweight management in a dog

A 7-year-old male, neutered Labrador retriever referred to the nutrition service for overweight management

Initial BW: 55 kg (121 lb)

Initial BCS: 9/9

Initial MCS: moderate muscle loss

History: bilateral hindlimb lameness, prior weight loss attempts unsuccessful

Initial diet: 705 kcal to 795 kcal (RERi*0.7), with 551 kcal from a commercial canine veterinary weight loss diet and 154 kcal to 244 kcal from treats; the estimate may have represented a minimum because it did not include occasional fruit and vegetables.

Target BCS: 4/9 to 5/9

Target BW: 37 to 39 kg (81–86 lb)

Prescribed daily calories: 766 kcal (RERi*0.7), with 95% coming from a commercial veterinary weight loss diet with the highest nutrient fortification per calorie and 5% allowance for treats; RERi*0.7 was chosen to balance the need to restrict calories while preventing malnutrition while considering 2 aspects:

- Initial calorie intake was below the author's traditional approach (RERi*1.0 for dogs) and likely underestimated because occasional fruit and vegetables were not included.
- The pet parent preferred to feed a commercial diet and even commercial veterinary/prescription weight loss diets have a limit to how little can be fed without underfeeding essential nutrients. Therefore, the author elected to start relatively conservatively (vs reducing to 80%–90% of initial kilocalories).

Updates (number of weeks since initial work-up)

- 11 wk: 51 kg (113 lb), increased activity
- 13 wk: 51 kg (111 lb), increased activity
- 23 wk: 52 kg (115 lb), increased activity, neighbor giving extra treats
- 47 wk: 58 kg (128 lb), pet parent had knee surgery approximately 5 months ago, pet parent's sister gave patient too many treats, pet parent concerned about weight gain
- 58 wk: patient developed a dermatopathy recently, referring veterinarian changed patient to a different veterinary weight loss diet, patient not active in the summer heat, pet parent suspects weight has not changed

Complicating factors

- Low initial calorie intake; thus, a typical approach (RERi*1.0 for dogs) would be successful.
- Compliance: treats
- Environmental/management factors that influenced energy expenditure: pet parent surgery and summer heat
- Health change: diet change secondary to dermatopathy
- Infrequent and irregular recheck intervals prevent timely adjustments/interventions.

OBESITY PREVENTION

Obesity prevention should be a priority. It likely is easier to establish healthy habits early in the pet's life compared with disrupting habits that contribute to overweight/obesity. As discussed previously, chronic positive energy imbalance is the primary risk factor for obesity. Causes of energy imbalance are numerous[96] and include conditions that reduce energy expenditure and enhance energy intake.

Pet-related risk factors include rapid growth,[97] age,[63,87] neutering,[18,44,87,98,99] reduced activity,[17,18] orthopedic disease,[55] hypothyroidism,[96] polyphagia (ie, secondary to disease or glucocorticoids),[96] food motivation,[88] and possibly low carnitine status.[100] Activity generally declines with age in both dogs[93] and cats.[101] Cats 5 years to 11 years old and dogs 6 years to 19 years old are more likely to be overweight than puppies, kittens, and senior cats.[102,103] Neutered dogs have lower daily energy requirements.[55] Working/active dogs are less likely to be overweight.[69] Pedrinelli and colleagues[55] reported the daily energy requirement for dogs with orthopedic disease to be 60 kcal/kg metabolic BW, which is below the author's general energy goal for overweight dogs (100% of RER for ideal/target BW) and may be due to limited activity. As discussed previously, carnitine is not considered an essential nutrient; however, Söder and colleagues[100] reported low plasma carnitine in overweight client-owned Labrador Retrievers. There is a link between gut microbes and obesity; however, effective gut microbe–related interventions in pets are uncertain.[104]

Pet parent–related risk factors include attitudes about diet, physical activity,[18] and the role of food in the human-animal bond.[105] Parents of overweight pets are more likely to underscore their pet's BCS,[106] more likely to value extra food (treats and table scraps)[18,69] over extra playtime,[69] more likely to interpret attention-seeking behavior as food-seeking behavior,[69] less likely to be strict with food,[87,88] and less likely to consider obesity a disease.[18] Veterinarians should be discussing obesity prevention with pet parents from the first visit. Obesity prevention, through establishment of healthy habits, may be most effective before a pet becomes an adult.

SUMMARY

Obesity has a negative influence on pet and pet parent quality of life and should be addressed intentionally, without shaming the pet or parent. The recommended diet could be a commercial pet food or a properly formulated homemade recipe and may include treats. The commercial diet or recipe should meet all of a pet's essential nutrient requirements (ie, only restrict calories) and treats should be limited to 10% of daily calories. Empower pet parents with details and clarity (eg, exactly what to feed and how much and specific goals). Monitoring should be strategic; if a plan is not successful, figure out why and ensure the plan is sustainable for the parent. Obesity management is important, but obesity prevention also should be focused on. It is likely easier to prevent, versus disrupt, daily routines that promote obesity.

CLINICS CARE POINTS

- Pet parent(s) goals should be clarified and the weight loss plan should be tailored to meet those goals.
- Evaluating the current/past diet can help tailor a weight loss plan to an individual pet.
- Provide a detailed plan; empower pet parents with tangible details, including exactly which food or food options and exactly how much of each option, exactly which treats, and exactly how much of each option.

- Monitoring is critical to determine if the plan is working.
  - If not, is the pet parent compliant? If not, figure out how to adjust the plan such that the pet parent(s) can implement.
  - If not, and pet parent(s) are compliant, then further energy restriction is needed.
- Manage satiety or perception of hunger. Cats, in particular, can display disruptive food-seeking behavior, which can cause pet parent(s) stress.

DISCLOSURE

The author's institution has gift-in-kind agreements with the following commercial pet food companies: Hill's Pet Nutrition, Nestle' Purina Petcar, and Royal Canin.

REFERENCES

1. Anon. Association for Pet Obesity Prevention. 2018. Available at: https://petobesityprevention.org/2018. Accessed July 6, 2020.
2. Anon. 2007-2013. Association for Pet Obesity Prevention. Available at: https://petobesityprevention.org/2007-2013. Accessed July 6, 2020.
3. German AJ, Holden SL, Wiseman-Orr ML, et al. Quality of life is reduced in obese dogs but improves after successful weight loss. Vet J 2012;192:428–34.
4. Salt C, Morris PJ, Wilson D, et al. Association between life span and body condition in neutered client-owned dogs. J Vet Intern Med 2019;33:89–99.
5. Kealy RD, Lawler DF, Ballam JM, et al. Effects of diet restriction on life span and age-related changes in dogs. J Am Vet Med Assoc 2002;220:1315–20.
6. Lawler DF, Evans RH, Larson BT, et al. Influence of lifetime food restriction on causes, time, and predictors of death in dogs. J Am Vet Med Assoc 2005;226:225–31.
7. Penell JC, Morgan DM, Watson P, et al. Body weight at 10 years of age and change in body composition between 8 and 10 years of age were related to survival in a longitudinal study of 39 Labrador retriever dogs. Acta Vet Scand 2019;61:42.
8. Glickman LT, Schofer FS, McKee LJ, et al. Epidemiologic study of insecticide exposures, obesity, and risk of bladder cancer in household dogs. J Toxicol Environ Health 1989;28:407–14.
9. Brunetto MA, Sá FC, Nogueira SP, et al. The intravenous glucose tolerance and postprandial glucose tests may present different responses in the evaluation of obese dogs. Br J Nutr 2011;106(Suppl 1):S194–7.
10. Backus RC, Cave NJ, Keisler DH. Gonadectomy and high dietary fat but not high dietary carbohydrate induce gains in body weight and fat of domestic cats. Br J Nutr 2007;98:641–50.
11. Hoenig M. The Cat as a Model for Human Obesity and Diabetes. J Diabetes Sci Technol 2012;6:525–33.
12. Verkest KR, Fleeman LM, Morton JM, et al. Association of postprandial serum triglyceride concentration and serum canine pancreatic lipase immunoreactivity in overweight and obese dogs. J Vet Intern Med 2012;26:46–53.
13. Brady RB, Sidiropoulos AN, Bennett HJ, et al. Evaluation of gait-related variables in lean and obese dogs at a trot. Am J Vet Res 2013;74:757–62.
14. Marshall WG, Hazewinkel HAW, Mullen D, et al. The effect of weight loss on lameness in obese dogs with osteoarthritis. Vet Res Commun 2010;34:241–53.
15. Marshall W, Bockstahler B, Hulse D, et al. A review of osteoarthritis and obesity: current understanding of the relationship and benefit of obesity treatment and prevention in the dog. Vet Comp Orthop Traumatol 2009;22:339–45.

16. Morrison R, Penpraze V, Beber A, et al. Associations between obesity and physical activity in dogs: a preliminary investigation. J Small Anim Pract 2013;54:570–4.
17. Warren BS, Wakshlag JJ, Maley M, et al. Use of pedometers to measure the relationship of dog walking to body condition score in obese and non-obese dogs. Br J Nutr 2011;106(Suppl 1):S85–9.
18. Muñoz-Prieto A, Nielsen LR, Dąbrowski R, et al. European dog owner perceptions of obesity and factors associated with human and canine obesity. Sci Rep 2018;8:13353. Available at: https://www.ncbi.nlm.nih.gov/pmc/articles/PMC6127309/. Accessed July 6, 2020.
19. de Godoy MR, Shoveller AK. Overweight adult cats have significantly lower voluntary physical activity than adult lean cats. J Feline Med Surg 2017;19:1267–73.
20. Wynn SG, Witzel AL, Bartges JW, et al. Prevalence of asymptomatic urinary tract infections in morbidly obese dogs. PeerJ 2016;4:e1711.
21. Mosing M, German AJ, Holden SL, et al. Oxygenation and ventilation characteristics in obese sedated dogs before and after weight loss: a clinical trial. Vet J 2013;198:367–71.
22. Pereira-Neto GB, Brunetto MA, Oba PM, et al. Weight loss improves arterial blood gases and respiratory parameters in obese dogs. J Anim Physiol Anim Nutr 2018;102:1743–8.
23. Manens J, Ricci R, Damoiseaux C, et al. Effect of body weight loss on cardiopulmonary function assessed by 6-minute walk test and arterial blood gas analysis in obese dogs. J Vet Intern Med 2014;28:371–8.
24. Belotta AF, Teixeira CR, Padovani CR, et al. Sonographic evaluation of liver hemodynamic indices in overweight and obese dogs. J Vet Intern Med 2018;32:181–7.
25. German AJ. Canine obesity–weighing on the mind of the owner? J Small Anim Pract 2011;52:619–20.
26. Bomberg E, Birch L, Endenburg N, et al. The financial costs, behaviour and psychology of obesity: a one health analysis. J Comp Pathol 2017;156:310–25.
27. Brooks D, Churchill J, Fein K, et al. 2014 AAHA weight management guidelines for dogs and cats. J Am Anim Hosp Assoc 2014;50:1–11.
28. Porsani MYH, Teixeira FA, Amaral AR, et al. Factors associated with failure of dog's weight loss programmes. Veterinary Medicine and Science n/a. Available at: https://onlinelibrary.wiley.com/doi/abs/10.1002/vms3.229. Accessed July 6, 2020.
29. Vega, V, Shepherd, ML. Multidisciplinary management of a morbidly obese dog. J Anim Physiol Anim Nutr 2019;103:404.
30. Vitger AD, Stallknecht BM, Nielsen DH, et al. Integration of a physical training program in a weight loss plan for overweight pet dogs. J Am Vet Med Assoc 2016;248:174–82.
31. Chandler M, Cunningham S, Lund EM, et al. Obesity and Associated Comorbidities in People and Companion Animals: A One Health Perspective. J Comp Pathol 2017;156:296–309.
32. Bjørnvad CR, Nielsen ME, Hansen SEM, et al. The effect of position on the precision of dual-energy X-ray absorptiometry and correlation with body condition score in dogs and cats. J Nutr Sci 2017;6:e20.
33. Anon. Global Nutrition Guidelines | WSAVA Global Veterinary Community. Available at: https://www.wsava.org/Guidelines/Global-Nutrition-Guidelines. Accessed January 13, 2020.

34. Flanagan J, Bissot T, Hours M-A, et al. Success of a weight loss plan for overweight dogs: The results of an international weight loss study. PLoS One 2017;12:e0184199.
35. Anon. PNA: Nutritional Calculators. Available at: https://www.petnutritionalliance.org/. Accessed July 6, 2020.
36. Wilson SA, Villaverde C, Fascetti AJ, et al. Evaluation of the nutritional adequacy of recipes for home-prepared maintenance diets for cats. J Am Vet Med Assoc 2019;254:1172–9.
37. MacMartin C, Wheat HC, Coe JB, et al. Conversation analysis of veterinarians' proposals for long-term dietary change in companion animal practice in Ontario, Canada. J Vet Med Educ 2018;45(4):514–33.
38. MacMartin C, Wheat HC, Coe JB, et al. Effect of question design on dietary information solicited during veterinarian-client interactions in companion animal practice in Ontario, Canada. J Am Vet Med Assoc 2015;246:1203–14.
39. Coe JB, O'Connor RE, MacMartin C, et al. Effects of three diet history questions on the amount of information gained from a sample of pet owners in Ontario, Canada. J Am Vet Med Assoc 2020;256:469–78.
40. Phillips AM, Coe JB, Rock MJ, et al. Feline obesity in veterinary medicine: insights from a thematic analysis of communication in practice. Front Vet Sci 2017;4:117.
41. Vandendriessche VL, Picavet P, Hesta M. First detailed nutritional survey in a referral companion animal population. J Anim Physiol Anim Nutr (Berl) 2017; 101(Suppl 1):4–14.
42. Shaw JR. Evaluation of communication skills training programs at North American veterinary medical training institutions. J Am Vet Med Assoc 2019;255:722–33.
43. Churchill J, Ward E. Communicating with pet owners about obesity: roles of the veterinary health care team. Vet Clin North Am Small Anim Pract 2016;46: 899–911.
44. Sapowicz SA, Linder DE, Freeman LM. Body condition scores and evaluation of feeding habits of dogs and cats at a low cost veterinary clinic and a general practice. ScientificWorldJournal 2016;2016:1901679.
45. Pearl RL. Effects of Dog and Owner Body Weight on Veterinarian Perceptions. J Anim Physiol Anim Nutr 2020;104:1587.
46. Jessica Vogelsang. The irresistible magic of story. In: Hill's Global Symposium Proceedings. Toronto, Canada, 2019.
47. Cornell KK, Kopcha M. Client-veterinarian communication: skills for client centered dialogue and shared decision making. Vet Clin North Am Small Anim Pract 2007;37:37–47.
48. Abood SK. Increasing adherence in practice: making your clients partners in care. Vet Clin North Am Small Anim Pract 2007;37:151–64.
49. Laflamme DP, Abood SK, Fascetti AJ, et al. Pet feeding practices of dog and cat owners in the United States and Australia. J Am Vet Med Assoc 2008;232: 687–94.
50. Michel KE, Willoughby KN, Abood SK, et al. Attitudes of pet owners toward pet foods and feeding management of cats and dogs. J Am Vet Med Assoc 2008; 233:1699–703.
51. DACVN RLRPD. Out-of-the-blue diet and nutrition queries: Pick your battles carefully. *dvm360.com*. Available at: http://veterinarymedicine.dvm360.com/out-blue-diet-and-nutrition-queries-pick-your-battles-carefully. Accessed May 29, 2019.

52. staff dvm360 com. Client handout: Forget the packaging, read the ingredient list. *dvm360.com.* Available at: http://veterinaryteam.dvm360.com/forget-packaging-read-ingredient-list. Accessed May 29, 2019.
53. Scheidegger J. Get pet food savvy and bring the pet food conversation back to the veterinary clinic. *dvm360.com.* Available at: http://veterinaryteam.dvm360.com/get-pet-food-savvy-and-bring-pet-food-conversation-back-veterinary-clinic. Accessed May 29, 2019.
54. Anon. Dog Food Reviews and Ratings. Dog Food Advisor. Available at: https://www.dogfoodadvisor.com/. Accessed May 29, 2019.
55. Pedrinelli V, Porsani MYH, Lima DM, et al. Predictive equations of maintenance energy requirement for healthy and chronically ill adult dogs. J Anim Physiol Anim Nutr (Berl) 2019. https://doi.org/10.1111/jpn.13184.
56. Linder DE, Freeman LM, Morris P, et al. Theoretical evaluation of risk for nutritional deficiency with caloric restriction in dogs. Vet Q 2012;32:123–9.
57. NRC. Nutrient requirements of dogs and cats. Washington, DC: The National Academies Press; 2006.
58. Floerchinger AM, Jackson MI, Jewell DE, et al. Effect of feeding a weight loss food beyond a caloric restriction period on body composition and resistance to weight gain in cats. J Am Vet Med Assoc 2015;247:365–74.
59. Yoo S, Ramsey JJ, Havel PJ, et al. Resting energy expenditure and body composition of Labrador Retrievers fed high fat and low fat diets. J Anim Physiol Anim Nutr (Berl) 2006;90:185–91.
60. Gooding MA, Minikhiem DL, Shoveller AK. Cats in positive energy balance have lower rates of adipose gain when fed diets containing 188 versus 121 ppm L-Carnitine. ScientificWorldJournal 2016;2016:2649093.
61. Courcier EA, Thomson RM, Mellor DJ, et al. An epidemiological study of environmental factors associated with canine obesity. J Small Anim Pract 2010;51:362–7.
62. Zejmis, S, Werre, SR, Hosig, K, et al. Survey of Food and Treat Choices of US Dog Owners. J Anim Physiol Anim Nutr 2019;103:404–5.
63. Wall M, Cave NJ, Vallee E. Owner and cat-related risk factors for feline overweight or obesity. Front Vet Sci 2019;6:266.
64. Slingerland LI, Fazilova VV, Plantinga EA, et al. Indoor confinement and physical inactivity rather than the proportion of dry food are risk factors in the development of feline type 2 diabetes mellitus. Vet J 2009;179:247–53.
65. German AJ, Holden SL, Serisier S, et al. Assessing the adequacy of essential nutrient intake in obese dogs undergoing energy restriction for weight loss: a cohort study. BMC Vet Res 2015;11:253.
66. Casna, B, Delaney, SJ, Shepherd ML. Cost Comparison of Homemade Versus Commercial Adult Maintenance Canine Diets. J Anim Physiol Anim Nutr 2017;101:1071–2.
67. Jung, H, Delaney, SJ, Shepherd, ML. Cost Comparison of Homemade versus Commercial Weight Loss Canine Diets. J Anim Physiol Anim Nutr 2020;104:1594.
68. German AJ, Luxmore J, Holden SL, et al. Feeding obese dogs during weight loss is on average cost-neutral. J Small Anim Pract 2015;56:366–9.
69. Kienzle E, Bergler R, Mandernach A. A comparison of the feeding behavior and the human-animal relationship in owners of normal and obese dogs. J Nutr 1998;128:2779S–82S.
70. Donfrancesco BD, Koppel K, Swaney-Stueve M, et al. Consumer acceptance of dry dog food variations. Animals (Basel) 2014;4:313–30.

71. Boya UO, Dotson MJ, Hyatt EM. A comparison of dog food choice criteria across dog owner segments: an exploratory study. Int J Consum Stud 2015; 39:74–82.
72. Conway DMP, Saker KE. Consumer attitude toward the environmental sustainability of grain-free pet foods. Front Vet Sci 2018;5:170.
73. Carter RA, Bauer JE, Kersey JH, et al. Awareness and evaluation of natural pet food products in the United States. J Am Vet Med Assoc 2014;245:1241–8.
74. Buff PR, Carter RA, Bauer JE, et al. Natural pet food: a review of natural diets and their impact on canine and feline physiology. J Anim Sci 2014;92:3781–91.
75. Elizabeth Sloan A. People and pets go more gourmet. Food Technol 2014;68: 24–35.
76. Lp W. Focus on Nutrition: Home-prepared Diets for Dogs and Cats. Compendium (Yardley, PA) 2013;35. Available at: http://pubmed.ncbi.nlm.nih.gov/23532921/. Accessed July 11, 2020.
77. Parr JM, Remillard RL. Handling alternative dietary requests from pet owners. Vet Clin North Am Small Anim Pract 2014;44:667–88, v.
78. Oliveira MCC, Brunetto MA, da Silva FL, et al. Evaluation of the owner's perception in the use of homemade diets for the nutritional management of dogs. J Nutr Sci 2014;3:e23.
79. Nemser SM, Doran T, Grabenstein M, et al. Investigation of Listeria, Salmonella, and toxigenic Escherichia coli in various pet foods. Foodborne Pathog Dis 2014; 11:706–9.
80. Finley R, Ribble C, Aramini J, et al. The risk of salmonellae shedding by dogs fed Salmonella-contaminated commercial raw food diets. Can Vet J 2007;48: 69–75.
81. O'Halloran C, Ioannidi O, Reed N, et al. Tuberculosis due to Mycobacterium bovis in pet cats associated with feeding a commercial raw food diet. J Feline Med Surg 2019;21(8):667–81.
82. CollegeGuelph OV. Guelph “legalName”:"University of, College" “name”:"Ontario Veterinary, et al. E. coli O157 Outbreak From Raw Pet Food: Canada. Worms & Germs Blog 2020. Available at: https://www.wormsandgermsblog.com/2020/06/articles/animals/dogs/e-coli-o157-outbreak-from-raw-pet-food-canada/. Accessed July 11, 2020.
83. Hutchinson D, Freeman LM, McCarthy R, et al. Seizures and severe nutrient deficiencies in a puppy fed a homemade diet. J Am Vet Med Assoc 2012;241: 477–83.
84. A L, E TB, S K, et al. Remarkable Frequency of a History of Liver Disease in Dogs Fed Homemade Diets With Buckwheat. Tierarztliche Praxis Ausgabe K, Kleintiere/Heimtiere 2019;47. Available at: http://pubmed.ncbi.nlm.nih.gov/31434124/. Accessed July 11, 2020.
85. Pedrinelli V, Mos G, Carciofi AC. Analysis of Recipes of Home-Prepared Diets for Dogs and Cats Published in Portuguese. J Nutr Sci 2017;6. Available at: http://pubmed.ncbi.nlm.nih.gov/29152237/. Accessed July 11, 2020.
86. White GA, Ward L, Pink C, et al. “Who's been a good dog?” - Owner perceptions and motivations for treat giving. Prev Vet Med 2016;132:14–9.
87. Russell K, Sabin R, Holt S, et al. Influence of feeding regimen on body condition in the cat. J Small Anim Pract 2000;41:12–7.
88. Raffan E, Smith SP, O'Rahilly S, et al. Development, factor structure and application of the Dog Obesity Risk and Appetite (DORA) questionnaire. PeerJ 2015;3:e1278.

89. Dodd L, Shepherd M, Werre S. Effect of personalized weight loss plans on weight loss in cats. J Anim Physiol Anim Nutr 2019;103:400.
90. Murphy M, Lusby AL, Bartges JW, et al. Size of food bowl and scoop affects amount of food owners feed their dogs. J Anim Physiol Anim Nutr (Berl) 2012; 96:237–41.
91. de Godoy MRC, Ochi K, de Oliveira Mateus LF, et al. Feeding frequency, but not dietary water content, affects voluntary physical activity in young lean adult female cats. J Anim Sci 2015;93:2597–601.
92. Herron ME, Buffington CAT. Environmental enrichment for indoor cats: implementing enrichment. Compend Contin Educ Vet 2012;34:E3.
93. Su DK, Murphy M, Hand A, et al. Impact of feeding method on overall activity of indoor, client-owned dogs. J Small Anim Pract 2019;60:438–43.
94. Robertson ID. The influence of diet and other factors on owner-perceived obesity in privately owned cats from metropolitan Perth, Western Australia. Prev Vet Med 1999;40:75–85.
95. Schmalberg J. Treatment of obesity in cats and dogs. Todays Vet Pract 2013;60–5.
96. German AJ. Obesity prevention and weight maintenance after loss. Vet Clin North Am Small Anim Pract 2016;46:913–29.
97. Serisier S, Feugier A, Venet C, et al. Faster growth rate in ad libitum-fed cats: a risk factor predicting the likelihood of becoming overweight during adulthood. J Nutr Sci 2013;2:e11.
98. Simpson M, Albright S, Wolfe B, et al. Age at gonadectomy and risk of overweight/obesity and orthopedic injury in a cohort of Golden Retrievers. PLoS One 2019;14:e0209131.
99. Lefebvre SL, Yang M, Wang M, et al. Effect of age at gonadectomy on the probability of dogs becoming overweight. J Am Vet Med Assoc 2013;243:236–43.
100. Söder J, Wernersson S, Dicksved J, et al. Indication of metabolic inflexibility to food intake in spontaneously overweight Labrador Retriever dogs. BMC Vet Res 2019;15:96. Available at: https://www.ncbi.nlm.nih.gov/pmc/articles/PMC6425671/. Accessed July 6, 2020.
101. Naik R, Witzel A, Albright JD, et al. Pilot study evaluating the effect of feeding method on overall activity of neutered indoor pet cats. J Vet Behav 2018;25:9–13.
102. Lund E, Armstrong P, Kirk C, et al. Prevalence and risk factors for obesity in adult dogs from private US veterinary practices. Intern J Appl Res Vet Med 2006;4:177–86.
103. Lund EM, Armstrong PJ, Kirk CA, et al. Prevalence and risk factors for obesity in adult cats from private US veterinary practices. Intern J Appl Res Vet Med 2005; 3(2):88–96.
104. Rollins AW, Shepherd M. Pathophysiology of obesity: Metabolic effects and inflammation mediators. In: Obesity in the Dog and Cat. First edition. Taylor & Francis; 2009. Available at: https://www.taylorfrancis.com/chapters/pathophysiology-obesity-metabolic-effects-inflammation-mediators-angela-witzel-rollins-megan-shepherd/e/10.1201/9781315151625-2.
105. Luño I, Palacio J, García-Belenguer S, et al. Emotional eating in companion dogs: Owners' perception and relation with feeding habits, eating behavior, and emotional state. J Vet Behav 2018;25:17–23.
106. Eastland-Jones RC, German AJ, Holden SL, et al. Owner misperception of canine body condition persists despite use of a body condition score chart. J Nutr Sci 2014;3:e45. Available at: https://www.ncbi.nlm.nih.gov/pmc/articles/PMC4473163/. Accessed July 6, 2020.

Nutritional Management for Dogs and Cats with Gastrointestinal Diseases

Catherine E. Lenox, DVM

KEYWORDS

• Gastrointestinal disease • Nutrition • Canine nutrition • Feline nutrition
• Nutritional management • GI nutrition

KEY POINTS

- Diet selection and a dog's or cat's feeding plan should be based on the patient's nutritional assessment and problem list.
- Nutrients of concern that are important when selecting a diet for a dog or cat with gastrointestinal (GI) disease include digestibility, energy, protein, fat, fiber, and cobalamin.
- Nutritional supplements may benefit certain patients with GI disease, but the supplement's quality control and the evidence of its efficacy should be investigated prior to use.
- Patients with GI disease should be treated as individuals, because not all dietary strategies work for all patients with similar disease processes.

INTRODUCTION

The gastrointestinal (GI) tract includes the oral cavity, esophagus, stomach, small intestine, and large intestine in addition to ancillary organs, such as the pancreas and liver. GI disease is a broad term, encompassing disorders anywhere in the GI tract. Although an individual canine or feline patient may have any of a variety of GI conditions that have an impact on 1 or more organs, patients with GI diseases often present with similar clinical signs, such as vomiting, diarrhea, constipation, dysrexia, and abdominal pain. Although some clinical signs are more indicative of disease in a particular location, such as regurgitation with esophageal disease, the similarities in clinical signs among many GI diseases mean that these diseases can be difficult to diagnose and medically manage and be challenging to manage with nutrition.

Nutritional modification is integral in the management of GI diseases, both in prevention of recurrence and in reduction of clinical signs. For example, dogs with chronic pancreatitis can benefit from being on a highly digestible and lower-fat diet long term, helping to prevent recurrence even when there may be predisposing factors, such as hyperlipidemia.[1] For dogs and cats with acute gastroenteritis, nutritional management

Royal Canin USA, 500 Fountain Lakes Boulevard, Suite 100, St Charles, MO 63301, USA
E-mail address: Catherine.Lenox@royalcanin.com

Vet Clin Small Anim 51 (2021) 669–684
https://doi.org/10.1016/j.cvsm.2021.01.006 vetsmall.theclinics.com

can help manage clinical signs, such as vomiting, by reducing meal volume with small, frequent meals.[2] There is no single diet or nutritional approach, however, that meets the needs of every patient with GI signs.

In order to select a nutritional plan for a dog or cat with GI disease, the patient's nutritional assessment (**Table 1**),[3,4] clinical signs, history and physical examination findings, laboratory findings, imaging, medication history, and other factors must be considered. Once a patient is evaluated from both nutritional and medical perspectives, the general nutritional case approach (**Box 1**) can be followed to select an appropriate diet and feeding plan for the dog or cat. This includes making a problem list, selecting nutrients of concern for the individual patient, and using that information in addition to the nutritional assessment to choose a diet and make feeding recommendations. Because there are a variety of nutritional options for GI disease, it is important to follow this process for all patients to create an individualized approach for dogs and cats with GI disease.

This review focuses on factors to consider when making a nutritional plan for a dog or cat with GI disease. This includes the nutrients of concern, nutritional approaches for common GI diseases, feeding management strategies, dietary options, dietary supplements, and diet selection for a small animal patient with GI disease.

NUTRIENTS OF CONCERN FOR GASTROINTESTINAL DISEASE IN DOGS AND CATS

After a problem list is made, there are a variety of different nutrients to consider when selecting a diet for GI disease in dogs and cats. These nutrients, which should be increased or decreased relative to the current diet, are called nutrients of concern or key nutritional factors. For many nutrients, there also is a target maximum level or minimum level to strive for when selecting a diet.

Nutrients and other factors to consider for patients with GI disease include digestibility, energy, protein, fat, fiber, and cobalamin. Not every nutrient of concern for GI disease is relevant for every patient. For example, cobalamin is not a nutrient of concern for a dog or cat with a single episode of acute gastroenteritis due to dietary indiscretion, but it is a key nutrient to consider for patients with chronic enteropathy. The nutrients of concern vary depending on the patient's clinical status, the nutritional assessment, the clinical signs present, the nature of the GI disease, and the chronicity of disease.

Digestibility

Although digestibility is a diet characteristic and not an actual nutrient, it is an important consideration in the selection of a diet for patients with GI disease. Digestibility

Table 1
Components of a nutritional assessment[3,4]

Patient assessment	Body weight BCS Muscle condition score Physical examination Laboratory and other diagnostic findings
Diet assessment	Complete diet history (including treats and supplements), including any recent changes in diet Dietary evaluation
Feeding management assessment	Feeding methods and feeding management Environmental factors that could contribute to nutritional needs

Box 1
General approach to nutrition cases

1. Assess the patient, including BCS and muscle condition score.
2. Assess the current diet and feeding management plan.
3. Assess the patient for signs of disease.
4. Make a problem list.
5. Identify aspects of disease to modify through dietary change.
6. Identify goals for nutritional modification
7. Identify nutrients of concern for the patient.
8. Identify goals for feeding management.
9. Select a diet and feeding plan for the patient.
10. Reassess the patient and make modifications as necessary.

refers to the ability of a diet to be digested by an animal, which has an impact on nutrient absorption in the GI tract and ultimately nutrient utilization. Digestibility is impacted by mechanical, enzymatic, chemical, and bacterial breakdown of the diet.[5] Digestibility considerations can be applied to the diet as a whole or to individual nutrients in the diet, such as the dietary protein.

The goal for patients with GI disease is to provide a highly digestible diet, except in cases of fiber-responsive disease. Overall digestibility and fecal quality have been better when dogs were fed highly digestible proteins compared with proteins with lower digestibility.[6] Fat and carbohydrate digestibility, however, also are important for the digestibility of the diet as a whole. Many patients with GI disease have difficulty digesting and tolerating dietary fat, such as those with exocrine pancreatic insufficiency. Varying the starch or soluble carbohydrate sources also can have a significant impact on diet digestibility,[7,8] although processing of raw materials also can have a major impact. Finally, the overall diet digestibility is impacted by the amount and type of dietary fiber,[9] which vary for GI patients depending on the condition managed and the chosen diet. Because digestibility is not listed on pet food labels, veterinarians may need to contact a manufacturer to ask about the digestibility of a given diet.

The ability of animals with GI disease to digest food and absorb dietary nutrients can be compromised, so a more digestible diet is used to compensate for this. All animals with GI disease can benefit from a highly digestible diet, unless the dog's or cat's condition is fiber-responsive. When a higher-fiber diet is needed, special attention should be paid to the digestibility of the ingredients providing dietary protein, fat, and soluble carbohydrate to ensure that these nutrients are easy to digest and absorb. Higher-fiber diets are lower in total digestibility, but it still is important to have highly digestible proteins, fats, and soluble carbohydrates.

Energy

Providing adequate energy allows an animal to continue normal physiologic processes while ill.[10] Energy requirements may vary depending on many factors, including age, spay/neuter status, life stage, breed, illness, activity level, and other factors.[11] For most patients, the goal when providing energy and estimating or calculating energy requirements is to achieve and maintain ideal body condition. In sick patients with GI or other diseases, however, this may not be a primary goal. Daily energy intake for hospitalized patients should be calculated as resting energy requirement (RER) × 1.0 (with RER = 70 × [current body weight in kg]$^{0.75}$) for most patients, and daily energy intake should be increased gradually up to this amount in malnourished patients.[10] For patients that are discharged, the energy intake typically is increased to maintenance energy requirements (MERs) (also called daily energy requirement), which are calculated as RER × the appropriate factor based on life stage and activity. This calculation can be performed using current or ideal weight, depending on the patient. Animals with decreased digestive capacity may need more energy than the average animal. For patients that are underweight at discharge, or for patients with compromised digestion, a starting point for calorie intake can be obtained by calculating RER for ideal weight and then multiplying by 1.4 to 1.6 (adult dogs) or 1.2 to 1.4 (adult cats) to calculate MER for weight gain. These MER factors are derived from the factors used to maintain weight in adult dogs and cats,[12,13] so it is important to calculate ideal weight and use ideal weight in the RER and MER calculations to allow for weight gain. One method to calculate estimated ideal weight for underweight patients is to divide current body weight by the percent of ideal weight the patient currently is at, which is based on body condition score (BCS). For BCS 4/9, divide by 90% (0.9); for BCS 3/9, divide by 80% (0.8); for BCS 2/9, divide by 70% (0.7); and for BCS 1/9, divide by 60% (0.6).

In addition to the amount of energy provided to the patient, the energy density of the chosen diet should be considered. Many patients with GI disorders have dysrexia, and using a more energy-dense diet can help reduce meal volume. If fat restriction is desired, however, it is more difficult to feed a high energy density to the patient, because protein and carbohydrates are lower in energy density than dietary fat.[11]

Protein

Both the amount of protein and the type of dietary protein should be considered when selecting a GI diet. Unless there are concurrent diseases, the amount of dietary protein most profoundly has an impact on patients with pancreatitis. High levels of dietary protein and/or fat can stimulate pancreatic secretions. In both cats and dogs, diet can increase pancreatic secretions due to stimulation of cholecystokinin and other GI hormones by luminal nutrients, such as long-chain fatty acids, amino acids, peptides, and protein.[14–17]

The type of protein in the diet also can have an impact on GI health. All patients with GI disease benefit from highly digestible protein sources. In patients with chronic enteropathy or adverse food reactions, however, the source of dietary protein is extremely important in the management of clinical signs. Options for patients needing a specific protein type to manage chronic enteropathy and/or adverse food reactions include hydrolyzed proteins or novel proteins.[5] Hydrolyzed proteins are broken down enzymatically with the intent of decreasing stimulation of the immune system.[18] Novel proteins are proteins to which the patient never has been exposed, and selection is based on a comprehensive diet history.[5]

Increasing dietary protein can be beneficial for palatability reasons or for helping replenish the dog's or cat's body's protein supplies after or during GI protein malabsorption or loss. This could occur with maldigestion and protein-losing enteropathies. Decreasing dietary protein relative to the current diet is not necessary for patients with GI disease unless they have concurrent conditions, such as hepatic encephalopathy.

Fat

The level of fat in a GI patient's diet is important for previously mentioned reasons, including the stimulation of pancreatic secretions in both dogs and cats and the impact of dietary fat on the energy density of a diet. Increasing dietary fat can help patients gain weight and can allow for small meal volumes in dysrexic patients. Dietary fat typically is not difficult to digest unless the fat digestion process is impaired.[5] When fat malabsorption occurs, there can be steatorrhea and/or significant weight loss. Dogs with pancreatitis or protein-losing enteropathies, such as lymphangiectasia, however, can benefit from fat restriction.[2] Dogs with pancreatitis benefit from fat restriction because this helps minimize hyperlipidemia and because high dietary fat can stimulate the onset of pancreatitis as well as pancreatic secretions,[19] whereas dogs with lymphangiectasia benefit from fat restriction because it helps reduce lacteal dilation and lymphatic flow.[20] Cats with GI disease seem to have more tolerance of dietary fat compared with dogs,[21] and fat restriction should not be a focus for the majority of cats with GI disease.

Fish oil omega-3 fatty acids, eicosapentaenoic acid (EPA) and docosahexaenoic acid (DHA), may be beneficial for patients with GI disease. EPA and DHA are long-chain polyunsaturated fatty acids with beneficial therapeutic effects demonstrated in patients with skin disease, renal disease, and other inflammatory and noninflammatory conditions.[22] EPA and DHA are thought to have anti-inflammatory effects.[23] Up to this point, no clinical trial has been done using EPA and DHA in canine or feline patients with intestinal inflammation or other GI diseases, but the anti-inflammatory nature of EPA and DHA suggests that patients with inflammatory GI diseases, such as inflammatory bowel disease may benefit from fish oil supplementation.[22,24,25]

Although some patients benefit from fat restriction, others can benefit from increased dietary fat. In dogs with GI disease, but without pancreatitis or lymphangiectasia, or if the patient is a cat, increasing dietary fat can be beneficial for patients that cannot tolerate large meal sizes, underweight patients, or dysrexic patients.

Fiber

Moderate amounts of fiber can be used for multiple GI conditions and to improve GI health, including to manage constipation and to potentially alter the microbiome.[26] Excessive amounts of fiber, however, are not beneficial for patients with GI disease. Increasing dietary fiber can reduce both the energy density and overall digestibility of the diet.[27] In patients with impaired digestive capacity, poor appetites, or low BCSs, high levels of dietary fiber may be contraindicated. In addition, the type of dietary fiber, not just the total amount of fiber, can have an impact on the digestibility of the diet.[28]

All fibers are classified as nondigestible carbohydrates and can be classified further as fermentable or nonfermentable and as soluble or insoluble. Fermentability refers to the ability of the fiber to be fermented by microbes in the colon of the dog and cat. Fermentation results in short-chain fatty acid production, which can benefit the host.[29] Solubility is a measure of the ability of the fiber to dissolve in water. In general, soluble fibers tend to be more fermentable than insoluble fibers.[29] Soluble fibers, such as pectins, gums, and psyllium, dissolve in water, which can result in softer and wetter feces, whereas insoluble fibers, such as cellulose, provide bulk and do not dissolve in water.[26,30] Many diets formulated for patients with GI disease are formulated with a small amount of dietary fiber but contain mixed fiber, meaning there are both soluble and insoluble fiber sources in the diet.

In patients that can tolerate fiber, it is important to look at both the amount of fiber and the type of fiber. When evaluating a diet for fiber content, it is important to look at both the soluble and insoluble fiber content of a diet. A veterinarian may need to contact the company regarding these values if they are not available in the product guide or other manufacturer materials. The measurement of total dietary fiber represents both soluble and insoluble fiber, whereas the crude fiber content refers to mostly insoluble fibers.[31,32] In patients with GI disease, soluble fiber can increase fecal moisture by dissolving in water in the GI tract and forming a viscous gel. Soluble fiber also can slow gastric emptying.[33] Insoluble fibers can decrease GI transit time[33] in addition to increasing fecal bulk. Overall, the balance of fibers in a diet influences GI health and fecal quality.[34]

Prebiotics are fermentable fibers that support the animal by stimulating growth of beneficial bacteria in the GI tract.[29] Prebiotics can be included in GI diets and other therapeutic or nontherapeutic diets and potentially can help benefit the dog or cat by altering the GI microbial populations.[30,35] Examples of prebiotics used in pet foods include fructooligosaccharides, beet pulp, and inulin.

Although all patients with GI disease can benefit from small amounts of mixed fiber sources, some patients need moderate to high amounts of fiber. Patients that can benefit from diets with higher fiber content include those with colitis, with fiber-responsive diarrhea, and some with constipation.

Cobalamin

Cobalamin, or vitamin B_{12}, can become deficient in dogs and cats with GI disease. Although cobalamin deficiency has multiple potential causes, 1 potential mechanism by which vitamin B_{12} deficiency occurs in dogs and cats with GI disease is poor absorption of cobalamin. Many of the GI conditions that result in hypocobalaminemia are chronic versus acute. Examples of conditions that can be associated with cobalamin deficiency include exocrine pancreatic insufficiency, chronic enteropathies, hepatobiliary diseases, and GI lymphoma.[36,37] In dogs with chronic diarrhea, hypocobalaminemia was found associated with more severe disease.[38] Cobalamin is absorbed exclusively in the ileum, so the presence of inflammation or other signs of disease having an impact on the ileum can have a significant impact on cobalamin status. Intrinsic factor, which binds vitamin B_{12} and promotes ileal absorption, is produced primarily in the pancreas in dogs and cats. Pancreatic disease may result in decreased intrinsic factor production and release, which can cause decreased absorption of cobalamin and hypocobalaminemia.[36,39] In many cases of dogs and cats with hypocobalaminemia, supplementation of vitamin B_{12} can result in partial or complete resolution of GI signs, and signs of the primary disease may not resolve without cobalamin supplementation.[36,39]

Patients with chronic GI signs should be tested for cobalamin deficiency and supplemented if deficient. One example of a cobalamin supplementation protocol[40] includes both oral and parenteral supplementation recommendations. In this commonly used parenteral protocol, cobalamin (250 μg for cats and 250–1500 μg for dogs, depending on body weight) is given subcutaneously weekly for 6 weeks and then repeated in a month. Testing should be repeated 1 month after the last dose to determine if further supplementation or work-up is needed.[40] The alternative oral supplementation protocol involves cobalamin (250 μg for cats and 250–1000 μg for dogs, depending on body weight) given daily for 12 weeks and then testing 1 week later to determine the next course of action.[40]

NUTRITIONAL APPROACHES FOR COMMON GASTROINTESTINAL DISEASES IN DOGS AND CATS

Once a patient is assessed for medical and nutritional issues, diagnostics are performed, and a final or tentative problem list is established, it is important to identify which problems in the patient's problem list can be managed by nutritional modification. Although many diseases have a nutritional component of management, there are some that do not. It is important to identify which problems are addressed with diet.

Once a clinician narrows down the problem list and includes aspects of the nutritional assessment in that problem list (problems like an abnormal BCS or decreased muscle condition), it is important to identify goals for nutritional modification and the nutrients of concern that help the clinician manage the disease with nutrition. One example of a goal for nutritional modification is providing supportive care for recovery in patients with pancreatitis. The nutrients of concern are increased digestibility, decreased dietary fiber, the use of moderate levels of dietary protein, and reduced dietary fat.[1]

Examples of common GI diseases in dogs and cats include pancreatitis, acute gastroenteritis, chronic enteropathy and inflammatory bowel disease, protein-losing enteropathy and lymphangiectasia, and chronic constipation. **Table 2** outlines the key nutrients of concern for these conditions and the levels of these nutrients that are beneficial for these patients.[1,5,26,41–50] Often, these goals for nutrients of concern are in relation to a pet's current diet. For example, a patient that develops pancreatitis while consuming a low-fat diet (less than 30 g of fat per 1000 kcal of food) may need to be switched to an ultra–low-fat diet (less than 20 g of fat per 1000 kcal) to help manage clinical signs of pancreatitis. The diet history of the dog or cat is essential when making a dietary recommendation for a pet with GI disease, because it is important to know what levels of the key nutrients of concern the patient currently is being fed. In addition, the problem list of the patient is important to ensure that these recommendations for diet selection are appropriate. If the patient has another major systemic disease, such as chronic kidney disease, recommendations and nutrients of concern may change depending on the dog's or cat's diagnoses.

DIETARY OPTIONS FOR PATIENTS WITH GASTROINTESTINAL DISEASE

There is a vast selection of diets that can be used for dogs and cats with GI disease. **Box 2** includes a comprehensive list of different diet options for patients with GI disease. There is no specific diet option that works for all patients with a single disease. Patients should be evaluated and managed as individuals. For example, some dogs and cats with chronic enteropathy respond well to elimination diets (novel or hydrolyzed protein), whereas others do not. Another example is cats with pancreatitis, which may but does not always occur in conjunction with intestinal inflammation and cholangiohepatitis.[42] In cases of feline pancreatitis with concurrent intestinal inflammation, a novel or hydrolyzed protein diet may be beneficial, whereas cases without intestinal inflammation may benefit from a highly digestible GI diet.

One important consideration when selecting a diet is that calories have to come from some combination of the 3 macronutrients: protein, fat, and carbohydrate. If the primary goal is fat restriction, then the relative amount of protein and carbohydrate in the diet increases to provide calories to the patient. Because many GI diets are fat restricted, they have higher levels of soluble carbohydrate and/or protein.

Home-cooked diets should be used with caution. They can be beneficial in cases of multiple disease processes present and there is no commercial option available for the patient and in cases of a dog's or cat's appetite that is poor and the patient will not consume a commercial diet. Home-cooked diets must be properly formulated, however, in order to provide complete and balanced nutrition for the patient as well as address the pet's medical issues. There are several reports of nutritional inadequacy of home-cooked diet recipes that have been found in books and on the Internet.[51–54]

Table 2
Target levels of nutrients of concern for common gastrointestinal diseases[a]

Condition	Energy Density[b]	Protein Amount	Protein Type	Fat	Fiber	Fiber type[c]	Cobalamin Supplementation Needed?	Benefit of *Common* Supplements Discussed?
Pancreatitis (dogs)[1]	Moderate	Moderate	Highly digestible	Low to ultralow	Low	Mixed	No	No
Pancreatitis (cats)[1,41,42]	Moderate to high	Moderate	Highly digestible, novel, or hydrolyzed[d] (depending on the presence of concurrent inflammatory conditions)	Moderate	Low	Mixed	Yes, after testing (especially if occurring in conjunction with inflammatory bowel disease)	Probiotics or synbiotics may be helpful, depending on clinical signs (especially if occurring in conjunction with inflammatory bowel disease)
Acute gastroenteritis[2]	Moderate to high	Moderate	Highly digestible	Low to high[e]	Low	Mixed	No	Probiotics or synbiotics may be helpful, depending on clinical signs
Chronic enteropathy/ inflammatory bowel disease[5,43–46]	High	Moderate	Highly digestible, novel, or hydrolyzed[d]	Low to moderate (can go high in patients with low BCS)	Low (some animals may respond to higher fiber)	Mixed	Yes, after testing	Probiotics or synbiotics may be helpful, depending on clinical signs

Colitis[2,47]	Moderate	Moderate to high	Highly digestible, novel, or hydrolyzed[d]	Moderate	High (if fiber is tolerated) or low (if fiber is not tolerated)	Mixed	No, unless concurrent ileal inflammation is suspected	Probiotics or synbiotics may be helpful, depending on clinical signs
Protein-losing enteropathy/ lymphangiectasia[2,48]	Moderate	Moderate to high	Highly digestible, novel, or hydrolyzed[d]	Low to ulra-low	Low	Mixed	Yes, after testing	Probiotics or synbiotics may be helpful, depending on clinical signs
Chronic constipation[26,49,50]	Low to moderate	Moderate	Highly digestible	Moderate	Low to high	Mixed, mostly soluble	No	Fiber supplementation may be helpful, depending on selected diet, response, and clinical signs

[a] The definition of the values associated with "low" or "high" or other values used in this table may vary among nutritionists. The values provided here are those used by the author.For the purposes of this table, energy density greater than 4000 kcal/kg is considered high, whereas low is less than 3100 kcal/kg for dogs and 3250 kcal/kg for cats (according to the Association of American Feed Control Officials definition of "low calorie").[66]For protein, less than 45 g/1000 kcal can be considered low for a dog, whereas greater than 70 g/1000 kcal can be considered high. For cats, a protein less than 70 g/1000 kcal is considered low, and greater than 100 g/1000 kcal is considered high.For dogs, ultralow can refer to a fat level less than 20 g/1000 kcal, low can refer to a fat level less than 30 g/1000 kcal, and high can refer to anything greater than 45 g/1000 kcal. In cats, under 30 g/1000 kcal to 35 g/1000 kcal can be considered low fat and high can refer to anything greater than 50 g/1000 kcal.For total dietary fiber (soluble fiber + insoluble fiber), less than 30 g/1000 kcal can be considered low whereas greater than 45 g/1000 kcal to 50 g/1000 kcal can be considered high. When selecting a diet, however, there are many factors to consider.Veterinarians may not be able to select a diet that fits all parameters at the same time. In these cases, prioritizing the problem list is important and making nutritional decisions based on priorities may be necessary.

[b] Energy density depends on the nutrient composition of the diet, including the dietary fat and fiber.

[c] Fiber type can be mainly soluble, mainly insoluble, or mixed soluble/insoluble.

[d] The protein type depends on the response to a food trial and the presence of intestinal inflammation.

[e] The ideal level of dietary fat for dogs and cats with acute gastroenteritis remains to be determined. Sources say that low fat can be beneficial for these patients,[2] but there is no study investigating the benefits of fat restriction versus the benefits of providing a diet with high energy density to reduce meal volume.

Box 2
Dietary options for dogs and cats with gastrointestinal disease

- "Sensitive digestion" over-the-counter diets
- Low-fat commercial veterinary therapeutic GI diets
- High-fiber GI diets
- Hydrolyzed protein diets
- Novel protein diets
- Moderate-calorie commercial veterinary therapeutic GI diets
- Moderate-fat to high-fat commercial veterinary therapeutic GI diets
- Commercial veterinary therapeutic GI diets formulated or Association of American Feed Control Officials feeding trial-tested for growth
- Home-cooked diets

There also is a report of lack of owner compliance with home-cooked diets.[55] If a home-cooked diet is needed for an individual patient, it is recommended that the diet be formulated by a board-certified veterinary nutritionist and that regular client follow-up is done to ensure that the home-cooked diet recipe is fed as intended. A board-certified veterinary nutritionist can be found at www.acvn.org/directory.

FEEDING MANAGEMENT STRATEGIES FOR PATIENTS WITH GASTROINTESTINAL DISEASE

Because patients with GI disease frequently have dysrexia in addition to clinical signs, such as vomiting or diarrhea, it is recommended that most patients be fed small, frequent meals when food is introduced. Most patients can be started at 25% to 50% of their RER for current weight, depending on the degree and duration of anorexia, clinical signs, and underlying disease.[2,10] If a patient has more severe clinical signs, complete anorexia, and/or a long duration of dysrexia, it is wise to start at the lower end of this range (ie, 25% of RER) and gradually work up to 100% of RER over 3 days to 7 days. Once the patient has stabilized, clinical signs have resolved, and the patient has been discharged, it usually is safe to work up to the patient's MER over the course of a week or 2.

Assisted feeding also may be beneficial for patients with GI disease. In patients lacking a gag reflex, or in patients with intractable vomiting or severe malabsorption, partial parenteral nutrition may be warranted. Most patients respond well, however, to antiemetics and assisted enteral nutrition can be used. Enteral nutrition is more physiologic versus parenteral nutrition and can benefit the GI tract by providing luminal nutrients for the enterocytes.[56] Early enteral nutrition has been shown to improve morbidity and mortality in dogs with pancreatitis,[57,58] be well tolerated in cats with pancreatitis,[59] and improve clinical outcome and weight gain in dogs with parvovirus enteritis.[60]

Patients do not need to be fasted through periods of vomiting and diarrhea, especially if the vomiting can be controlled with antiemetic therapy. Several studies have shown the benefit of early enteral nutrition, and it is well tolerated, even in both canine and feline patients with pancreatitis.[57,59] Patients with diarrhea do not benefit from fasting, and gut barrier function may be impaired by fasting.[61] Feeding through the GI tract, even if feeding small, frequent meals, is easy, safe, and physiologic for most patients.[62]

For any patient that benefits from an elimination diet, either novel or hydrolyzed protein, a food elimination trial is required to make a diagnosis of food-responsive enteropathy.[45] Food trials require strict elimination of all known dietary antigens. A full diet history (**Box 3**) is necessary to select a diet for the trial, especially if utilizing a novel protein diet. Once a diet is selected, that diet alone should be fed for the duration of the trial, which generally is recommended to be 1 weeks to 4 weeks in patients with GI signs alone and up to 12 weeks in patients with signs of cutaneous adverse food reactions in addition to GI signs. A diet challenge should be done at the end of the trial to confirm the diagnosis of adverse food reactions.

COMMON DIETARY SUPPLEMENTS FOR GASTROINTESTINAL DISEASE

There are many dietary supplements available for dogs and cats, some of which are marketed for patients with GI disease or GI signs. Some common dietary supplements for dogs and cats with GI disease include probiotics, synbiotics, and fiber supplements. Dietary supplements are not closely regulated, so caution should be used when veterinarians are recommending them.

Probiotics are live microorganisms that may provide the animal with a beneficial health effect.[63] Synbiotics contain both prebiotics and probiotics, which provide an animal with similar benefits but in different ways. Although probiotic and synbiotic supplements are used frequently in veterinary medicine, and may have some benefits, there is limited evidence that these supplements have a strong positive benefit in dogs and cats with specific GI diseases.[64] As with all supplements, it is important to use a quality probiotic or synbiotic supplement from a trusted brand or reputable company with published research on its products as well as to investigate the quality control of the supplement.

Fiber supplements also are utilized in patients with GI disease. In general, fiber supplementation is most beneficial for dogs with constipation or fiber-responsive diarrhea, cats with constipation,[50] or cats with large bowel signs due to inflammatory bowel disease or other conditions.[42] Some investigators recommend pure psyllium supplementation at 1.25 mL or 0.25 tsp per meal,[13] but the ideal dosing strategy for psyllium or other fiber supplements has not been determined at this time.[32] Severely constipated cats with additional conditions, such as chronic kidney disease, who cannot consume a high fiber GI diet due to concurrent diseases, may require more

Box 3
Components of a full diet history

- Diet type, amount, and frequency + duration of feeding + how it is measured
- All treat types, amounts, and frequency
- Table scraps/human foods amounts and frequency
- Food for medication administration
- Food for training
- Other pets' food (if any access)
- Any other food or treats the pet may consume
- Dietary supplements
- Flavored medications
- Flavored toothpaste

Box 4
Clinics care points

- When selecting a diet for a patient with GI disease, consider the problem list, and prioritize it if there are multiple problems. Some problems may be of equal priority, but others may not be as important to manage as others.
- In addition to the problem list, factor in the nutrients of concern for that patient and look at the dog's or cat's nutritional assessment, including the diet history. This helps determine if the nutrients of concern should be increased, maintained, or decreased relative to current intake.
- Diet selection should be individualized for the specific patient in question. Not all patients with chronic enteropathy, for example, respond to the same nutritional strategy.
- Reassessment is equally as important as diet selection for nutritional management. Performing regular medical and nutritional assessments for patients with GI disease is important for long-term management, when needed.

than a 1.25 mL or 0.25 tsp twice daily. When veterinarians recommend fiber supplementation, ensuring adequate water intake is essential.

Some veterinarians also recommend canned pumpkin as a fiber supplement. Canned pumpkin is mostly water (90 g water per 100 g canned pumpkin) with little fiber (2.9 g total dietary fiber per 100 g canned pumpkin).[65] It may, however, be beneficial for some patients.

SUMMARY

Although there are many factors to consider when managing dogs and cats with GI diseases with nutrition, the most important things to keep in mind are the primary priorities for the patient (which usually are 1 to 2 items on the patient's problem list that require the most attention) and that an individualized approach should be taken for all patients. Not all patients with 1 disease process benefit from a single diet. There are many dietary options for GI disease because different patients benefit from different diets and nutritional strategies. **Box 4** contains guidelines for selecting a GI diet. Diet selection should be tailored to the individual patient, and, because nutrition is an iterative process, the dog or cat should be reassessed to ensure that the diet selection and nutrition plan is ideal for that patient.

DISCLOSURE

Dr C.E. Lenox discloses that she is a full-time associate of Royal Canin.

REFERENCES

1. Villaverde C. Nutritional management of exocrine pancreatic diseases. In: Fascetti AJ, Delaney SJ, editors. Applied veterinary clinical nutrition. Ames (IA): John Wiley & Sons; 2012. p. 221–33.
2. Cave N. Nutritional management of gastrointestinal diseases. In: Fascetti AJ, Delaney SJ, editors. Applied veterinary clinical nutrition. Ames (IA): John WIley & Sons; 2012. p. 175–220.
3. Baldwin K, Bartges J, Buffington T, et al. AAHA nutritional assessment guidelines for dogs and cats. J Am Anim Hosp Assoc 2010;46(4):285–96.

4. Freeman L, Becvarova I, Cave N, et al. WSAVA nutritional assessment guidelines. Compend Contin Educ Vet 2011;33(8):E1–9.
5. Rudinsky AJ, Rowe JC, Parker VJ. Nutritional management of chronic enteropathies in dogs and cats. J Am Vet Med Assoc 2018;253(5):570–8.
6. Nery J, Biourge V, Tournier C, et al. Influence of dietary protein content and source on fecal quality, electrolyte concentrations, and osmolarity, and digestibility in dogs differing in body size. J Anim Sci 2010;88(1):159–69.
7. Carciofi AC, Takakura FS, de-Oliveira LD, et al. Effects of six carbohydrate sources on dog diet digestibility and post-prandial glucose and insulin response. J Anim Physiol Anim Nutr (Berl) 2008;92(3):326–36.
8. de-Oliveira LD, Carciofi AC, Oliveira MC, et al. Effects of six carbohydrate sources on diet digestibility and postprandial glucose and insulin responses in cats. J Anim Sci 2008;86(9):2237–46.
9. Kienzle E, Biourge V, Schonmeier A. Prediction of energy digestibility in complete dry foods for dogs and cats by total dietary fiber. J Nutr 2006;136(7 Suppl): 2041S–4S.
10. Chan DL, Freeman LM. Nutrition in critical illness. Vet Clin North Am Small Anim Pract 2006;36(6):1225–41, v–vi.
11. National Research Council. Energy. In: Nutrient requirements of dogs and cats. Washington, DC: The National Academies Press; 2006. p. 28–48.
12. Debraekeleer J, Gross KL, Zicker SC. Feeding young adult dogs: before middle age. In: Hand MS, Thatcher CD, Remillard RL, et al, editors. Small animal clinical nutrition. 5th edition. Topeka (KS): Mark Morris Institute; 2010. p. 257–72.
13. Gross KL, Becvarova I, Armstrong PJ, et al. Feeding young adult cats: before middle age. In: Hand MS, Thatcher CD, Remillard RL, et al, editors. Small animal clinical nutrition. 5th edition. Topeka (KS): Mark Morris Institute; 2010. p. 373–88.
14. Backus RC, Rosenquist GL, Rogers QR, et al. Elevation of plasma cholecystokinin (CCK) immunoreactivity by fat, protein, and amino acids in the cat, a carnivore. Regul Pept 1995;57(2):123–31.
15. Meyer JH, Kelly GA. Canine pancreatic responses to intestinally perfused proteins and protein digests. Am J Physiol 1976;231(3):682–91.
16. Meyer JH, Kelly GA, Spingola LJ, et al. Canine gut receptors mediating pancreatic responses to luminal L-amino acids. Am J Physiol 1976;231(3):669–77.
17. Sun G, Chang TM, Xue WJ, et al. Release of cholecystokinin and secretin by sodium oleate in dogs: molecular form and bioactivity. Am J Physiol 1992;262(1 Pt 1):G35–43.
18. Cave NJ. Hydrolyzed protein diets for dogs and cats. Vet Clin North Am Small Anim Pract 2006;36(6):1251–68, vi.
19. Lem KY, Fosgate GT, Norby B, et al. Associations between dietary factors and pancreatitis in dogs. J Am Vet Med Assoc 2008;233(9):1425–31.
20. Olson NC, Zimmer JF. Protein-losing enteropathy secondary to intestinal lymphangiectasia in a dog. J Am Vet Med Assoc 1978;173(3):271–4.
21. Laflamme DP, Xu H, Long GM. Effect of diets differing in fat content on chronic diarrhea in cats. J Vet Intern Med 2011;25(2):230–5.
22. Bauer JE. Therapeutic use of fish oils in companion animals. J Am Vet Med Assoc 2011;239(11):1441–51.
23. Calder PC. n-3 polyunsaturated fatty acids, inflammation, and inflammatory diseases. Am J Clin Nutr 2006;83(6 Suppl):1505S–19S.
24. Hickman MA. Interventional nutrition for gastrointestinal disease. Clin Tech Small Anim Pract 1998;13(4):211–6.

25. Trepanier L. Idiopathic inflammatory bowel disease in cats. Rational treatment selection. J Feline Med Surg 2009;11(1):32–8.
26. Wara A, Datz C. Cats and dietary fiber. Vet Focus 2014;24(3):26–32.
27. Fekete S, Hullar I, Andrasofszky E, et al. Reduction of the energy density of cat foods by increasing their fibre content with a view to nutrients' digestibility. J Anim Physiol Anim Nutr (Berl) 2001;85(7–8):200–4.
28. Fekete SG, Hullar I, Andrasofszky E, et al. Effect of different fibre types on the digestibility of nutrients in cats. J Anim Physiol Anim Nutr (Berl) 2004;88(3–4):138–42.
29. National Research Council. Carbohydrates and fiber. In: Nutrient requirements of dogs and cats. Washington, DC: The National Academies Press; 2006. p. 7.
30. Barry KA, Wojcicki BJ, Middelbos IS, et al. Dietary cellulose, fructooligosaccharides, and pectin modify fecal protein catabolites and microbial populations in adult cats. J Anim Sci 2010;88(9):2978–87.
31. Farcas AK, Larsen JA, Fascetti AJ. Evaluation of fiber concentration in dry and canned commercial diets formulated for adult maintenance or all life stages of dogs by use of crude fiber and total dietary fiber methods. J Am Vet Med Assoc 2013;242(7):936–40.
32. Linder DE. Featuring fiber: understanding types of fiber & clinical uses. Today's Vet Pract 2017;7:69–74.
33. de Godoy MR, Kerr KR, Fahey GC Jr. Alternative dietary fiber sources in companion animal nutrition. Nutrients 2013;5(8):3099–117.
34. Weber MP, Biourge VC, Nguyen PG. Digestive sensitivity varies according to size of dogs: a review. J Anim Physiol Anim Nutr (Berl) 2017;101(1):1–9.
35. Swanson KS, Grieshop CM, Flickinger EA, et al. Fructooligosaccharides and Lactobacillus acidophilus modify gut microbial populations, total tract nutrient digestibilities and fecal protein catabolite concentrations in healthy adult dogs. J Nutr 2002;132(12):3721–31.
36. Kather S, Grutzner N, Kook PH, et al. Review of cobalamin status and disorders of cobalamin metabolism in dogs. J Vet Intern Med 2020;34(1):13–28.
37. Simpson KW, Fyfe J, Cornetta A, et al. Subnormal concentrations of serum cobalamin (vitamin B12) in cats with gastrointestinal disease. J Vet Intern Med 2001;15(1):26–32.
38. Volkmann M, Steiner JM, Fosgate GT, et al. Chronic diarrhea in dogs - retrospective study in 136 cases. J Vet Intern Med 2017;31(4):1043–55.
39. Ruaux CG, Steiner JM, Williams DA. Early biochemical and clinical responses to cobalamin supplementation in cats with signs of gastrointestinal disease and severe hypocobalaminemia. J Vet Intern Med 2005;19(2):155–60.
40. Texas A&M University Gastrointestinal Laboratory. Cobalamin Information. Available at: https://vetmed.tamu.edu/gilab/research/cobalamin-information/. Accessed May 29, 2020.
41. Bazelle J, Watson P. Pancreatitis in cats: is it acute, is it chronic, is it significant? J Feline Med Surg 2014;16(5):395–406.
42. Jergens AE. Feline idiopathic inflammatory bowel disease: what we know and what remains to be unraveled. J Feline Med Surg 2012;14(7):445–58.
43. Allenspach K, Culverwell C, Chan D. Long-term outcome in dogs with chronic enteropathies: 203 cases. Vet Rec 2016;178(15):368.
44. Allenspach K, Wieland B, Grone A, et al. Chronic enteropathies in dogs: evaluation of risk factors for negative outcome. J Vet Intern Med 2007;21(4):700–8.
45. Guilford WG, Jones BR, Markwell PJ, et al. Food sensitivity in cats with chronic idiopathic gastrointestinal problems. J Vet Intern Med 2001;15(1):7–13.

46. Mandigers PJ, Biourge V, German AJ. Efficacy of a commercial hydrolysate diet in eight cats suffering from inflammatory bowel disease or adverse reaction to food. Tijdschr Diergeneeskd 2010;135(18):668–72.
47. Witzel A. Diarrhea, vomiting, and food, oh my! Nutritional management for gastrointestinal disease. Today's Vet Pract 2018;8:18–20.
48. Okanishi H, Yoshioka R, Kagawa Y, et al. The clinical efficacy of dietary fat restriction in treatment of dogs with intestinal lymphangiectasia. J Vet Intern Med 2014; 28(3):809–17.
49. Davenport DJ, Remillard RL, Carroll M. Constipation/obstipation/megacolon. In: Hand MS, Thatcher CD, Remillard RL, et al, editors. Small animal clinical nutrition. 5th edition. Topeka (KS): Mark Morris Institute; 2010. p. 1117–26.
50. Freiche V, Houston D, Weese H, et al. Uncontrolled study assessing the impact of a psyllium-enriched extruded dry diet on faecal consistency in cats with constipation. J Feline Med Surg 2011;13(12):903–11.
51. Heinze CR, Gomez FC, Freeman LM. Assessment of commercial diets and recipes for home-prepared diets recommended for dogs with cancer. J Am Vet Med Assoc 2012;241(11):1453–60.
52. Larsen JA, Parks EM, Heinze CR, et al. Evaluation of recipes for home-prepared diets for dogs and cats with chronic kidney disease. J Am Vet Med Assoc 2012; 240(5):532–8.
53. Stockman J, Fascetti AJ, Kass PH, et al. Evaluation of recipes of home-prepared maintenance diets for dogs. J Am Vet Med Assoc 2013;242(11):1500–5.
54. Wilson SA, Villaverde C, Fascetti AJ, et al. Evaluation of the nutritional adequacy of recipes for home-prepared maintenance diets for cats. J Am Vet Med Assoc 2019;254(10):1172–9.
55. Johnson LN, Linder DE, Heinze CR, et al. Evaluation of owner experiences and adherence to home-cooked diet recipes for dogs. J Small Anim Pract 2016; 57(1):23–7.
56. Michel KE. Interventional nutrition for the critical care patient: optimal diets. Clin Tech Small Anim Pract 1998;13(4):204–10.
57. Harris JP, Parnell NK, Griffith EH, et al. Retrospective evaluation of the impact of early enteral nutrition on clinical outcomes in dogs with pancreatitis: 34 cases (2010-2013). J Vet Emerg Crit Care (San Antonio) 2017;27(4):425–33.
58. Mansfield CS, James FE, Steiner JM, et al. A pilot study to assess tolerability of early enteral nutrition via esophagostomy tube feeding in dogs with severe acute pancreatitis. J Vet Intern Med 2011;25(3):419–25.
59. Klaus JA, Rudloff E, Kirby R. Nasogastric tube feeding in cats with suspected acute pancreatitis: 55 cases (2001-2006). J Vet Emerg Crit Care (San Antonio) 2009;19(4):337–46.
60. Mohr AJ, Leisewitz AL, Jacobson LS, et al. Effect of early enteral nutrition on intestinal permeability, intestinal protein loss, and outcome in dogs with severe parvoviral enteritis. J Vet Intern Med 2003;17(6):791–8.
61. Qin HL, Su ZD, Gao Q, et al. Early intrajejunal nutrition: bacterial translocation and gut barrier function of severe acute pancreatitis in dogs. Hepatobiliary Pancreat Dis Int 2002;1(1):150–4.
62. Remillard RL. Nutritional support in critical care patients. Vet Clin North Am Small Anim Pract 2002;32(5):1145–64, viii.
63. Jugan MC, Rudinsky AJ, Parker VJ, et al. Use of probiotics in small animal veterinary medicine. J Am Vet Med Assoc 2017;250(5):519–28.

64. Jensen AP, Bjornvad CR. Clinical effect of probiotics in prevention or treatment of gastrointestinal disease in dogs: A systematic review. J Vet Intern Med 2019; 33(5):1849–64.
65. USDA FoodData Central. Pumpkin, canned, without salt 2019. Available at: https://fdc.nal.usda.gov/fdc-app.html#/food-details/168450/nutrients. Accessed May 29, 2020.
66. Association of American Feed Control Officials. Model bill and regulations. In: Lueders D, editor. 2020 Official Publication. Champaign (IL): Association of American Feed Control Officials, Inc.; 2020. p. 109–233.

Nutritional Management for Dogs and Cats with Chronic Kidney Disease

Valerie J. Parker, DVM

KEYWORDS

• Dysrexia • Phosphorus • Protein • Body condition score • Proteinuria • Potassium • Vitamin D

KEY POINTS

- Dogs and cats with kidney disease commonly develop dysrexia and exhibit weight loss.
- Body composition measurements (ie, body weight, body condition score) can have diagnostic and prognostic implications for dogs and cats with kidney disease.
- The optimal nutritional management of kidney disease varies by disease type (eg, chronic kidney disease, protein-losing nephropathy).
- Assisted enteral nutrition can alleviate the stress that owners feel with hyporexic animals and can allow for the provision of optimal nutritional support.

INTRODUCTION

Nutritional management is a crucial component of veterinary care provided to dogs and cats with kidney disease. It has the potential to slow progression of disease and also prolong survival. This article reviews the nutritional goals for dogs and cats with chronic kidney disease (CKD) and protein-losing nephropathy (PLN). Beyond the impressive body of evidence already in existence to support these recommendations, additional research will continue to refine and enhance the ways in which we provide optimal nutrition to our patients.

CHRONIC KIDNEY DISEASE

Body Composition

An animal's body composition (body weight [BW], body condition score [BCS], and muscle condition score)[1] may yield clues about the impending diagnosis of CKD, and it has also been shown to affect survival in dogs and cats with CKD. A loss of BW may precede a diagnosis of CKD in cats by up to 3 years, and weight loss often increases after diagnosis.[2] Cats with CKD and a BW of less than 4.2 kg at diagnosis

The Ohio State University, 601 Vernon L. Tharp Street, Columbus, OH 43210, USA
E-mail address: parker.888@osu.edu

Vet Clin Small Anim 51 (2021) 685–710
https://doi.org/10.1016/j.cvsm.2021.01.007

had a shorter survival than cats with CKD that had a BW of 4.2 kg or more.[2] Thin dogs (BCS of <4/9) with CKD had a shorter survival than dogs with a BCS of 4 or more out of 9,[3] and overweight dogs (ie, BCS of >5/9) had longer survival than ideal and underweight dogs.[4]

Muscle loss seen in patients with CKD is likely multifactorial, related to (1) sarcopenia, an age-related loss of muscle; (2) cachexia, muscle loss affected by inflammatory cytokines; and/or (3) decreased protein and amino acid (AA) intake, whether owing to specific dietary manipulation and/or decreased caloric intake.[5,6] Protein-energy wasting, a cachectic state characterized by nutritional and metabolic derangements, is commonly identified in people with CKD, and it contributes to decreased quality of life and increased morbidity and mortality[7,8] (**Fig. 1**). Dogs with CKD that had normal muscle mass scores had longer survival than dogs with muscle loss.[4]

Research is ongoing in both human and veterinary medicine to better identify and understand cachexia in a variety of conditions. Several studies have validated the usefulness of ultrasound examination and computed tomography scans to measure muscle mass in dogs and cats, which may have greater clinical usefulness compared with other research methods.[9–12] If we can better define cachexia and its effects on morbidity and mortality, we may be able to identify methods by which to lessen cachexia or its deleterious effects.

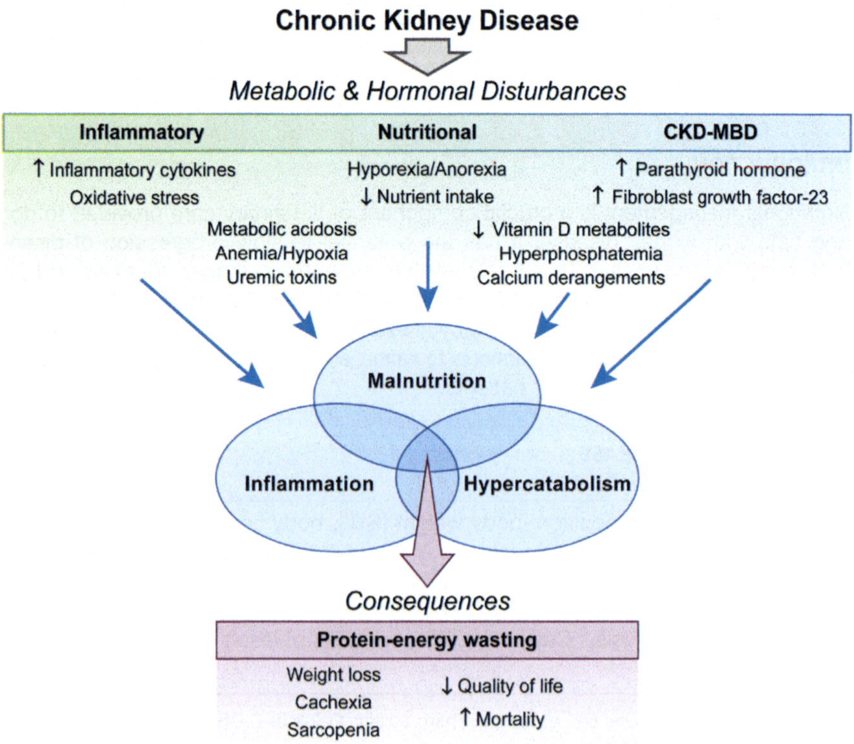

Fig. 1. Contributors and consequences of protein–energy wasting (PEW) syndrome associated with CKD. CKD-MBD, CKD–mineral and bone disorder. (Reproduced with permission of The Ohio State University.)

Maintaining adequate caloric intake is imperative to maintaining BW, BCS, and muscle condition scores. Some animals will maintain weight eating their resting energy requirement – $70 \times BW_{kg}^{0.75}$; however, others will require multiplication of a maintenance energy requirement factor.[13] If an animal is losing weight despite eating more than 2 times the resting energy requirement, it should be evaluated for other diseases that can contribute to increased energy needs (eg, hyperthyroidism), maldigestion (eg, exocrine pancreatic insufficiency), or malabsorption (eg, inflammatory bowel disease).

Appetite Dysregulation

Animals with CKD are often hyporexic or anorexic, reported in up to 92% of cats.[2] It can be helpful to offer a variety of both dry and canned diet options to increase intake. Medications to ameliorate nausea may be useful (eg, maropitant, ondansetron); however, the bioavailability and efficacy of these drugs is variable across species.[14,15] Acid-reducing agents are not generally recommended because dogs and cats rarely develop uremic gastropathy.[16,17] The exception to this would be if there is evidence of gastrointestinal bleeding,[18] which is more common in advanced CKD.[19]

Appetite stimulants can be useful in dogs and cats with CKD. Capromorelin, a ghrelin receptor agonist, has been approved by the US Food and Drug Administration for both dogs and cats. It is labeled to increase appetite and body weight in dogs[20] and for management of weight loss in cats, respectively.[21] Mirtazapine can be effective in both oral and transdermal forms to aid in weight gain, decrease vomiting, and improve appetite in cats.[22,23] The transdermal form has been approved by the US FDA for weight gain. Anecdotally, many animals respond well to these medications. See **Table 1** for medications and dosages.

Assisted Enteral Nutrition

When an animal will not eat enough to maintain BW, the placement of a feeding tube may be a viable option to provide enteral nutritional support and a good route for additional water and medications.[24] The feeding tube will likely be in place for the remainder of the animal's life; thus, placement of either esophagostomy or gastrostomy tubes is appropriate.[25,26] With proper maintenance, these tubes can be used for months to years.[24,26] Canned veterinary therapeutic renal diets can be blended with water (or a liquid enteral diet designed for kidney disease) to achieve appropriate consistency to be fed via tubes (**Box 1**).

Nutritional Modification

Phosphorus

There is strong evidence for dietary modification in dogs and cats with CKD. Feeding a veterinary therapeutic renal diet can prolong survival and decrease the risks of uremic crises in dogs and cats with naturally occurring CKD.[4,27–29] The primary nutrient of concern for CKD is dietary phosphorus. Decreasing dietary phosphorus intake slowed the progression of renal disease and prolonged survival in dogs with induced CKD.[30] Hyperphosphatemia is related to reduced survival in cats with CKD.[31–33] In 1 study, for every 1 mg/dL (0.32 mmol/L) increase in serum phosphorus, there was an 11.8% increased risk of death.[32] The plasma phosphate concentration is a potent stimulator of fibroblast growth factor-23 (FGF-23), a phosphatonin that affects the development of CKD mineral and bone disorder (CKD-MBD).[34,35] Feeding a reduced phosphorus diet decreased plasma phosphate and FGF-23 in cats with CKD.[36]

The 2019 International Renal Interest Society treatment guidelines suggest maintaining plasma (or serum) phosphate concentrations in dogs and cats with CKD between 2.7 and 4.6 mg/dL (0.87–1.49 mmol/L), although a target of less than 5.0 mg/dL

Table 1
Medications and supplements commonly prescribed for dogs and cats with CKD and PLN

Medication or Supplement	Canine Dose	Feline Dose	Comments
Appetite stimulants			
Capromorelin	3 mg/kg PO q24 h	2 mg/kg PO q24 h	Hypersalivation may be observed with administration in dogs and cats.
Mirtazapine	3.75–30 mg per dog q12–24 h 1 mg/kg PO q12–24 h	1.88 mg per cat PO q48 h ~2 mg (1.5-inch strip TD q24–48 h	The half-life of mirtazapine is prolonged in cats with CKD and/or liver disease. Cats that exhibit excitation may require dose reduction. Prokinetic effect observed in healthy dogs dosed with 2.0 mg/kg PO once.
Antiemetics			
Maropitant	1 mg/kg SC or IV q24 h 2 mg/kg PO q24 h	1 mg/kg IV or PO q24 h	Refrigeration may reduce pain associated with SC injection.
Ondansetron	0.2–0.5 mg/kg IV or SC q6-12h 0.5–1.0 mg/kg PO q6–8h	0.2–0.5 mg/kg IV or SC q6–12h 0.5–1.0 mg/kg PO q6–8h	Oral bioavailability is low (<10%) in dogs. Oral bioavailability is moderate (32%) in cats. Half-lives are short in dogs and cats, with SC half-life longest in cats (3.2 ± 0.5 h).[15] Oral ondansetron is rarely cost-effective in larger dogs. Give 30 min before meals.
Antihypertensive and antiproteinuric medications			

Telmisartan (antihypertensive and antiproteinuric)	0.5–1.0 mg/kg PO q24 h, up to 3.0 mg/kg/d	0.5–1.0 mg/kg PO q24 h, up to 3.0 mg/kg/d	Labeled for cats to initially start with a higher dose (1.5 mg/kg PO q12 h × 14 d), then taper to minimum dose of 0.5 mg/kg PO q24 h. Monitor for azotemia, hyperkalemia, and hypotension.
Amlodipine (antihypertensive)	0.1–0.5 mg/kg PO q12–24h, up to 1.0 mg/kg PO q12 h	0.625–1.25 mg per cat PO q12–24 h	
Enalapril (antihypertensive and antiproteinuric)	0.5–1.0 mg/kg PO q12–24 h	0.25–0.5 mg/kg PO q12–24 h	Monitor for azotemia, hyperkalemia, and hypotension.
Benazepril (antihypertensive and antiproteinuric)	0.5 mg/kg PO q12–24 h, up to 2.0 mg/kg PO/d	0.5–1.0 mg/kg mg/kg PO q12–24 h, up to 2.0 mg/kg/d	
Acid-reducing medications			
Famotidine	1 mg/kg PO q12 h 1 mg/kg IV loading dose, then 8 mg/kg/d IV CRI (up to 3 d)	1 mg/kg PO q12 h	Famotidine has poor potency relative to proton pump inhibitors.
Omeprazole	1 mg/kg PO q12 h	1 mg/kg PO q12 h	Only indicated if overt evidence of GI bleeding. Prolonged administration of acid suppressants have been associated with calcium and parathyroid hormone derangements in humans.
Phosphate binders			
Aluminum hydroxide	30–100 mg/kg/d PO	30–100 mg/kg/d PO	Must be given with food.
Lanthanum carbonate	10-40 mg/kg/d PO	30 mg/kg/d PO, up to 95 mg/kg/d PO	Divide daily dose into multiple meals. Titrate to effect.
Sevelamer	30–50 mg/kg PO q8 h	30–50 mg/kg PO q8 h 40–80 mg/kg PO q12 h	Monitor for ionized hypercalcemia with use of calcium salts.
Calcium carbonate Calcium acetate	60–90 mg/kg/d PO 90–150 mg/kg/d PO	60–90 mg/kg/d PO 90–150 mg/kg/d PO	
Epakitin (8% chitosan, 10% calcium carbonate)	1 g per 5 kg BW PO q12 h	1 g per 5 kg BW PO q12 h	
Erythropoietic medication			

(*continued on next page*)

Table 1
(*continued*)

Medication or Supplement	Canine Dose	Feline Dose	Comments
Darbepoetin	0.25–1.0 μg/kg SC per week until target PCV attained	0.25–1.0 μg/kg SC per week until target PCV attained	Monitor packed cell volume, blood pressure. Once target PCR met, increase dose interval to once every 2–3 wk OR decrease dose to maintain PCV. Give iron dextran: 50 mg per cat OR 10 mg/kg (dog) IM once to ensure adequate iron stores.
Antithrombotic medication			
Clopidogrel	1–5 mg/kg PO q24 h	18.75 mg per cat PO q24 h	Recommended to reduce hypercoagulability associated with proteinuria.
Vitamins and minerals			
Potassium gluconate, potassium citrate	2 mEq per 4.5 kg q12 h	1–4 mEq per cat q12 h	Titrate based on individual animal's response.
Calcitriol	2–2.5 ng/kg PO q24 h, up to 5 ng/kg/d	1.5–3.5 ng/kg PO q24 h	Monitor for ionized hypercalcemia. Use cautiously in animals with hyperphosphatemia.
Calcifediol			Not currently labeled for use in dogs or cats.

			Providing ~2 μg/kg PO 3 times weekly increased 25(OH) and 1,25$(OH)_2$D concentrations in dogs with CKD.
Vitamins C and E			Supplementation with antioxidants may reduce renal oxidative stress. Use caution with vitamin C in animals prone to calcium oxalate urolithiasis production. Dogs with CKD had higher concentrations of plasma vitamin C and several B vitamins, and no difference in plasma vitamin E compared with healthy dogs.
Additional supplements			
Fish oil (EPA and DHA)	140 mg/kg $BW^{0.75}$ 66 mg/kg/d	200–300 mg EPA/DHA per cat per day	Liquid (eg, pump) and twist-off capsule options are useful for cats who cannot ingest larger capsules. Double or triple strength capsules are useful for large dogs to reduce the number of capsules, and subsequent calories, provided.
Azodyl (symbiotic)	1–3 capsules per day	1–2 capsules per day	Capsules should be given whole. Limited evidence for use in azotemic animals.

Abbreviations: GI, gastrointestinal; IV, intravenously; PO, by mouth; SC, subcutaneously.

Box 1
Equation to determine caloric density of blended canned diet

$$\frac{(\text{kcal per can} + \text{kcal liquid added})}{\text{mL of can} + \text{mL added liquid}} = \frac{\text{kcal}}{\text{mL}}$$

Example: Blend (1) 5.5 oz (156 g) can of Hill's Prescription Diet k/d with Chicken (177 kcal per can). Because 1 g is approximately equal to 1 mL, assume that 1 can = 156 mL. Through some trial and error, by adding small increments of water at a time, if you determine that it takes 25 mL water to achieve a smooth consistency to be fed via a 14-F esophagostomy feeding tube, that means the following:

$$\frac{177 \text{ kcal } (1 \text{ can k/d}) + 0 \text{ kcal (water)}}{156 \text{ mL } (1 \text{ can k/d}) + 25 \text{ mL (water)}} = \frac{177 \text{ kcal}}{181 \text{ mL}} = 0.98 \text{ kcal per mL}$$

* If a higher caloric density were required, a liquid enteral diet appropriate for feline CKD could be substituted for water. For example, if Royal Canin Veterinary Diet Feline Renal Support Liquid (0.9 kcal/mL) were used to blend the canned Hill's Prescription Diet k/d diet, it would add an additional 22.5 kcal, increasing the resultant kcal/mL to 1.10 kcal/mL. However, when only a small volume of water is required to prepare a canned diet for provision via a feeding tube, this difference is fairly insignificant, and the cost-to-benefit ratio is low.

* Commercial formulas, caloric density, and consistency of diets may change. Thus, the caloric density of a diet should always be confirmed, and the amount of liquid needed to blend with the diet may vary over time to ensure the consistency of the slurry remains appropriate.

(1.62 mmol/L) for patients with stage 3 CKD and less than 6.0 mg/dL (1.94 mmol/L) for patients with stage 4 CKD was deemed more realistic.[37] Controlling the circulating phosphate concentrations is first addressed by decreasing the dietary phosphorus intake, then adding oral phosphate binders with food, if needed.[38] Currently available canine and feline veterinary therapeutic renal diets are shown in **Tables 2** and **3**.

Evidence suggests that not only the amount of phosphorus, but also the form of dietary phosphorus, as well as the dietary calcium:phosphorus ratio, may influence renal health.[39–42] Phosphorus from organic sources (eg, meat, bone meal, grains) is less bioavailable than phosphorus from certain inorganic sources (eg, sodium or potassium phosphate salts). Feeding these highly available phosphate salts, especially in a diet with too little calcium, resulted in renal damage in previously healthy cats.[39,41,42] Some of this damage is alleviated by maintaining a dietary calcium:phosphorus intake of 1.0 or more.[42]

Protein

It is controversial if and/or when protein should be restricted in animals, especially cats, with CKD.[43–45] In people with CKD, providing adequate protein, including essential AAs, can decrease the risk of the development of protein-energy wasting and loss of lean body mass (LBM).[7,46,47] In dogs and cats, dietary protein intake has been shown to influence LBM.[48,49] In dogs with CKD, feeding a diet with protein concentration of more than 51 g/Mcal (>5.1 g/100 kcal) better allowed dogs to maintain body condition.[50] Feeding higher protein diets may then be preferable, because it has been shown that dogs with CKD and a BCS of 4 or more out of 9 had longer survival than dogs with a thin BCS.[3,4]

Protein requirements have conventionally been determined based on the maintenance of nitrogen balance.[51,52] This factor differs from using maintenance of LBM as a marker of protein adequacy. To maintain nitrogen balance in 20 healthy cats,

Table 2
Comparison of selected nutrients of concern (per 100 kcal) for currently available veterinary therapeutic renal diets for dogs

Canine Renal Diets	Calories (kcal)	Phosphorus (mg)	Protein (g)	Potassium (mg)	Sodium (mg)	Vit D (IU)	Calcium (mg)	EPA & DHA (mg)
Royal Canin Canine Renal Support + Hydrolyzed Protein (dry)	385/cup	50	3.4	150	90	19.5	70	120
Royal Canin Canine Renal Support A (dry)	352/cup	50	3.5	150	90	25.0	100	120
Hill's Prescription Diet k/d Canine Chicken & Vegetable Stew (5.5 or 12.5 oz can)	158 or 358/can	61	3.6	226	35	16.3	170	156
Hill's Prescription Diet k/d Canine (13 oz can)	422/can	62	3.6	201	45	18.9	180	129
Hill's Prescription Diet k/d Canine with Lamb (13 oz can)	421/can	64	3.6	204	45	19.2	184	132
Hill's Prescription Diet k/d + Mobility Canine (dry)	496/cup	65	3.5	155	43	33.5	140	157
Hill's Prescription Diet k/d Canine Beef & Vegetable Stew (5.5 or 12.5 oz can)	145 or 330/can	65	3.8	235	38	19.0	188	136
Royal Canin Canine Renal Support S (dry)	365/cup	70	3.1	150	90	24.8	140	120
Royal Canin Canine Renal Support E (13.5 oz can)	598/can	70	3.5	160	80	20.1	110	100
Hill's Prescription Diet k/d + Mobility Canine Chicken & Vegetable Stew (12.5 oz can)	352/can	72	3.6	217	40	37.5	171	417
Hill's Prescription Diet k/d Canine (dry)	402/cup	73	3.5	186	40	30.4	188	117
Hill's Prescription Diet k/d Canine with Lamb (dry)	459/cup	74	3.6	154	38	30.5	165	120
Royal Canin Canine Renal Support F (dry)	356/cup	30	3.4	150	90	25.3	150	110
Purina Pro Plan Veterinary Diets NF Kidney Function Canine Formula (dry)	478/cup	30	3.4	170	60	31.8	150	120

(continued on next page)

Table 2
(continued)

Canine Renal Diets	Calories (kcal)	Phosphorus (mg)	Protein (g)	Potassium (mg)	Sodium (mg)	Vit D (IU)	Calcium (mg)	EPA & DHA (mg)
Royal Canin Canine Renal Support + Advanced Mobility Support (dry)	332/cup	80	3.5	150	100	25.3	150	150
Royal Canin Canine Renal Support T (13.5 oz can)	595/can	80	3.8	160	90	22.0	160	110
Purina Pro Plan Veterinary Diets NF Kidney Function Canine Formula (13.3 oz can)	483/can	80	4.1	230	40	36.1	160	120
Royal Canin Canine Renal Support Liquid (237 mL bottle)	1.3/mL	90	3.7	160	100	16.0	140	110
BLUE Natural Veterinary Diet KS Kidney Support (dry)	404/cup	90	4.0	220	50	39.5	110	190
Royal Canin Canine Renal Support + Advanced Mobility Support (13 oz can)	374/can	100	4.0	170	100	19.6	160	100
BLUE Natural Veterinary Diet KS Kidney Support (12.5 oz can)	354/can	100	4.7	480	50	17.4	230	120
Royal Canin Canine Renal Support D (13.5 oz can)	344/can	110	4.0	170	100	19.1	160	100
Royal Canin Renal Support Early Consult (5.2 oz can)	156/can	120	6.0	170	90	19.4	160	110
Royal Canin Renal Support Early Consult (dry)	316/cup	130	5.7	150	90	25.1	200	130
2020 AAFCO Canine adult maintenance minimum		100	4.5	150	20	12.5	125	–
2020 AAFCO Canine adult maintenance maximum		400	–	–	–	75.0	625	–

Diets are listed by ascending phosphorus concentrations. Association of American Feed Control Officials (AAFCO) minimum and maximum (when applicable) nutrient requirements for canine adult maintenance are provided for reference.

*Note that nutrient profiles can change approximately every 6 to 12 mo.

Table 3
Comparison of selected nutrients of concern (per 100 kcal) for currently available veterinary therapeutic renal diets for cats

Feline Renal Diets	Calories (kcal)	Phosphorus (mg)	Protein (g)	Potassium (mg)	Sodium (mg)	Vit D (IU)	Calcium (mg)	EPA & DHA (mg)
Royal Canin Feline Renal Support D (3 oz can)	98/can	80	6.8	190	80	17.8	130	140
Royal Canin Feline Renal Support Liquid (237 mL bottle)	0.9/mL	80	7.5	180	90	31.2	130	150
Purina Pro Plan Veterinary Diets NF Early Care (dry)	494/cup	90	9.0	350	70	86.0	150	120
Purina Pro Plan Veterinary Diets NF Advanced Care (dry)	536/cup	90	6.9	350	70	79.0	150	120
Purina Pro Plan Veterinary Diets NF Advanced Care (5.5 oz can)	165/can	90	6.7	370	80	24.8	160	110
Royal Canin Feline Renal Support E (5.1 oz can)	151/can	90	7.0	180	90	23.2	150	130
Royal Canin Feline Renal Support S (dry)	397/cup	100	5.9	210	100	16.7	170	100
Royal Canin Feline Renal Support + Hydrolyzed Protein (dry)	402/cup	100	6.3	220	90	19.4	160	100
Royal Canin Feline Renal Support T (3 oz can)	82/can	100	6.6	190	100	26.0	160	140
Hill's Prescription Diet k/d Feline with Tuna (5.5 oz can)	170/can	104	6.6	247	56	26.3	174	140
Hill's Prescription Diet k/d + Mobility Chicken & Vegetable Stew (2.9 oz can)	68/can	108	6.6	234	54	43.4	198	180
BLUE Natural Veterinary Diet KM Kidney + Mobility Support (5.5 oz can)	156/can	110	6.1	560	50	55.0	160	150

(continued on next page)

Table 3
(continued)

Feline Renal Diets	Calories (kcal)	Phosphorus (mg)	Protein (g)	Potassium (mg)	Sodium (mg)	Vit D (IU)	Calcium (mg)	EPA & DHA (mg)
Purina Pro Plan Veterinary Diets NF Early Care (5.5 oz can)	162/can	110	9.7	380	100	22.3	150	120
Royal Canin Feline Renal Support A (dry)	347/cup	110	5.8	230	90	20.3	210	100
Royal Canin Feline Renal Support F (dry)	376/cup	110	6.5	230	100	22.5	160	100
Hill's Prescription Diet k/d Feline Chicken & Vegetable Stew (2.9 oz can)	70/can	111	6.8	239	53	44.2	176	133
Hill's Prescription Diet k/d + Mobility Feline (dry)	483/cup	115	6.6	188	63	17.5	160	191
Hill's Prescription Diet k/d Vegetable & Tuna Stew (2.9 oz can)	77/can	115	7.1	247	57	36.8	193	145
Hill's Prescription Diet k/d Feline (dry)	541/cup	116	6.8	169	58	28.8	163	115
Hill's Prescription Diet k/d Feline with Ocean Fish (dry)	444/cup	118	6.7	168	59	43.3	167	131
Hill's Prescription Diet k/d Feline with Chicken (5.5 oz can)	177/can	120	7.6	279	61	28.3	215	155
Royal Canin Feline Renal Support Early Consult (3 oz can)	82/can	120	8.4	180	90	17.8	160	170
Hill's Prescription Diet k/d Early Support Feline Chicken (dry)	536/cup	127	7.7	170	57	23.7	170	112
BLUE Natural Veterinary Diet KM Kidney + Mobility Support (dry)	425/cup	130	6.9	220	70	43.4	140	220
Royal Canin Feline Renal Support Early consult (dry)	299/cup	130	7.3	210	100	20.9	180	200

Hill's Prescription Diet k/d Early Support Feline Chicken, Vegetable & Rice Stew (2.9 oz can)	79/can	133	7.6	210	61	31.5	198	174
2020 AAFCO Feline adult maintenance minimum		125	6.5	150	50	7.0	150	–
2020 AAFCO Feline adult maintenance maximum		–	–	–	–	75.2	–	–

Diets are listed by ascending phosphorus concentrations. Association of American Feed Control Officials (AAFCO) minimum and maximum (when applicable) nutrient requirements for feline adult maintenance are provided for reference.

*Note that nutrient profiles can change approximately every 6 to 12 mo.

1.5 g protein per kilogram BW (2.1 g/kg BW)$^{0.75}$ was needed. However, to maintain LBM, 5.2 g protein per kilogram BW (7.8 g/kg BW)$^{0.75}$ was required.[49] Another consideration is that dietary AA profiles can differ between diets even if crude protein is similar.[48,53] Diets enhanced with essential AAs may be able to better maintain LBM.[53,54]

There are diets available that provide lower phosphorus concentrations (ie, <1.00–1.35 g/Mcal; <100–135 mg/100 kcal) and higher protein concentrations, which may be preferable in some instances (eg, to better allow the maintenance of LBM, for young dog with renal dysplasia). For both dogs and cats, there may be additional diets that are not specifically marketed for kidney disease that meet these nutritional goals (**Table 4**).

One exception to feeding a higher protein diet is when proteinuria is present. Proteinuria can be diagnosed in dogs and cats with kidney disease as a primary disease process, most commonly glomerular disease or as a sequela of tubulointerstitial kidney disease. Typically the term PLN is reserved for cases of glomerular disease, and most clinicians consider a urine protein:creatinine ratio of 2.0 or more to be significant. Recommendations for when to initiate therapy for dogs and cats with proteinuria may vary depending on the presence of azotemia, but the importance of addressing proteinuria should be apparent, because it has been associated with decreased survival in dogs and cats with kidney disease.[31,33,55–59] Although most of the veterinary literature on PLN relates to dogs, cats may also be diagnosed with significant proteinuria.[60] The management of proteinuria relies on both medical and dietary interventions, including decreasing protein intake.[61]

The goal of nutritional modification with PLN is to decrease dietary protein enough to decrease proteinuria, but not so much as to contribute to LBM loss. The proposed mechanism for the benefit of protein restriction is a decreased glomerular filtration rate and subsequent decrease in structural damage to the remaining glomeruli.[62] Given the tremendous variability in protein concentration among commercially available diets, the recommended degree of protein reduction is highly dependent on the individual animal's diet. It is extremely important to obtain a complete and thorough diet history, including information about treats, dietary supplements, and foods used for medication administration. If the animal's diet is very high in protein when PLN is diagnosed, it may be unnecessary to transition that animal to a veterinary renal diet. If the animal is receiving a large percentage of calories from high-protein treats (eg, chicken breast, rawhides, dental chews), modification of the treats alone may sufficiently decrease the animal's protein intake.[63]

This author recommends initially decreasing the total dietary protein by 25% to 50%, depending on the severity of proteinuria, azotemia, and clinical signs. Dietary protein restriction typically results in a decrease in proteinuria within 1 month. If the animal's diet already is low to moderate in protein concentration (near the AAFCO minimum recommendation for adult maintenance), it may be preferable to allow medical management time to decrease proteinuria before further restricting dietary protein.

A possible approach to optimize dietary restriction of protein without contributing to LBM loss is to strategically supplement AAs. In people with PLN, feeding low-protein diets with concurrent supplementation of keto acids or essential AAs is advantageous because it can improve protein status while minimizing nitrogen load.[64–67] This concept is related to the ability of keto acids to stimulate protein synthesis while inhibiting protein breakdown. This dietary regimen can improve hypoalbuminemia and decrease proteinuria.[64]

Dogs with PLN have decreased concentrations of several AAs as compared with healthy controls.[68] Oral essential AA supplementation for 4 to 8 weeks in dogs with

Table 4
Nonrenal diets that may be appropriate for dogs and cats with CKD

	Calories (kcal)	Phosphorus (mg)	Protein (g)	Sodium (mg)	Potassium (mg)	Vitamin D (IU)	Calcium (mg)	EPA and DHA (mg)
Canine Diets								
Hill's Prescription Diet t/d Canine (dry)	248/cup	107	4.5	58	173	15.2	157	1
Hill's Prescription Diet g/d Canine (can)	388/can	109	4.9	56	188	53.9	200	3
Hill's Prescription Diet g/d Canine (dry)	361/cup	110	4.6	50	179	25.2	149	6
Royal Canin Canine Hepatic (14.4 oz can)	527/can	110	4.6	60	200	12.7	170	80
Hill's Prescription Diet j/d Canine (dry)	353/cup	117	4.6	47	190	14	151	200
Feline diets								
Royal Canin Feline Health Nutrition Aging 12+ thin slices in gravy (3 oz)	71/can	115	11.0	94	178	23.0	146	167
Royal Canin Feline Health Nutrition Aging 12+ loaf in sauce (5.8 oz)	139/can	116	10.5	105	2.00	22.1	158	158
Hill's Science Diet Adult Tender Tuna Dinner Cat Food (5.5 oz can)	162/can	127	10.1	117	172	79.6	194	187
Hill's Science Diet Adult 7+ Tender Tuna Dinner Cat Food (5.5 oz)	152/can	129	9.9	112	174	78.4	203	50
Hill's Science Diet Adult 11+ Healthy Cuisine Seared Tuna and Carrot Medley Cat Food (2.8 oz)	66/can	135	8.9	90	213	45.3	187	152

Diets are listed by ascending phosphorus concentrations. Nutrients are listed on a per 100 kcal basis. This is not an all-inclusive list.
*Note that nutrient profiles can change approximately every 6 to 12 mo.

renal proteinuria resulted in increased serum albumin concentrations and BW with no effect on the urine protein:creatinine ratio.[69] It remains unclear whether the lack of decrease in the urine protein:creatinine ratio is clinically as important as the increase in albumin and BW.

Potassium

Serum potassium concentrations may be abnormal owing to underlying kidney disease, dietary intake, acid–base abnormalities, gastrointestinal complications, or medications. It is reported that 20% to 30% of cats with CKD will develop hypokalemia.[70,71] Hypokalemia may result in muscle weakness, polyuria, polydipsia, and constipation.[72] There is a wide range of potassium currently available in veterinary renal diets (see **Tables 1** and **2**). Thus, if hypokalemia is present, it may be helpful to offer a higher potassium-containing diet or oral potassium supplementation with either potassium gluconate or potassium citrate.[73,74]

Dogs with CKD can develop either hypokalemia or hyperkalemia.[74,75] Medications that influence the renin–angiotensin–aldosterone system (eg, angiotensin-converting enzyme inhibitors, angiotensin receptor antagonists) may contribute to hyperkalemia and the doses may need to be adjusted.[61] Additionally, the dietary intake of potassium may exceed renal excretory capability. In these cases, choosing a lower potassium-containing diet may alleviate the hyperkalemia. If feeding a commercial diet is ineffective, then a decreased potassium home-prepared diet may be considered.[75] It is also important to ensure that pseuduohyperkalemia (eg, from thrombocytosis) is not falsely affecting therapeutic recommendations.[76]

Sodium

The role of dietary sodium restriction for dogs and cats with CKD is controversial. Studies in people and experimental canine models suggest that high sodium intake contributes to hypertension, nephrotoxicity, and progression of proteinuria.[77,78] In 1 study that included 6 cats with renal insufficiency, feeding a high sodium diet (2.9 g/Mcal; 290 mg/100 kcal), increased the serum concentrations of creatinine, urea nitrogen, and phosphorus. There was no effect noted on blood pressure.[79] Given these findings, it has generally been recommended to avoid high sodium intake in dogs and cats with CKD. Conversely, in other larger long-term studies, there have been no adverse effects on renal function noted in cats fed high sodium diets (2.9–3.1 g/Mcal; 290–310 mg/100 kcal).[80,81]

In contrast, there are several studies in rats, dogs, and cats that demonstrate adverse effects from excessive restriction of sodium, including activation of the renin–angiotensin–aldosterone system and subsequent kaliuresis.[82–84] Some evidence in people suggests that the dietary sodium to potassium ratio plays a larger role in determination of hypertension or relative risk of CKD than either nutrient alone.[85,86] An inverse relationship between hypokalemia and systemic hypertension has been documented in cats,[87] and consideration is given to the prevalence of a relative or absolute hyperaldosteronism contributing to both.[88]

One of the biggest issues with regards to recommendations for dietary sodium intake is the lack of standardization for what is considered a high, moderate, or low sodium intake. Diets that are typically promoted as reduced in sodium for dogs and cats can provide up to 2 to 5 times the AAFCO minimums for cats and dogs, respectively. This author does not currently specifically aim to feed a reduced sodium diet to animals with CKD; however, this is often a moot point because all veterinary therapeutic renal diets exceed AAFCO minimums (see **Tables 2** and **3**).

Metabolic acidosis

Metabolic acidosis is a common complication observed with CKD.[70,89] In people, metabolic acidosis decreases the glomerular filtration rate, induces muscle wasting, and decreases muscle protein synthesis.[90] In cats, overt metabolic acidosis may not be recognized until late-stage disease, and there are minimal data to specifically suggest that metabolic acidosis precedes worsening renal function.[91] It is likely, however, that the blood pH is remaining normal in many animals with CKD at the expense of bone health because increased dietary acid loads cause bone to resorb calcium.[92] In dogs and cats with CKD, bone quality is affected, likely owing to a complex relationship between metabolic acidosis and other hormonal derangements observed with CKD-MBD (eg, hyperparathyroidism, increased FGF-23).[93,94] Veterinary therapeutic renal diets are typically fortified with alkalinizing agents (eg, potassium citrate). For animals that develop metabolic acidosis, treatment with additional potassium citrate or sodium bicarbonate may be considered.[89]

Vitamin D

Derangements in vitamin D metabolism are commonly identified in dogs and cats with CKD. Dogs with both CKD and nonazotemic PLN tend to have lower serum 25-hydroxyvitamin D (25[OH]D) and 1,25-dihydroxyvitamin D (1,25[OH]$_2$D; calcitriol) concentrations than healthy dogs.[95,96] These metabolites decrease with increasing International Renal Interest Society stage.[95] Cats with CKD have lower calcitriol concentrations than healthy cats, and cats with end-stage CKD show significantly lower concentrations than cats with compensated disease.[97] Derangements in vitamin D metabolism likely influence the development of CKD-MBD (**Fig. 2**).[35]

For several decades, calcitriol treatment has been recommended to reduce parathyroid hormone concentrations and improve quality of life in dogs and cats with CKD.[98,99] However, the cost, monitoring, and potential for toxicity (eg, hypercalcemia) are sometimes limiting factors for pet owners. Additional research is needed to determine the manner in which supplementation with various forms of vitamin D influences vitamin D repletion, parathyroid hormone, and FGF-23 concentrations, quality of life, preservation of renal function, and survival.

There does not seem to be a clear relationship between dietary vitamin D$_3$ (ie, cholecalciferol) intake and subsequent serum 25(OH)D concentrations in dogs[100,101]; thus, simply increasing cholecalciferol intake is not likely by itself to improve vitamin D status based on 25(OH)D concentration. However, in 1 study that investigated the usefulness of cholecalciferol supplementation for treatment of canine atopy, very high doses (range, 300–2700 IU/kg) did increase serum 25(OH)D concentrations by 250% (a mean increase of 80 μg/mL).[102] It is important to note that these doses exceed the AAFCO maximum recommendations for vitamin D intake.

Providing an extended-release formulation of 25(OH)D (calcifediol) to dogs with CKD rapidly increased serum 25(OH)D concentrations.[103] Additional studies are underway to elucidate appropriate dosing recommendations and to determine effects on the complex pathophysiology of CKD-MBD. It has yet to be determined if increased 25(OH)D concentrations will translate to improved survival or quality of life for dogs with CKD.

Calcium

Dogs and cats with CKD may develop derangements in calcium homeostasis.[95,97,104,105] There is a risk of soft tissue mineralization when the calcium × phosphorus product exceeds 60 to 70 mg^2/dL.[106] An increased calcium × phosphorus product has been associated with decreased survival in dogs with CKD.[59,106] Ionized hypercalcemia is often present in cats with CKD.[105] Some cats may have concurrent

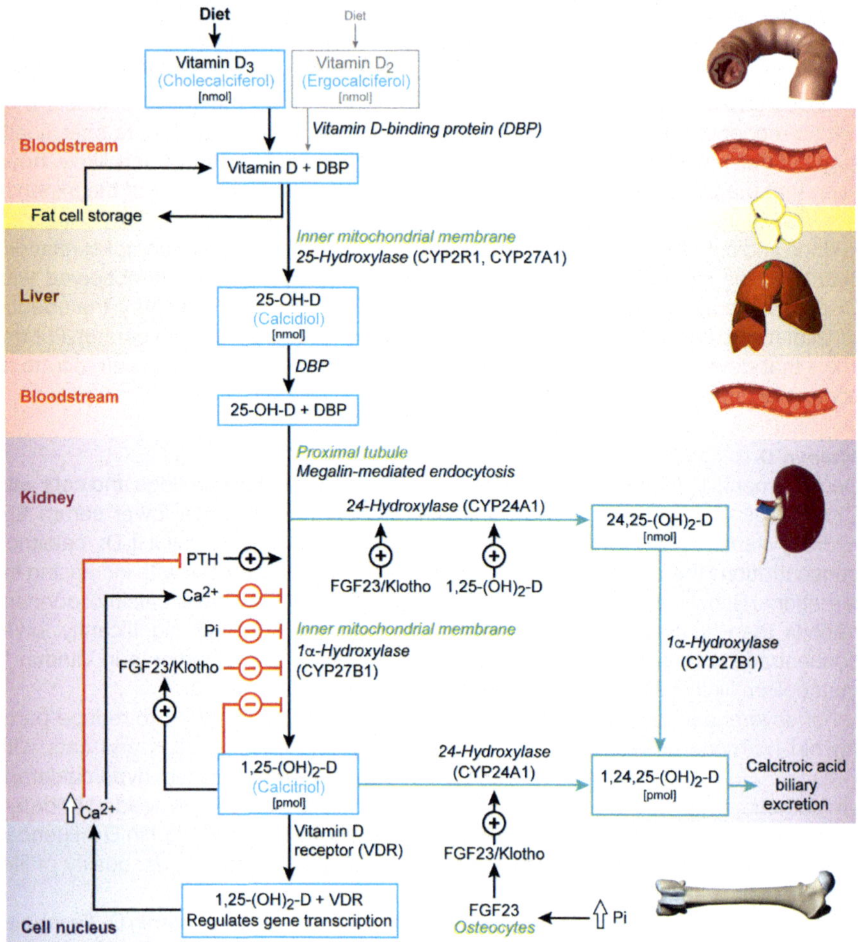

Fig. 2. Comprehensive overview of vitamin D metabolism, starting with dietary intake and progressing through hepatic and renal transformation. Also notice the influences of phosphate (Pi), ionized calcium (Ca^{2+}), FGF-23, Klotho, and parathyroid hormone (PTH). CYP, cytochrome P450. (Reproduced with permission of The Ohio State University.)

CKD and idiopathic hypercalcemia; however, there may be additional pathophysiologic mechanisms by which cats with CKD develop ionized hypercalcemia. Feeding a reduced phosphorus diet may contribute to the development of ionized hypercalcemia, and hypercalcemia may subsequently be managed by feeding a higher phosphorus diet and by manipulating the dietary calcium to phosphorus ratio.[107] Several other nutritional strategies have been suggested for addressing ionized hypercalcemia in cats (eg, increasing fiber, decreasing dietary calcium intake, and limiting the intake of vitamins A and D).[108] However, additional research is needed to understand the pathophysiology and treatment of hypercalcemia in CKD.

Omega-3 fatty acids and supplement use

Many pet owners have the desire to provide additional dietary supplements and nutraceuticals to their pets with CKD. In 1 study, 38% of pet owners administered vitamins, minerals, or other supplements to their cats with CKD.[109] There are a plethora of supplements marketed for patients with kidney disease. Careful selection of type, dose, and brand is important to avoid toxicities or lack of efficacy.[110] This process entails a consideration of the specific brand (eg, reputable, tested by an independent company), potential benefits (research driven vs hypothetical), risks (known or hypothetical), and interaction with other medications and supplements. Some supplements provide unwanted calories and added nutrients that may be nominal or, alternatively, toxic. Additionally, for an animal that is already wary of taking its necessary medication(s), forcing it to take unnecessary (or even potentially harmful) supplements may add undue stress.

This author routinely recommends omega-3 fatty acid supplementation with eicosopentaenoic acid (EPA) and docosahexaenoic acid (DHA) for their anti-inflammatory properties. In experimental models, EPA/DHA supplementation reduced proteinuria; however, this finding has not been demonstrated clearly in naturally occurring disease. Although an optimal dose of EPA/DHA for animals with kidney disease has not been determined, general dose recommendations for dogs include 50 to 75 mg/kg or up to 140 mg EPA and DHA/kg $(BW)^{0.75}$.[111,112] Many veterinary therapeutic renal diets have added EPA/DHA, and the amounts provided should be determined based on the pet's caloric intake (ie, mg EPA/DHA per 100 kcal ingested daily). It can then be decided whether or not to add to the total dose.

Other diet options

If the animal will not eat, or if the owner is unwilling to feed, any available veterinary therapeutic renal diet options, there may be some other diets (either veterinary therapeutic diets marketed for other diseases or over-the-counter commercial diets) that still provide acceptable nutrient profiles. The author typically considers phosphorus as the primary nutrient of concern for CKD, and subsequently aims to provide less than 1.5 g phosphorus/Mcal (150 mg/100 kcal) to dogs and cats with CKD (see **Table 4**). Not all senior diets are appropriate options for animals with CKD, and careful attention must be paid to specific nutrient profiles.

Comorbid patients and home-cooked diets

Choosing an appropriate diet for dogs and cats with comorbid conditions can be challenging, because each patient's needs are unique. Nutritional management goals must be identified and prioritized to achieve the results most favorable to the patient's overall health and quality of life. For example, in the case of a dog with relatively mild CKD and chronic, recurrent pancreatitis, there may be preference to prioritize feeding a low fat diet that is moderate in phosphorus (eg, <2.0 g/Mcal; 200 mg/100 kcal). In a cat with concurrent CKD and inflammatory bowel disease, feeding a low to moderate phosphorus limited antigen diet would be recommended. Even when appropriate commercial diet options are available, pet owners may elect to feed home-prepared diets to their pets.

Studies have shown that most recipes that pet owners will find online or in books, including those designed for pets with CKD, do not provide complete and balanced nutrition.[113–115] Thus, for owners who prefer to feed a home-prepared diet, or if a suitable diet cannot be identified, a board certified veterinary nutritionist should be consulted (http://acvn.org). It is imperative that owners follow instructions closely to avoid contributing to nutritional deficiencies or toxicities. Many pet owners have trouble following explicit instructions over time, so monitoring is important.[116]

SUMMARY

Dogs and cats are affected by different forms of kidney disease, and nutritional management will vary accordingly. It is best practice when determining a nutritional plan for any dog or cat to consider that animal as an individual. The animal's energy needs and specific nutrients of concern should be determined first. Using that information, appropriate diet options can be chosen and offered. Maintaining adequate energy intake is of utmost importance in CKD patients. Concurrent medical management may be required in many cases, and assisted enteral nutritional support can offer sustenance for hyporexic patients.

CLINICS CARE POINTS

- Dogs and cats with kidney disease commonly develop dysrexia and exhibit weight loss.
- Body composition measurements (ie, BW, BCS, MCS) can have diagnostic and prognostic implications for dogs and cats with kidney disease.
- Optimal nutritional management of kidney disease varies by disease type (eg, CKD, PLN).
- Assisted enteral nutrition can alleviate the stress that owners feel with hyporexic animals and can allow for provision of optimal nutritional support.

DISCLOSURE

The author has received research funding from Purina, Hill's and Royal Canin.

REFERENCES

1. Baldwin K, Buffington T, Freeman LM, et al. AAHA nutritional assessment guidelines for dogs and cats. J Am Anim Hosp Assoc 2010;46:285–96.
2. Freeman LM, Lachaud MP, Matthews S, et al. Evaluation of weight loss over time in cats with chronic kidney disease. J Vet Intern Med 2016;30:1661–6.
3. Parker VJ, Freeman LM. Association between body condition and survival in dogs with acquired chronic kidney Disease. J Vet Intern Med 2011;25:1306–11.
4. Pedrinelli V, Lima DM, Duarte CN, et al. Nutritional and laboratory parameters affect the survival of dogs with chronic kidney disease. PLoS One 2020;15:e0234712.
5. Mak RH, Ikizler AT, Kovesdy CP, et al. Wasting in chronic kidney disease. J Cachexia Sarcopenia Muscle 2011;2:9–25.
6. Wang XH, Mitch WE. Mechanisms of muscle wasting in chronic kidney disease. Nat Rev Nephrol 2014;10:504–16.
7. Obi Y, Qader H, Kovesdy CP, et al. Latest consensus and update on protein-energy wasting in chronic kidney disease. Curr Opin Clin Nutr 2015;18:254–62.
8. Carrero JJ, Thomas F, Nagy K, et al. Global prevalence of protein-energy wasting in kidney disease: a meta-analysis of contemporary observational studies from the international society of renal nutrition and metabolism. J Ren Nutr 2018;28:380–92.
9. Hutchinson D, Sutherland-Smith J, Watson AL, et al. Assessment of methods of evaluating sarcopenia in old dogs. Am J Vet Res 2012;73:1794–800.
10. Freeman LM, Sutherland-Smith J, Cummings C, et al. Evaluation of a quantitatively derived value for assessment of muscle mass in clinically normal cats. Am J Vet Res 2018;79:1188–92.

11. Freeman LM, Michel KE, Zanghi BM, et al. Evaluation of the use of muscle condition score and ultrasonographic measurements for assessment of muscle mass in dogs. Am J Vet Res 2019;80(6):595–600.
12. Rayhel LH, Quimby JM, Green EM, et al. Intra- and inter-rater reliability in the cross-sectional area of feline lumbar epaxial musculature evaluated via abdominal CT scan. J Feline Med Surg 2020;22(8):721–8.
13. Ramsey JJ. Determining energy requirements. In: Fascetti AJ, Delaney SJ, editors. Applied veterinary clinical nutrition. 1st edition. West Sussex: Wiley-Blackwell; 2012. p. 23–45.
14. Quimby JM, Brock WT, Moses K, et al. Chronic use of maropitant for the management of vomiting and inappetence in cats with chronic kidney disease: a blinded, placebo-controlled clinical trial. J Feline Med Surg 2015;17:692–7.
15. Quimby JM, Lake RC, Hansen RJ, et al. Oral, subcutaneous, and intravenous pharmacokinetics of ondansetron in healthy cats. J Vet Pharmacol Ther 2014; 37:348–53.
16. Peters RM, Goldstein RE, Erb HN, et al. Histopathologic features of canine uremic gastropathy: a retrospective study. J Vet Intern Med 2005;19:315–20.
17. McLeland SM, Lunn KF, Duncan CG, et al. Relationship among serum creatinine, serum gastrin, calcium-phosphorus product, and uremic gastropathy in cats with chronic kidney disease. J Vet Intern Med 2014;28:827–37.
18. Marks SL, Kook PH, Papich MG, et al. ACVIM consensus statement: support for rational administration of gastrointestinal protectants to dogs and cats. J Vet Intern Med 2018;32:1823–40.
19. Crivellenti LZ, Borin-Crivellenti S, Fertal KL, et al. Occult gastrointestinal bleeding is a common finding in dogs with chronic kidney disease. Vet Clin Pathol 2017;46:132–7.
20. Rhodes L, Zollers B, Wofford JA, et al. Capromorelin: a ghrelin receptor agonist and novel therapy for stimulation of appetite in dogs. Vet Med Sci 2018;4:3–16.
21. Wofford JA, Zollers B, Rhodes L, et al. Evaluation of the safety of daily administration of capromorelin in cats. J Vet Pharmacol Ther 2018;41:324–33.
22. Quimby JM, Lunn KF. Mirtazapine as an appetite stimulant and anti-emetic in cats with chronic kidney disease: a masked placebo-controlled crossover clinical trial. Vet J 2013;197:651–5.
23. Poole M, Quimby JM, Hu T, et al. A double-blind, placebo-controlled, randomized study to evaluate the weight gain drug, mirtazapine transdermal ointment, in cats with unintended weight loss. J Vet Pharmacol Ther 2019;42:179–88.
24. Ross S. Utilization of feeding tubes in the management of feline chronic kidney disease. Vet Clin North Am 2016;46:1099–114.
25. Ireland LM, Hohenhaus AE, Broussard JD, et al. A comparison of owner management and complications in 67 cats with esophagostomy and percutaneous endoscopic gastrostomy feeding tubes. J Am Anim Hosp Assoc 2003;39:241–6.
26. Campbell SJ, Marks SL, Yoshimoto SK, et al. Complications and outcomes of one-step low-profile gastrostomy devices for long-term enteral feeding in dogs and cats. J Am Anim Hosp Assoc 2006;42:197–206.
27. Elliott J, Rawlings JM, Markwell PJ, et al. Survival of cats with naturally occurring chronic renal failure: effect of dietary management. J Small Anim Pract 2000;41: 235–42.
28. Jacob F, Polzin DJ, Osborne CA, et al. Clinical evaluation of dietary modification for treatment of spontaneous chronic renal failure in dogs. J Am Vet Med Assoc 2002;220:1163–70.

29. Ross SJ, Osborne CA, Kirk CA, et al. Clinical evaluation of dietary modification for treatment of spontaneous chronic kidney disease in cats. J Am Vet Med Assoc 2006;229:949–57.
30. Finco DR, Brown SA, Crowell WA, et al. Effects of dietary phosphorus and protein in dogs with chronic renal failure. Am J Vet Rew 1992;53:2264–71.
31. King JN, Tasker S, Gunn-Moore DA, et al. Prognostic factors in cats with chronic kidney disease. J Vet Intern Med 2007;21:906–16.
32. Boyd LM, Langston C, Thompson K, et al. Survival in cats with naturally occurring chronic kidney disease. J Vet Intern Med 2008;22:1111–7.
33. Kuwahara Y, Ohba Y, Kitoh K, et al. Association of laboratory data and death within one month in cats with chronic renal failure. J Small Anim Pract 2006; 47(8):446–50.
34. de Brito Galvao JF, Nagode LA, Schenck PA, et al. Calcitriol, calcidiol, parathyroid hormone, and fibroblast growth factor-23 interactions in chronic kidney disease. J Vet Emerg Crit Care 2013;23:134–62.
35. Foster JD. Update on mineral and bone disorders in chronic kidney disease. Vet Clin North Am 2016;46:1131–49.
36. Geddes RF, Elliott J, Syme HM. The effect of feeding a renal diet on plasma fibroblast growth factor 23 concentrations in cats with stable azotemic chronic kidney disease. J Vet Intern Med 2013;27:1354–61.
37. IRIS Treatment Recommendations for CKD. Available at: http://www.iris-kidney.com/guidelines/recommendations.shtml. Accessed July 6, 2020.
38. Kidder AC, Chew D. Treatment options for hyperphosphatemia in feline CKD: what's out there? J Feline Med Surg 2009;11:913–24.
39. Alexander J, Stockman J, Atwal J, et al. Effects of the long-term feeding of diets enriched with inorganic phosphorus on the adult feline kidney and phosphorus metabolism. Br J Nutr 2018;121:1–21.
40. Böswald LF, Kienzle E, Dobenecker B. Observation about phosphorus and protein supply in cats and dogs prior to the diagnosis of chronic kidney disease. J Anim Phys Anim Nutr 2018;102(Suppl 1):31–6.
41. Dobenecker B, Webel A, Reese S, et al. Effect of a high phosphorus diet on indicators of renal health in cats. J Feline Med Surg 2018;20:339–43.
42. Dobenecker B, Hertel-Böhnke P, Webel A, et al. Renal phosphorus excretion in adult healthy cats after the intake of high phosphorus diets with either calcium monophosphate or sodium monophosphate. J Anim Phys Anim Nutr 2018;102: 1759–65.
43. Scherk MA, Laflamme DP. Controversies in veterinary nephrology: renal diets are indicated for cats with international renal interest society chronic kidney disease stages 2 to 4: the con view. Vet Clin North Am 2016;46:1067–94.
44. Polzin DJ, Churchill JA. Controversies in veterinary nephrology: renal diets are indicated for cats with international renal interest society chronic kidney disease stages 2 to 4: the pro view. Vet Clin North Am 2016;46:1049–65.
45. Larsen JA. Controversies in veterinary nephrology: differing viewpoints: role of dietary protein in the management of feline chronic kidney disease. Vet Clin North Am 2016;46:1095–8.
46. Hanna RM, Ghobry L, Wassef O, et al. A practical approach to nutrition, protein-energy wasting, sarcopenia, and cachexia in patients with chronic kidney disease. Blood Purif 2020;49:202–11.
47. Ikizler TA, Cano NJ, Franch H, et al. Prevention and treatment of protein energy wasting in chronic kidney disease patients: a consensus statement by the international society of renal nutrition and metabolism. Kidney Int 2013;84:1096–107.

48. Wakshlag JJ, Barr SC, Ordway GA, et al. Effect of dietary protein on lean body wasting in dogs: correlation between loss of lean mass and markers of proteasome-dependent proteolysis. J Anim Physiol Anim Nutr 2003;87:408–20.
49. Laflamme DP, Hannah SS. Discrepancy between use of lean body mass or nitrogen balance to determine protein requirements for adult cats. J Feline Med Surg 2013;15(8):691–7.
50. Sanderson SL, Tetrick M, Brown SA, et al. Effect of dietary approach on clinical outcome measures in dogs with naturally occurring chronic kidney disease (abstract). J Anim Physiol Anim Nutr 2013;97:1198–9.
51. Wannemacher RW Jr, McCoy JR. Determination of optimal dietary protein requirements of young and old dogs. J Nutr 1966;88:66–74.
52. Wichert B, Schade L, Gebert S, et al. Energy and protein needs of cats for maintenance, gestation and lactation. J Feline Med Surg 2009;11:808–15.
53. Hall JA, Fritsch DA, Jewell DE, et al. Cats with IRIS stage 1 and 2 chronic kidney disease maintain body weight and lean muscle mass when fed food having increased caloric density, and enhanced concentrations of carnitine and essential amino acids. Vet Rec 2019;184:190–200.
54. Kovesdy CP, Kopple JD, Kalantar-Zadeh K. Management of protein-energy wasting in non-dialysis-dependent chronic kidney disease: reconciling low protein intake with nutritional therapy. Am J Clin Nutr 2013;97:1163–77.
55. Cook AK, Cowgill LD. Clinical and pathological features of protein-losing glomerular disease in the dog: a review of 137 cases. J Am Anim Hosp Assoc 1996;32:313–22.
56. Jacob F, Polzin DJ, Osborne CA, et al. Evaluation of the association between initial proteinuria and morbidity rate or death in dogs with naturally occurring chronic renal failure. J Am Vet Med Assoc 2005;226:393–400.
57. Syme HM, Markwell PJ, Pfeiffer D, et al. Survival of cats with naturally occurring chronic renal failure is related to severity of proteinuria. J Vet Intern Med 2006; 20:528–35.
58. Wehner A, Hartmann K, Hirschberger J. Associations between proteinuria, systemic hypertension and glomerular filtration rate in dogs with renal and nonrenal diseases. Vet Rec 2008;162:141–7.
59. Rudinsky AJ, Harjes LM, Byron J, et al. Factors associated with survival in dogs with chronic kidney disease. J Vet Intern Med 2018;32:1977–82.
60. Rayhel LH, Quimby JM, Cianciolo RE, et al. Clinicopathologic and pathologic characteristics of feline proteinuric kidney disease. J Feline Med Surg 2020. https://doi.org/10.1177/1098612X20921056.
61. Brown S, Wlliott J, Francey T, et al. Consensus recommendations for standard therapy for glomerular disease in dogs. J Vet Intern Med 2013;27:S27–43.
62. Valli VE, Baumal R, Thorer P, et al. Dietary modification reduces splitting of glomerular basement membranes and delays death due to renal failure in canine X-linked hereditary nephritis. Lab Invest 1991;65:67–73.
63. Parker VJ, Freeman LM. Nutritional management of protein-losing nephropathy in dogs. Compendium 2012;E1–5.
64. Walser M, Hill S, Tomalis EA. Treatment of nephrotic adults with a supplemented, very low-protein diet. Am J Kidney Dis 1996;28:354–64.
65. Aparicio M, Chauveau P, De Precigout V, et al. Nutrition and outcome on renal replacement therapy of patients with chronic renal failure treated by a supplemented very low protein diet. J Am Soc Nephrol 2000;11:708–16.

66. Aparicio M, Bellizzi V, Chauveau P, et al. Protein-restricted diets plus keto/amino acids - A valid therapeutic approach for chronic kidney disease patients. J Ren Nutr 2012;22:S1–21.
67. Koppe L, de Oliveira MC, Fouque D. Ketoacid analogues supplementation in chronic kidney disease and future perspectives. Nutrients 2019;11:2071.
68. Parker VJ, Fascetti AJ, Klamer BG. Amino acid status in dogs with protein-losing nephropathy. J Vet Intern Med 2019;33:680–5.
69. Zatelli A, D'Ippolito P, Roura X, et al. Short-term effects of dietary supplementation with amino acids in dogs with proteinuric chronic kidney disease. Can Vet J 2017;58:1287–93.
70. DiBartvalola SP, Rutgers HC, Zack PM, et al. Clinicopathologic findings associated with chronic renal disease in cats: 74 cases. J Am Vet Med Assoc 1987;190:1196–202.
71. Elliott J, Barber PJ. Feline chronic renal failure: clinical findings in 80 cases diagnosed between 1992 and 1995. J Small Anim Pract 1998;39:78–85.
72. Phillips SL, Polzin DJ. Clinical disorders of potassium homeostasis. Hyperkalemia and hypokalemia. Vet Clin North Am 1998;28:545–64.
73. Sieberg LG, Quimby JM. Retrospective study of the efficacy of oral potassium supplementation in cats with kidney disease. J Feline Med Surg 2020;22:539–43.
74. Bartges JW. Chronic kidney disease in dogs and cats. Vet Clin North Am 2012;42:669–92.
75. Segev G, Fascetti AJ, Weeth LP, et al. Correction of hyperkalemia in dogs with chronic kidney disease consuming commercial renal therapeutic diets by a potassium-reduced home-prepared diet. J Vet Intern Med 2010;24:546–50.
76. Woolcock AD, Keenan A, Cheung C, et al. Thrombocytosis in 715 Dogs. J Vet Intern Med 2017;31:1691–9.
77. Ritz E, Koleganova N, Piecha G. Role of sodium intake in the progression of chronic kidney disease. J Ren Nutr 2009;19:61–2.
78. Vogel JA. Salt-induced hypertension in the dog. Am J Physiol 1966;210:186–90.
79. Kirk CA, Jewell DE, Lowry SR. Effects of sodium chloride on selected parameters in cats. Vet Ther 2006;7:333–46.
80. Xu H, Laflamme DP, Long GL. Effects of dietary sodium chloride on health parameters in mature cats. J Feline Med Surg 2009;11:435–41.
81. Reynolds BS, Chetboul V, Nguyen P, et al. Effects of dietary salt intake on renal function: a 2-year study in healthy aged cats. J Vet Intern Med 2013;27:507–15.
82. Okamoto C, Hayakawa Y, Aoyama T, et al. Excessively low salt diet damages the heart through activation of cardiac (pro) renin receptor, renin-angiotensin-aldosterone, and sympatho-adrenal systems in spontaneously hypertensive rats. PLoS One 2017;12(12):e0189099.
83. Miller WL, Borgeson DD, Grantham JA, et al. Dietary sodium modulation of aldosterone activation and renal function during the progression of experimental heart failure. Eur J Heart Fail 2015;17:144–50.
84. Buranakarl C, Mathur S, Brown SA. Effects of dietary sodium chloride intake on renal function and blood pressure in cats with normal and reduced renal function. Am J Vet Res 2004;65:620–7.
85. Perez V, Chang ET. Sodium-to-potassium ratio and blood pressure, hypertension, and related factors. Adv Nutr 2014;5:712–41.
86. Mirmiran P, Nazeri P, Bahadoran Z, et al. Dietary Sodium to potassium ratio and the incidence of chronic kidney disease in adults: a longitudinal follow-up study. Prev Nutr Food Sci 2018;23:87–93.

87. Syme HM, Barber PJ, Markwell PJ, et al. Prevalence of systolic hypertension in cats with chronic renal failure at initial evaluation. J Am Vet Med Assoc 2002; 220:1799–804.
88. Syme H. Hypertension in small animal kidney disease. Vet Clin North Am 2011; 41(1):63–89.
89. Langston C. Managing fluid and electrolyte disorders in kidney disease. Vet Clin North Am 2017;47(2):471–90.
90. Kalantar-Zadeh K, Mehrotra R, Fouque D, et al. Metabolic acidosis and malnutrition-inflammation complex syndrome in chronic renal failure. Semin Dial 2004;17:455–65.
91. Elliott J, Syme HM, Reubens E, et al. Assessment of acid-base status of cats with naturally occurring chronic renal failure. J Small Anim Pract 2003;44:65–70.
92. Bushinsky DA. Acid-base imbalance and the skeleton. Eur J Nutr 2001;40: 238–44.
93. Shipov A, Segev G, Meltzer H, et al. The effect of naturally occurring chronic kidney disease on the micro-structural and mechanical properties of bone. PLoS One 2014;9:e110057.
94. Shipov A, Shahar R, Sugar N, et al. The influence of chronic kidney disease on the structural and mechanical properties of canine bone. J Vet Intern Med 2018; 32:280–7.
95. Parker VJ, Harjes LM, Dembek K, et al. Association of vitamin D metabolites with parathyroid hormone, fibroblast growth factor-23, calcium, and phosphorus in dogs with various stages of chronic kidney disease. J Vet Intern Med 2017; 31:791–8.
96. Miller MS, Klamer BG, Chew DJ, et al. Association between vitamin D metabolites, vitamin D binding protein, and proteinuria in dogs. J Vet Intern Med 2020; 34(6):2468–77.
97. Barber PJ, Elliott J. Feline chronic renal failure: calcium homeostasis in 80 cases diagnosed between 1992 and 1995. J Small Anim Pract 1998;39:108–16.
98. Hostutler RA, DiBartola SP, Chew DJ, et al. Comparison of the effects of daily and intermittent-dose calcitriol on serum parathyroid hormone and ionized calcium concentrations in normal cats and cats with chronic renal failure. J Vet Intern Med 2006;20:1307–13.
99. Nagode LA, Chew DJ, Podell M. Benefits of calcitriol therapy and serum phosphorus control in dogs and cats with chronic renal failure. Both are essential to prevent of suppress toxic hyperparathyroidism. Vet Clin North Am 1996;26: 1293–330.
100. Young LR, Backus RC. Oral vitamin D supplementation at five times the recommended allowance marginally affects serum 25-hydroxyvitamin D concentrations in dogs. J Nutr Sci 2016;5:e31.
101. Young LR, Backus RC. Serum 25-hydroxyvitamin D3 and 24R,25-dihydroxyvitamin D3 concentrations in adult dogs are more substantially increased by oral supplementation of 25-hydroxyvitamin D3 than by vitamin D3. J Nutr Sci 2017;6:e30.
102. Klinger CJ, Hobi S, Johansen C, et al. Vitamin D shows in vivo efficacy in a placebo-controlled, double-blinded, randomised clinical trial on canine atopic dermatitis. Vet Rec 2018;182:406–13.
103. Parker VJRA, Beizaei A, Chew DJ. Effects of calcifediol supplementation on markers of chronic kidney disease - mineral bone disorder (CKD-MBD) in dogs with CKD. J Vet Intern Med 2020;34(6):2497–506.

104. Cortadellas O, Fernandez del Palacio MJ, Talavera J, et al. Calcium and phosphorus homeostasis in dogs with spontaneous chronic kidney disease at different stages of severity. J Vet Intern Med 2010;24:73–9.
105. van den Broek DHN, Chang YM, Elliott J, et al. Chronic kidney disease in cats and the risk of total hypercalcemia. J Vet Intern Med 2017;31:465–75.
106. Lippi I, Guidi G, Marchetti V, et al. Prognostic role of the product of serum calcium and phosphorus concentrations in dogs with chronic kidney disease: 31 cases. J Am Vet Med Assoc 2014;245:1135–40.
107. Geddes RF, van den Broek DHN, Chang Y, et al. The effect of attenuating dietary phosphate restriction on blood ionized calcium concentrations in cats with chronic kidney disease and ionized hypercalcemia. J Vet Intern Med 2021. https://doi.org/10.1111/jvim.16050.
108. de Brito Galvão JF, Parker V, Schenck PA, et al. Update on feline ionized hypercalcemia. Vet Clin North Am 2017;47:273–92.
109. Markovich JE, Freeman LM, Labato MA, et al. Survey of dietary and medication practices of owners of cats with chronic kidney disease. J Feline Med Surg 2015;17:979–83.
110. Dzanis DA. Regulatory aspects of diets, supplements, and nutraceuticals. Clin Tech Small Anim Pract 1998;13:193–6.
111. Lenox CE. Role of dietary fatty acids in dogs & cats. Todays Vet Pract 2016; 6:83–8.
112. Bauer JE. Therapeutic use of fish oils in companion animals. J Am Vet Med Assoc 2011;239:1441–51.
113. Stockman J, Fascetti AJ, Kass PH, et al. Evaluation of recipes of home-prepared maintenance diets for dogs. J Am Vet Med Assoc 2013;242:1500–5.
114. Larsen JA, Parks EM, Heinze CR, et al. Evaluation of recipes for home-prepared diets for dogs and cats with chronic kidney disease. J Am Vet Med Assoc 2012; 240:532–8.
115. Wilson SA, Villaverde C, Fascetti AJ, et al. Evaluation of the nutritional adequacy of recipes for home-prepared maintenance diets for cats. J Am Vet Med Assoc 2019;254:1172–9.
116. Johnson LN, Linder DE, Heinze CR, et al. Evaluation of owner experiences and adherence to home-cooked diet recipes for dogs. J Small Anim Pract 2016; 57:23–7.

Nutritional Management of Behavior and Brain Disorders in Dogs and Cats

Valarie V. Tynes, DVM[a,*], Gary M. Landsberg, DVM[b]

KEYWORDS

• Cognition • Epilepsy • Seizures • Anxiety • Aggression • Nutraceutical • Supplement • Diet

KEY POINTS

- Evidence supporting the role of nutritional supplements and dietary ingredients in cognitive and behavioral health has grown over the last few years. Although much of the research is in laboratory animals and humans, extrapolation of the data, combined with the studies in dogs and cats, makes this mode of therapy promising.
- Cognitive dysfunction, as with most health and behavior problems, is most successfully managed when identified early in the course of the problem; therefore, clinicians should be proactive in screening patients for these conditions.
- Although interactions with other medications are unlikely, clinicians should become familiar with each ingredient's mode of action and patient history, before combining with other medications or supplements.
- Diet and nutritional supplementation should be used in conjunction with a comprehensive program of environmental management, enrichment, and/or behavior modification.

INTRODUCTION

Nutrition plays a fundamental role in the structural and functional development of the brain from before birth, through adolescence, and into adulthood. Poor nutrition in a gestating female has detrimental effects on the developing offspring, both in physical abilities and mental or emotional development. Deficiencies of vitamins and minerals have been associated with behavioral disorders in both humans and animals, including anxiety and aggression, and there is increasing evidence that gut microbiota can influence behavior.[1–5] Behavior is regulated by neurotransmitters and hormones. Any changes in the availability of their precursors can affect production of these compounds and the behaviors influenced by them.

[a] Ceva Animal Health, LLC 8735 Rosehill Road, Suite 300 Lenexa, KS 66215, USA; [b] Richmond Hill, Ontario, Canada
* Corresponding author.
E-mail address: pigvet@hughes.net

Vet Clin Small Anim 51 (2021) 711–727
https://doi.org/10.1016/j.cvsm.2021.01.011

Studies have examined the role of different nutrients, including amino acids, fatty acids, and medium-chain triglycerides (MCTs), on cognitive and behavioral disorders in many species, including humans.[1,6–8] Several other natural products, such as plant extracts, protein hydrolysates, and probiotics, have also shown promise in the treatment of problem behaviors.[5,9–13] Although research in dogs and cats is limited, with the preponderance of evidence supporting many of these products in other species, some extrapolation may be warranted.

Every year, millions of dogs and cats are relinquished to shelters and/or euthanized because of behavior problems.[1] This euthanasia often occurs after training, behavior modification, and sometimes even psychotropic drugs have been attempted, but rarely is the role of diet and nutrition considered. Although nutritional supplements may be beneficial, they must be used in conjunction with environmental management and behavior modification for a successful outcome.

NUTRITION AND BEHAVIOR

All behavior occurs as a result of the activity of chemical messengers in the form of neurotransmitters and hormones, in the central nervous system (CNS).[1] Researchers have hypothesized for years as to how changing the availability of the precursors to these chemicals could influence behavior.[1] Tryptophan and tyrosine are the precursors to serotonin and dopamine, two of the neurotransmitters that play important roles in learning, emotions, and impulse control.

Lower levels of serotonin have been shown to be associated with aggression in many species, including dogs.[1] A diet high in tryptophan has been found to aid in decreasing aggression in some species in experimental conditions and to increase aggression in others.[1] It has also been suggested that tryptophan supplementation can improve an individual's ability to cope with stress.[9]

The rate-limiting step in the synthesis of serotonin is conversion of tryptophan by tryptophan hydroxylase to 5-hydroxytryptophan. Tryptophan is found in nearly all protein-containing foods but in small concentrations in many, compared with the other large neutral amino acids (LNAAs). Tryptophan must compete with the other LNAAs for a shared transporter system in order to cross the blood-brain barrier. This system is saturable, so increasing the blood or plasma concentration of 1 LNAA increases the brain uptake of that one but decreases brain uptake of others[14]; therefore, by simply increasing the protein levels in the diet, the concentration of tryptophan uptake into the brain can be markedly reduced (depending on the type of protein).[14] The result can be markedly reduced levels of serotonin synthesis and subsequent effects on mood and cognition. However, some proteins, such as lactalbumin from whey, or chicken and turkey, are much higher in tryptophan than others. If feeding a source of protein that is higher in tryptophan than the other LNAAs, then the results can be increased levels of central tryptophan concentrations and increased serotonin synthesis.[14] Other aspects of meal composition can also affect tryptophan uptake into the brain. Carbohydrate-rich meals and subsequent insulin secretion enhance peripheral and skeletal muscle uptake of LNAAs. Because it is largely albumin bound, tryptophan is protected from this, and some studies have shown significant increases in tryptophan/LNAA ratios (compared with baseline) after a meal high in carbohydrates. This finding has also been associated with improved mood and better cognitive performance when in stressed human patients.[9,15,16]

Few studies have looked for an association between protein or tryptophan levels and behavior in dogs. One early study attempted to evaluate the effect of protein and tryptophan on aggression in dogs.[15] Twelve dogs, each with a diagnosis of dominance aggression, territorial aggression, or hyperactivity, and 14 control dogs were fed diets with low (49.5 g/1000 kcal), medium (70.8 g/1000 kcal), or high (92.8 g/1000 kcal) levels of protein for 2 weeks each. Low and medium protein levels resulted in a significant decrease in dogs showing territorial aggression that was attributed to fear.[17]

In a follow-up study, each of 11 dogs with dominance aggression, territorial aggression, or hyperactivity was fed for 1 week on 4 different diets; low or high protein, with or without added tryptophan.[18] Dogs fed high protein without tryptophan supplementation had the highest scores for dominance aggression, whereas dogs on the low-protein diet with tryptophan had the lowest scores for territorial aggression. The investigators concluded that adding tryptophan or decreasing protein might reduce dominance aggression, whereas a low-protein diet with added tryptophan might help reduce territorial aggression.[18] However, the first study does not include an assessment of tryptophan/LNAA ratios and, in the second study, the carbohydrate/protein ratio is not clearly reported. Typically, when protein is reduced in a diet, carbohydrate content is increased, thus further affecting tryptophan availability to the brain and presenting a potential confounding factor in this study. An additional concern with both of these studies is that 1 to 2 weeks may be insufficient to determine whether diet will alter behavior. Although doses of 10 to 15 mg/kg/d of L-tryptophan were recommended in another more recent study,[19] further studies with varying levels of tryptophan supplementation in dogs have not shown a behavioral effect. However, tryptophan/LNAA ratios were also not assessed in that study.[20] It is still only hypothesized that increasing tryptophan availability to the brain results in increased levels of serotonin. Much more research is needed in dogs to confirm what percentage increase in tryptophan may be needed to lead to clinically significant increases in serotonin levels and subsequent improvement in any problem behavior (**Box 1**).

NUTRITION AND ANXIETY

Most problem behaviors in dogs and cats are a result of fear and anxiety (**Box 2**). The causes of fear and anxiety are multifactorial, including genetic effects, perinatal effects, poor socialization, and experience.

Although scientific evidence of effect is limited, several nutraceuticals have shown some promising results for the treatment of signs of fear, stress, or anxiety in dogs and cats, including alpha-casozepine (Zylkene) and L-theanine (Anxitane)[10–12,21,22] either alone or in combination with other ingredients, including L-theanine with *Magnolia officinalis*, *Phellodendron amurense*, and concentrated whey protein (Solliquin),[13] or functional foods supplemented with alpha-casozepine (Royal Canin Canine and Feline Calm Diets, Hills Prescription Diets: Feline Urinary Stress and Canine i/d Stress).[24,25]

Box 1
Clinical pearl: Diet and Aggression

Until more information is available, clinicians should ensure that patients with a diagnosis of aggression are not on diets that contain higher than necessary protein levels for the individual's stage of growth, reproduction, and health, especially if the protein sources are those typically low in tryptophan. If desiring to increase tryptophan availability to the brain, increasing carbohydrate to protein ratios may be more effective than simply decreasing protein content or adding tryptophan to the diet. In addition, when switching diets to observe for behavior change, clients should be counseled that change may be seen within 1 to 2 weeks but 6 to 8 weeks may be needed to fully assess any therapeutic effect.

Box 2
Clinical pearl: The Physical Effects of Stress

Patients with chronic, recurring, soft stools are common in veterinary practice. Clinicians must consider all of the potential medical problems that might be causing the signs, as well as the role of stress and anxiety in causing or contributing to the problem. Many skin and urinary conditions can also be stress related. In these cases, some form of dietary intervention may aid the patient while diagnostics are pursued and appropriate behavioral management is implemented.

(**Table 1**) Purina ProPlan Veterinary Supplements Calming Care, a probiotic supplement BL999 (*Bifidobacterium longum*) has also shown efficacy at decreasing signs of anxiety in dogs.[5]

Other functional foods that have shown some efficacy in reducing anxiety and stress in dogs include a fish hydrolysate–supplemented diet and a diet supplemented with fish and vegetable hydrolysates, minerals, and nutraceuticals including *Valeriana*, but these are not yet commercially available.[26,27]

Although there is no published evidence supporting a cause and effect, dietary ingredients have been reported to cause behavior problems, with exclusion or avoidance of the ingredients leading to an improvement in behavior. In 1 case report, behavioral changes including aggression were resolved with a hydrolyzed protein, gluten-free diet. Diagnosis was a suspected nonceliac gluten hypersensitivity.[28]

THE GUT MICROBIOME AND BEHAVIOR

It has been recognized for some time that the brain regulates gut activity but, over the past decade, numerous studies have begun to uncover the myriad ways in which gut microbes influence the brain.[2,29] The brain-gut-microbiota axis includes the CNS, the neuroendocrine system and the neuroimmune system, the sympathetic and parasympathetic branches of the autonomic nervous system, and the enteric nervous system (ENS) in addition to the intestinal microbiota.[29] The nerve fibers that integrate all of these structures as well as the smooth muscle of the gastrointestinal (GI) system result in bidirectional communication that allows the brain to influence the GI tract and conversely for messages from the GI tract to influence the brain.

When the hypothalamic-pituitary-adrenal (HPA) axis is triggered under a situation of physical or psychological stress, it results in altered gut permeability and changes in gut motility and secretion.[29] These changes can subsequently result in an imbalance in

Table 1
Nutritional supplements for fear, anxiety, and stress

Ingredient	Purported Mode of Action	Dose (mg/kg/d)
Alpha-casozepine[10–13,24,25]	• Tryptic hydrolysate of bovine alpha 1 casein • Affinity for GABA receptors • Benzodiazepine-like effects without side effects	15–25
L-Theanine[21–23]	• Structure similar to glutamic acid • Inhibits excitatory neurotransmission by binding to glutamate receptors • Neuroprotective effects	10–15

Abbreviation: GABA, gamma-aminobutyric acid.

the microbiome population or dysbiosis, by changing the environment in which the bacteria reside. The resulting dysbiosis can lead to diarrhea (ie, stress diarrhea) and other signs of GI distress. Psychosocial stress resulting in increased gut permeability can also result in pathogenic bacteria and their antigens crossing the epithelial barrier and activating an inflammatory immune response that further activates the HPA.[29] However, changes in gut permeability also allow bacteria to cross the intestinal mucosa and directly access immune cells and neuronal cells of the ENS, providing a potential pathway by which the microbiota can influence the CNS.[2]

A growing body of evidence in humans and animals shows that a healthy gut microbiota is critical to the normal development of the HPA axis as well as its future functioning.[29] It has been determined that the microbiota can influence CNS function directly by activating stress circuits, thus contributing to anxiety and depression.[2]

The exact role that the microbiome plays in dog behavior has yet to be fully elucidated, but, in 1 study, an analysis of fecal microbiome samples from 31 dogs found significantly different populations of gut bacteria in dogs that showed conspecific aggression compared with the dogs that did not.[3]

A more recent study of 42 dogs from a shelter in Italy compared gut microbiome populations among dogs diagnosed by a veterinary behaviorist as aggressive (11), phobic (13), or normal (18) behavioral phenotypes.[4] The gut microbiome of the aggressive dogs was found to differ significantly from both the normal dogs and the phobic dogs. Although it is unknown whether these unique gut microbiomes are a cause of the behavioral phenotype or a result, the findings support continued study into the role that the gut microbiome plays in behavior.

Probiotic supplementation in both rodents and humans has been shown to significantly change behavior.[30] A meta-analysis of trials investigating probiotics supplementation in humans identified beneficial effects from some probiotics in reducing anxiety and depression.[30] One probiotic supplement has shown efficacy in decreasing anxiety in dogs.[5] In a placebo-controlled blinded, crossover study of 24 anxious Labrador retrievers over 12 weeks, dogs treated with BL999 (*Bifidobacterium longum*) showed a significant decrease in anxious behaviors, reduced salivary cortisol concentrations, decreased heart rate, and increased heart rate variability in response to both exercise and anxiety-inducing situations.[5]

POLYUNSATURATED FATTY ACIDS

Omega-3 long-chain, polyunsaturated fatty acids (PUFAs) are considered fundamental to brain function, with eicosapentaenoic acid (EPA) and docosahexaenoic acid (DHA) considered most important. They play a vital role in maintaining cell membrane structure, fluidity, and cell-to-cell communication.[31]

Studies in humans providing DHA and EPA together in the form of fish oils have shown an ability to improve cognition in healthy adults and slow cognitive decline in those with mild impairment.[32]

For aging dogs and cats, PUFAs are frequently combined with other supplements or in diets for brain health, so it may be impossible to know the exact role individual fatty acids play in preventing or slowing cognitive decline; however, based on evidence from other species, they are likely to be helpful.

Higher levels of DHA have been shown to support improved neurologic development in dogs.[33] At least 1 study showed a positive correlation between serum concentrations of DHA and improved discrimination learning, as well as electroretinogram-measured retinal function in puppies fed a diet high in DHA.[33,34] Puppies fed the diet high in DHA also had significantly better performance in cognition and psychomotor performance. However, the diet was also enriched with several other vitamins and antioxidants that could have contributed to the results.[34]

In 1 study comparing fearful and nonfearful Great Danes, the fearful dogs had lower levels of several phospholipids, including phosphatidylcholine.[35] Two studies in dogs have identified an association between hypocholesterolemia and aggression.[36,37] To date, only 1 study in dogs has found evidence of lower levels of DHA in aggressive dogs compared with controls. This study also showed that the aggressive dogs had significantly lower levels of cholesterol and higher omega-6/omega-3 ratios than controls.[37] These studies only support association, and not causation.

Like any drug or supplement, there is the potential for adverse effects if a patient receives omega-3 fatty acids in very large amounts. These adverse effects include altered platelet function, GI effects (diarrhea, pancreatitis), detrimental effects on wound healing, and lipid peroxidation.[38] The National Research Council publication on nutrient requirements of dogs and cats indicates a safe upper limit of the combined amounts of EPA and DHA as 2800 mg/1000 kcal of diet, equivalent to 370 mg/(kg body weight)$^{0.75}$ for dogs. This amount is equivalent to 2080 mg for a 10-kg dog. Presently, not enough published data are available to set a safe upper limit for cats. However, it is recommended that additional vitamin E be added to any feline diet supplemented with large amounts of fish oil.

Because of their many potential benefits, supplementation of omega-3 PUFAs should be considered in the management of behavior problems. Adverse events are likely to be dose dependent, so owners should be asked whether their pets are taking any other medications or supplements and to advise the clinician if there are any changes in the pet's condition (**Box 3**).

NUTRITION AND COGNITIVE DYSFUNCTION SYNDROME

Cognitive dysfunction syndrome (CDS) is a neurodegenerative disorder of senior dogs and cats characterized by a gradual, progressive cognitive decline. It is a result of irreversible brain disorder that is marked by the accumulation of β-amyloid plaques and perivascular infiltrates in the brain; a decrease in frontal and temporal lobe volume; an increase in ventricular size, meningeal calcification, and in free radicals; and a reduction in neurons.[39,40] Reduced brain glucose metabolism in aging dogs contributes to brain energy deprivation, leading to a decrease in neuronal function.[41] Reduced cholinergic function, a reduction in noradrenergic neurons in the locus coeruleus, and circulatory changes resulting in decreased blood flow to the brain also contribute to declining cognitive function, declining motor function, and sleep-wake cycle disruption.[42–44]

Treatment of CDS is aimed at prevention, slowing decline and improving clinical signs. This treatment relies on early recognition and intervention. Because cognitive therapeutics are most effective at maintaining brain health and preventing or slowing cognitive decline, early intervention is optimal. However, most pet owners do not

Box 3
Clinical pearl: PUFAs and Behavior

Omega-3 PUFAs are an easy, safe, and cost-effective addition to the management plan for many behavior problems. Clinicians need to be aware of the pet's diagnosis, medications, changes in physical or behavioral health, and the pet's current diet because many therapeutic diets for growth, cognitive, and dermatologic health are already fortified with additional PUFAs.

report signs until they are significantly advanced, at which point treatment may have minimal effect. Therefore, veterinarians should be proactive in educating their clients about CDS and screening for clinical signs (**Box 4**).

Strategies that might reduce the risk factors associated with cognitive decline, and slow the progression and improve signs of CDS, include drugs, functional foods, and nutritional supplements focused on reducing the effects of oxidative stress, correcting nutritional deficiencies and metabolic changes associated with cognitive decline, reducing inflammation, and improving mitochondrial function, neuronal health, and signaling. Although single-ingredient supplements may be beneficial, the greatest effect might be achieved with the combined effects of behavioral enrichment and a blend of ingredients.[46] This possibility is supported by human studies in which physical and mental activity and diets containing fruits, vegetables, seeds, legumes, nuts and fish oils, and a diet with both omega-3 fatty acids and B vitamins, have been shown to reduce cognitive decline.[6,47]

Nutritional Support for Cognitive Dysfunction Syndrome

Studies in both laboratory models and clinical trials have shown a beneficial effect of nutrition on improving signs and slowing progression of CDS in dogs. In 1 study, dogs fed high-quality commercial diets appropriate to their age, size, or health, were 2.8 times less likely to develop CDS than dogs fed low-quality commercial food or table scraps.[48]

A diet (Hills Prescription Diet b/d Canine) supplemented with fatty acids, antioxidants (vitamins C and E, β-carotene, selenium, flavonoids, carotenoids), and mitochondrial cofactors (DL-alpha-lipoic acid and L-carnitine) was evaluated in a laboratory study of beagles.[46] Over 2 years, discrimination learning was improved with behavioral enrichment, and reversal learning was improved by both behavioral enrichment and diet, whereas the 2 treatments together were more effective than either treatment alone.[46] A blinded, 60-day clinical trial in 125 dogs compared the total number of improved signs in the supplemented diet with the control group, and observed a significant difference in favor of the supplemented food[49] (**Table 2** provides a guide to screening for cognitive decline using the mnemonic DISHAA).

More recently, another diet (Purina ProPlan Neurocare) was evaluated in a clinical trial of dogs with CDS that were identified through screening with a DISHAA questionnaire for the 6 categories of signs.[50] The diet was supplemented with both a brain protection blend (BPB) containing arginine, antioxidants (vitamins C and E, and selenium), B vitamins, and fish oil containing DHA and EPA, as well as 6.5% MCTs. MCTs may improve energy metabolism in the brain as well as increase polyunsaturated fatty acid levels in the brain (**Box 5**). Dogs on the supplemented diet significantly improved in all 6 categories of DISHAA after 90 days compared with only 4 categories in the control diet.[50] Although improvement in the control diet group may have been a placebo

Box 4
Clinical pearl: Screening for CDS

Clinicians should begin screening all patients by at least 7 years of age, once to twice yearly for cognitive decline, using one of the many screening tools available. If clinicians wait until pet owners report signs of cognitive decline, it may be too late to effect significant improvement. In dogs more than 8 years of age, new signs may arise and existing signs are likely to progress over 6 to 12 months.[45] In 1 study, using a validated DISHAA questionnaire, after 6 months, 42% of dogs with no signs developed mild impairment, whereas 24% of dogs with mild signs progressed to moderate.[45]

Table 2
Clinical signs represented by the mnemonic DISHAA

D	Disorientation
I	Social interactions
S	Sleep-wake cycles
H	House soiling, learning, and memory
A	Activity
A	Anxiety

For a cognitive screening questionnaire, see https://www.purinainstitute.com/sites/g/files/auxxlc381/files/2018-08/DISHAA.pdf.

effect, the control diet also contained some of the BPB ingredients at levels greater than AAFCO requirements, which may have contributed to a therapeutic benefit.

In an 8-month laboratory study in beagles aged 7.5 to 11.6 years, a 5.5% MCT-supplemented diet led to a significant improvement in a variety of neuropsychological tasks as early as 30 days after beginning supplementation. The group supplemented with MCTs had significantly increased levels of the ketone body, β-hydroxybutyrate (BHB).[8] In another 6-month study in beagles aged 9 to 11.5 years, dogs fed the BPB-supplemented diet showed significantly better performance on complex discrimination tasks.[52]

A supplement containing phosphatidylserine (**Box 6**), *Ginkgo biloba*, antioxidants, and vitamin B_6 (Senilife) has been shown to improve cognition in dogs in both a clinical and a laboratory study.[56,57] In a double-blinded crossover study in 9 laboratory beagles, aged 7 to 12.7 years, dogs receiving the supplement were significantly improved in a visuospatial memory task compared with baseline.[56] In addition, dogs treated in the first arm of the study did not decline after crossover, indicating that their level of performance was maintained after supplementation was discontinued.[56] In an open-label clinical trial of 8 dogs diagnosed with CDS based on signs of disorientation, social interactions, sleep-wake cycles, house soiling, and activity , dogs administered Senilife once daily for 3 months showed a highly significant improvement in the 5 behavioral categories compared with the start of the trial.[57]

Aktivait (VetPlus Ltd), which contains phosphatidylserine, omega-3 fatty acids, vitamins E and C, L-carnitine, alpha-lipoic acid, coenzyme Q, and selenium, has also shown significant improvement in dogs with CDS. In a 42-day trial in dogs with

Box 5
Medium-chain triglycerides in brain health

- A significant decline in brain glucose metabolism has been documented in aging dogs.[41]
- In humans, cerebral glucose metabolism is significantly lower in patients with Alzheimer disease (AD) compared with healthy older controls.[51]
- Supplementation with MCTs can increase levels of ketones in the brain.[51]
- MCTs are converted by the liver and by astrocytes in the brain to ketone bodies.
- Ketones can then be used by neurons as an alternative source of energy, alleviating glucose deficits.
- Diets supplemented with MCTs have been shown to improve memory in humans with AD.[7]

Box 6
Phosphatidylserine in brain health

- Phosphatidylserine (PS) is found in the cell membrane of neurons and plays a critical role in activating signaling pathways in the neuronal system.[53]
- PS modulates the function of several membrane-bound receptors and the release of some neurotransmitters.[53]
- PS supplements have been reported to improve cognitive function in both humans and animals.[54]
- A significant decrease in DHA content in PS has been reported in patients with AD.[32]
- DHA in the brain plays a pivotal role in PS production. When DHA level is high in the brain, PS levels are high; when DHA levels are low, PS levels are low.[55]

behavioral symptoms of cognitive dysfunction related to disorientation, social interactions, sleep-wake cycles, and house soiling, there was significant improvement in all 4 categories compared with placebo, and significant improvements in age-related behavior and quality of life reported by both owners and veterinary staff.[58]

S-adenosyl–L-methionine (SAMe) is a metabolite found in all cells, where it functions as a methyl donor. SAMe-dependent methylation reactions are particularly important in the CNS, where they play an important role in maintaining the integrity of cellular membranes and are required for the synthesis and inactivation of neurotransmitter monoamines such as noradrenaline, adrenaline, dopamine, serotonin, and histamine.[59] Decreased levels of SAMe have been found in the brains of patients with Alzheimer disease (AD).[59] There is evidence that SAMe crosses the blood-brain barrier intact, with oral administration increasing cerebrospinal fluid concentrations in dogs.

In a double-blind, placebo-controlled clinical trial, the SAMe (Novifit, Virbac)-treated dogs showed significantly improved activity levels, awareness, and mental impairment scores compared with placebo.[60] In a blinded, placebo-controlled laboratory study of 14 aged beagle dogs, executive function but not short-term working memory was enhanced with SAMe.[61]

There are limited data currently available on the effects of cognitive therapeutics in cats.

In a laboratory trial, assessing the effects of the BPB over 1 year in cats aged 5.5 to 8.7 years, cats on the therapeutic diet performed significantly better than controls on discrimination and reversal learning tasks.[62]

In a 30-day study of cats aged 10 years and older, the cats fed a test diet containing antioxidants, DHA, cysteine, and methionine had significantly improved activity compared with before 8 years of age and compared with controls.[63] Although neither of these cat formulations is commercially available, these studies provide some insight as to the potential effect of these ingredient blends on cognition and behavior in senior cats.

SAMe (Novifit) has also been studied in aged cats in a blinded, placebo-controlled laboratory study.[61] Compared with placebo, cats that were least impaired had a significant reduction in reversal learning errors; however, no effect was seen in the most impaired cats.[61]

For further description of nutrients that have been found to be beneficial to brain health, see **Table 3**. However, no comparative studies have been done to compare the relative value of any of these proven supplements or diets, nor is there any evidence for potential additive, synergistic, or competitive interactions if multiple options are used concurrently.

Table 3
The role of nutrients for brain aging and cognitive dysfunction in senior pets

Ingredient/Supplement	Purported Mechanism of Action
Arginine[64]	• Precursor to nitrous oxide enhanced nitrous oxide synthesis for maintaining normal blood pressure, circulation, and cognition • Antioxidant • Regulation of glucose metabolism • Supports neurogenesis
Alpha-lipoic acid[46,49,65,66]	• Improves mitochondrial function; cofactor for mitochondrial respiratory chain enzymes • Reduces production of reactive oxygen species (antioxidant) • Increases intracellular glutathione levels • Neuroprotective • Improves nerve blood flow and nerve conduction • May attenuate the decrease in neurotransmitter levels that occurs with age
B_6, B_{12}, and folic acid[6,52,63,67,68]	• All 3 are essential to the health of the CNS ○ Deficiencies of vitamin B_{12} and folic acid lead to impaired methylation and increased plasma homocysteine level ○ Correct for B vitamin deficiency and minimize risk of increased homocysteine level ○ Increased homocysteine level associated with renal and heart disease in dogs ○ Low concentrations of B vitamins and increased homocysteine level associated with cardiovascular disease and risk of cognitive impairment in humans ○ Improvements in cognitive impairment with good omega 3 fatty acid status • Pyridoxine (vitamin B_6) ○ Normal brain development, function, and neuronal health; neuroprotective ○ Cofactor in the synthesis of serotonin, noradrenaline, and dopamine. • Vitamin B_{12} ○ Required to form methionine, which undergoes methylation to SAMe
β-Carotene[69]	• Antioxidant • Improves immune function
L-Carnitine[46,49,63,67,70]	• Mitochondrial lipid metabolism and required for the maintenance of normal mitochondrial functioning • Transport of long-chain fatty acids through inner mitochondrial membrane • Regulates ketogenesis • Neuroprotective • Increases levels of antioxidants

(*continued on next page*)

Table 3
(*continued*)

Ingredient/Supplement	Purported Mechanism of Action
MCTs[7,51]	• May increase ketone levels in brain, providing alternative energy source • Have been shown to improve memory in humans with cognitive deficits
Omega-3 fatty acids (DHA and EPA)[31,32,49,52,71]	• Neuronal cell membrane plasticity and health • Neuroprotective • Antiinflammatory • Corrects for age-related DHA deficiencies contributing to cognitive decline • DHA increases brain-derived neurotrophic factor level • DHA enhances neurogenesis
Vitamin E[46,49,52,66,72]	• Antioxidant: protects cell membranes from oxidative damage • Antiinflammatory • Neuroprotective

NUTRITION AND EPILEPSY

Idiopathic epilepsy is a condition defined by chronic recurring seizures of unknown cause, which negatively affect quality of life for both patients and their caregivers. Dogs with epilepsy may have concurrent medical as well as behavioral conditions, and the medications used to treat seizures can increase the risk of complications associated with these other problems. Even with appropriate antiepileptic drug (ADE) therapy, approximately one-third of dogs and humans continue to experience seizures.[73,74] Differing nutritional strategies have been investigated for decreasing seizure frequency in humans, and a ketogenic diet has been found to be effective in some cases.[75]

Although dogs do not readily become ketotic, diets high in MCTs have been shown to increase BHB, a ketone body that may provide an alternative to glucose as a source of energy for the brain.[76] It has been hypothesized that MCTs may have direct antiseizure effects, but the exact mechanism of action remains unclear and a direct correlation between blood ketone bodies and seizure reduction has not been consistently found.[77] Diets high in MCTs increase plasma levels of decanoic acid (C10) and octanoic acid (C8), as well as BHB. Decanoic acid has been shown to have antiseizure effects, by acting as an α-amino-3-hydroxy-5-methyl-4-isoxazolepropionic acid (AMPA) receptor antagonist that inhibits excitatory neurotransmission.[78] AMPA receptors play the key role in generating and propagating epileptic activity. Although AMPA receptor antagonism by decanoic acid may be most relevant to providing the antiseizure effect of MCT-supplemented diets, octanoic acid (C8) may also enhance seizure control and neuroprotection.[79] MCTs may also act to improve brain metabolism and provide protection against mitochondrial dysfunction.[80]

In a clinical trial in dogs with epilepsy that were on at least 1 epileptic medication, a diet supplemented with 5.5% MCT was shown to reduce seizure frequency and number of days with seizures compared with a placebo diet.[81] Over the 3 months of treatment, seizure frequency was reduced in 71% of 21 dogs, whereas 14% became seizure free. The MCT diet resulted in significant increase of blood BHB level compared with the placebo diet, and did not significantly affect plasma levels of phenobarbital or potassium bromide (KBr).[81]

In a subsequent study in 28 dogs with epilepsy that were on at least 1 epileptic medication, dogs receiving a diet containing 9% MCT oil had significantly reduced seizure frequency and seizure days. Twelve of the dogs had an overall reduction in seizure frequency and 2 dogs became seizure free. However, 11 dogs showed no response to the supplementation.[82] The MCT oil contained octanoic acid (50%–65%) and decanoic acid (30%–50%). These studies provide evidence that diets high in MCTs (eg, Purina ProPlan Neurocare) may be useful for adjunctive management of seizures in dogs with epilepsy.

Several other dietary considerations may be important when dealing with patients with epilepsy. These considerations include body composition, dietary macronutrient distribution (the proportion of calories from protein, fats, and carbohydrates), omega-3 fatty acid supplementation, amounts of dietary chloride, and the possible role of food allergies. Dogs with epilepsy may be at an increased risk of developing pancreatitis and the use of potassium bromide and/or phenobarbital may play a role in the development of pancreatitis. High-fat foods should be avoided, especially if the dog has other risk factors for pancreatitis, such as obesity.[76]

Omega 3 PUFAs have also been postulated to have antiepileptic effects, but no controlled trials have supported a benefit with regard to reducing seizures or seizure frequency. However, PUFAs may be useful in decreasing the hypertriglyceridemia that is common in dogs on long-term treatment with phenobarbital.[83]

SUMMARY

All behavioral treatment plans should take a multimodal approach that includes environmental management and behavioral modification. Psychotropic medications may play a valuable role in many cases but are less preferred by some owners and not ideal for every patient, especially geriatric animals, or those with other medical conditions. Offering some nutritional management in conjunction with these other interventions appeals to many clients who prefer a more natural approach. Dietary management, when used appropriately, is likely to be safe, and chances for side effects minimal, especially compared with pharmacologic agents. Many of the supplements are also relatively palatable and thus make treatment easier for the client. All of these features can increase the likelihood of compliance and thus the chance of a successful outcome.

It is the clinician's role to remember that supplements and diets are not regulated by the US Food and Drug Administration. Quality and consistency can vary greatly between products and manufacturers. Clients should be given some guidance regarding the use of products so that, if they do wish to use supplements, they purchase those that are supported by evidence and can be acquired from reliable sources.

CLINICS CARE POINTS

- Tryptophan supplementation alone may be ineffective at increasing serotonin concentrations in the CNS; other components of the diet, such as protein type and carbohydrate content, affect tryptophan uptake to the brain.
- Limited studies have shown promising results for several different nutraceuticals and functional foods in controlling signs of anxiety in dogs and cats, but use of these products should always be combined with a complete behavioral management plan in order to increase the chance of successful treatment.
- CDS can progress rapidly, so screening of dogs should begin early (5–7 years, depending on breed) and patients should be screened every 6 months for new or worsening signs.

- Both the diets and supplements that have been studied for their roles in improving the signs of cognitive dysfunction have shown better results when initiated before clinical signs of the conditions have become severe.
- Dogs with epilepsy not adequately controlled by antiepileptic drugs may experience a decrease in seizure frequency when fed a diet high in MCTs.

DISCLOSURE

Dr V.V. Tynes is an employee of Ceva Animal Health, the manufacturer of Senilife. Dr G. Landsberg is employed by CanCog Inc, a contract research organization that conducted several of the referenced studies in cognitive dysfunction and behavior.

REFERENCES

1. Bosch G, Beerda B, Hendriks WH, et al. Impact of nutrition on canine behaviour: current status and possible mechanisms. Nutr Res Rev 2007;20:180–94.
2. Foster JA, Neufeld KAM. Gut–brain axis: how the microbiome influences anxiety and depression. Trends Neurosci 2013;36(5):305–12.
3. Kirchoff NS, Udell MAR, Sharpton TJ. The gut microbiome correlates with conspecific aggression in a small population of rescued dogs (Canis familiaris). PeerJ 2019;7:e6103.
4. Mondo E, Barone M, Soverini M. Gut microbiome structure and adrenocortical activity in dogs with aggressive and phobic behavioral disorders. Heliyon 2020;6(1):e03311.
5. McGowan RTS, Barnett HR, Czarnecku-Maulden G, et al. Tapping into those "gut feelings": Impact of BL99 (Bifidobacterium longum) on anxiety in dogs In: Proceedings of the American College of Veterinary Behaviorists Veterinary Behavior Symposium. Denver, CO, July 11–12, 2018.
6. Oulhaj A, Jernerén F, Refsum H, et al. Omega-3 fatty acid status enhances the prevention of cognitive decline by B vitamins in mild cognitive impairment. J Alzheimers Dis 2016;50:547–57.
7. Reger MA, Henderson ST, Hale C, et al. Effects of beta-hydroxybutyrate on cognition in memory-impaired adults. Neurobiol Aging 2004;25:311–4.
8. Pan Y, Larson B, Araujo JA, et al. Dietary supplementation with medium-chain TAG has long-lasting cognition-enhancing effects in aged dogs. Br J Nutr 2010;103:1746–54.
9. Markus CR, Olivier B, Panhuysen GE, et al. The bovine protein α-lactalbumin increases the plasma ratio of tryptophan to the other large neutral amino acids, and in vulnerable subjects raises brain serotonin activity, reduces cortisol concentration, and improves mood under stress. Am J Clin Nutr 2000;71:1536–44.
10. Miclo L, Perrin E, Driou A, et al. Characterization of α-casozepine, a tryptic peptide from bovine αs1-casein with benzodiazepine-like activity. FASEB J 2001;15: 1780–2.
11. Beata C, Beaumont-Graff E, Diaz C, et al. Effects of alpha-casozepine (Zylkene) versus selegiline hydrochloride (Selgian, Anipryl) on anxiety disorders in dogs. J Vet Behav 2007;2:175–83.
12. Beata C, Beaumont-Graff E, Coll V, et al. Effect of alpha casozepine (Zylkene) on anxiety in cats. J Vet Behav 2007;2:40–6.
13. DePorter TL, Bledsoe DL, Conley JR, et al. Case report series of clinical effectiveness and safety of Solliquin® for behavioral support in dogs and cats. In: American

College of Veterinary Behaviorists Veterinary Behavior Symposium Proceedings. San Antonio, TX, 2016. p. 27–8.
14. Fernstrom JD. Large neutral amino acids: dietary effects on brain neurochemistry and function. Amino Acids 2013;45:419–30.
15. Wurtman RJ, Wurtman JJ, Regan MM, et al. Effects of normal meals rich in carbohydrates or proteins on plasma tryptophan and tyrosine ratios. Am J Clin Nutr 2003;77:128–32.
16. Markus CR. Effects of carbohydrates on brain tryptophan availability and stress performance. Biol Psychol 2007;76:83–90.
17. Dodman NH, Reisner I, Shuster L, et al. Effect of dietary protein content on behavior in dogs. J Am Vet Med Assoc 1996;208(3):376–9.
18. DeNapoli JS, Dodman NH, Shuster L, et al. Effect of dietary protein content and tryptophan supplementation on dominance aggression, territorial aggression, and hyperactivity in dogs. J Am Vet Med Assoc 2000;217:504–8.
19. Pereira GG, Fragoso S, Pires E. Effect of dietary intake of L-tryptophan supplementation on working dogs demonstrating stress related behaviours. In: Proceedings 53rd BSAVA Congress. Birmingham, UK, April 8–11, 2010.
20. Templeman JR, Davenport GM, Cant JP, et al. The effect of graded concentrations of dietary tryptophan on canine behavior in response to the approach of a familiar or unfamiliar individual. Can J Vet Res 2018;82(4):294–305.
21. Wakabayashi C, Numakawa T, Ninomiya M, et al. Behavioral and molecular evidence for psychotropic effects in L-theanine. Psychopharmacology 2012;219: 1099–109.
22. Araujo JA, De Rivera C, Ethier JL, et al. ANXITANE tablets reduce fear of human beings in a laboratory model of anxiety-related behavior. J Vet Behav 2010;5: 268e275.
23. Dramard V, Kern L, Hofmans J, et al. Effect of l-theanine tablets in reducing stress-related emotional signs in cats: an open-label field study. Ir Vet J 2018. https://doi.org/10.1186/s13620-018-0130-4.
24. Landsberg GM, Milgram NW, Mougeot I, et al. Therapeutic effects of an α-casozepine and L-Tryptophan supplemented diet on fear and anxiety in the cat. J Feline Med Surg 2017;6:594–602.
25. Miyaji K, Kato M, Ohtani N, et al. Experimental verification of the effects on normal domestic cats by feeding Prescription diet for decreasing stress. J Appl Anim Welf Sci 2015;18:355–62.
26. Landsberg GM, Mougeot I, Kelly S, et al. Assessment of noise induced fear and anxiety in dogs: modification by a novel fish hydrolysate supplemented diet. J Vet Behav 2015;10:391–5.
27. Sechi S, Di Cerbo A, Canello S, et al. Effects in dogs with behavioural disorders of a commercial nutraceutical diet on stress and neuroendocrine parameters. Vet Rec 2017;180:18.
28. Sunol A, Perez-Accino J, Kelley M, et al. Successful dietary treatment of aggression and behavioral changes in a dog. J Vet Behav 2020;37:56–60.
29. Dinan TG, Cryan JF. Regulation of the stress response by the gut microbiota: implications for Psychoneuroendocrinology. Psychoneuroendocrinology 2012;37: 1369–78.
30. Pirbaglou M, Katz J, de Souza RJ, et al. Probiotic supplementation can positively affect anxiety and depressive symptoms: a systematic review of randomized controlled trials. Nutr Res 2016;36:889–98.
31. Kaur H, Singla A, Snehdep S, et al. Role of omega-3 fatty acids in canine health: a review. Int J Curr Microbiol Appl Sci 2020;9(3):2283–93.

32. Kidd PM. Omega-3 DHA and EPA for cognition, behavior, and mood: clinical findings and structural-functional synergies with cell membrane phospholipids. Altern Med Rev 2007;12(3):207–27.
33. Heinemann KM, Waldron MK, Bigley KE, et al. Long-chain (n-3) polyunsaturated fatty acids are more efficient than α-linolenic acid in Improving electroretinogram responses of puppies exposed during gestation, lactation, and weaning. Nutr Neurosci 2005;135:1960–6.
34. Zicker SC, Jewell DE, Yamka RM, et al. Evaluation of cognitive learning, memory, psychomotor, immunologic, and retinal functions in healthy puppies fed foods fortified with docosahexaenoic acid–rich fish oil from 8 to 52 weeks of age. J Am Vet Med Assoc 2012;241:583–94.
35. Puurunen J, Tiira K, Lehtonen M, et al. Non-targeted metabolite profiling reveals changes in oxidative stress, tryptophan and lipid metabolisms in fearful dogs. Behav Brain Funct 2016;12:7.
36. Sentürk S, Yalçin E. Hypocholesterolaemia in dogs with dominance aggression. J Vet Med A Physiol Pathol Clin Med 2003;50:339–42.
37. Re S, Zanoletti M, Emanuele E. Aggressive dogs are characterized by low omega-3 polyunsaturated fatty acid status. Vet Res Commun 2008;32:225–30.
38. Lenox CE, Bauer JE. Potential adverse effects of omega-3 fatty acids in dogs and cats. J Vet Intern Med 2013;27:217–26.
39. Tapp PD, Siwak CT, Gao FQ, et al. Frontal lobe volume, function, and beta-amyloid pathology in a canine model of aging. J Neurosci 2004;224:8205–13.
40. Rofina JE, van Ederen AM, Touissaint MJ, et al. Cognitive disturbances in old dogs suffering from the canine counterpart of Alzheimer's disease. Brain Res 2006;1069:216–26.
41. London ED, Ohata M, Takei H, et al. Regional cerebral metabolic rate for glucose in beagle dogs of different ages. Neurobiol Aging 1983;4:121–6.
42. Zhang JH, Sampogna S, Morales FR, et al. Age-related changes in cholinergic neurons in the laterodorsal and the pedunculo-pontine tegmental nuclei of cats: a combined light and electron microscopic study. Brain Res 2005;1052:47–55.
43. Araujo JA, Nobrega JN, Raymond R, et al. Aged dogs demonstrate both increased sensitivity to scopolamine and decreased muscarinic receptor density. Pharmacol Biochem Behav 2011;98:203–9.
44. Insua D, Suárez ML, Santamarina G, et al. Dogs with canine counterpart of Alzheimer's disease lose noradrenergic neurons. Neurobiol Aging 2010;31:625–35.
45. Madari A, Farbakova J, Katina S, et al. Assessment of severity and progression of canine cognitive dysfunction syndrome using the Canine Dementia Scale (CADES). Appl Anim Behav Sci 2015;17:138–45.
46. Milgram NW, Head E, Zicker SC, et al. Learning ability in aged beagle dogs is preserved by behavioral enrichment and dietary fortification: a two-year longitudinal study. Neurobiol Aging 2005;26:77–90.
47. Scarmeas N, Stern Y, Tang MX, et al. Mediterranean diet and risk for Alzheimer's disease. Ann Neurol 2006;59:912–21.
48. Katina S, Farbakova J, Madari A, et al. Risk factors for canine cognitive dysfunction syndrome in Slovakia. Acta Vet Scand 2016;58:17.
49. Dodd CE, Zicker SC, Jewell DE, et al. Can a fortified food affect the behavioral manifestations of age-related cognitive decline in dogs? Vet Med 2003;98:396–408.

50. Pan Y, Landsberg G, Mougeot I, et al. Efficacy of a therapeutic diet on dogs with signs of cognitive dysfunction syndrome (CDS): a prospective double blinded placebo controlled clinical trial. Front Nutr 2018;5:127.
51. Henderson ST. High carbohydrate diets and Alzheimer's disease. Med Hypotheses 2004;62:689–700.
52. Pan Y, Kennedy AD, Jönsson TJ, et al. Cognitive enhancement in old dogs from dietary supplementation with a nutrient blend containing arginine, antioxidants, B vitamins and fish oil. Br J Nutr 2018. https://doi.org/10.1017/S0007114517003464.
53. Kim H-Y, Huang BX, Spector AA. Phosphatidylserine in the brain: metabolism and function. Prog Lipid Res 2014;1–18. https://doi.org/10.1016/j.plipres.2014.06.002.
54. Delwaide PJ, Gyselynck-Mambourg AM, Hurlet A, et al. Double blind randomized controlled study of phosphatidylserine in senile demented patients. Acta Neurol Scand 1986;73:136–40.
55. Hamilton J, Greiner R, Salem N Jr, et al. N-3 Fatty acid deficiency decreases phosphatidylserine accumulation selectively in neuronal tissues. Lipids 2000;35:863–9.
56. Araujo JA, Landsberg GM, Milgram NW, et al. Improvement of short-term memory performance in aged beagles by a nutraceutical supplement containing phosphatidylserine, Ginkgo biloba, vitamin E, and pyridoxine. Can Vet J 2008;49(4):379–85.
57. Osella MC, Re G, Odore R, et al. Canine cognitive dysfunction: prevalence, clinical signs treatment with a nutraceutical. Appl Anim Behav Sci 2007;105:297–310.
58. Heath SE, Barabas S, Craze PG. Nutritional supplementation in cases of canine cognitive dysfunction - a clinical trial. Appl Anim Behav Sci 2007;105:274–83.
59. Bottiglieri T. S-Adenosyl-L-methionine (SAMe): from the bench to the bedside—molecular basis of a pleiotrophic molecule. Am J Clin Nutr 2002;76(suppl):1151S–7S.
60. Rème CA, Dramard V, Kern L, et al. Effect of S-adenosylmethionine tablets on the reduction of age-related mental decline in dogs: a double-blind placebo-controlled trial. Vet Ther 2008;9:69–82.
61. Araujo JA, Faubert ML, Brooks ML, et al. Novifit (NoviSAME) tablets improve executive function in aged dogs and cats: implications for treatment of cognitive dysfunction syndrome. Intern J Appl Res Vet Med 2012;10(1):90–8.
62. Pan Y, Araujo JA, Burrows J, et al. Cognitive enhancement in middle-aged and old cats with dietary supplementation with a nutrient blend containing fish oil, B vitamins, antioxidants and arginine. Br J Nutr 2013;10:1–10.
63. Houpt KA, Levine E, Landsberg GM, et al. Antioxidant fortified food improves owner perceived behavior in the aging cat. In: Proceedings ESFM Feline Conference, Prague, September 21-23, 2007.
64. Yi J, Horky LL, Freidlich AL, et al. L-arginine and Alzheimer's disease. Int J Clin Exp Pathol 2009;3:211–38.
65. Packer L, Tritschler HJ, Wessel K. Neuroprotection by the metabolic antioxidant a-lipoic acid. Free Radic Biol Med 1997;22:359–78.
66. Head E, Nukala VN, Fenoglio KA, et al. Effects of age, dietary, and behavioral enrichment on brain mitochondria in a canine model of human aging. Exp Neurol 2009;220(1):171–6.
67. Selhub J, Bagley LC, Miller J, et al. B vitamins, homocysteine, and neurocognitive function in the elderly. Am J Clin Nutr 2000;71(2):614S–20S.

68. Calderón-Ospina CA, Nava-Mesa MO. B Vitamins in the nervous system: current knowledge of the biochemical modes of action and synergies of thiamine, pyridoxine and cobalamin. CNS Neurosci Ther 2020;26:5–13.
69. Chew BP, Park JS, Wong TS, et al. Dietary beta-carotene stimulates cell-mediated and humoral immune response in dogs. J Nutr 2000;130:1910–3.
70. Rani PJA, Panneerselvam C. Effect of l-carnitine on brain lipid peroxidation and antioxidant enzymes in old rats. J Gerontol 2002;57:B134–7.
71. Cole GM, Ma QL, Frautschy SA. Omega-3 fatty acids and dementia. Prostaglandins Leukot Essent Fatty Acids 2009;81:213–21.
72. La Fata G, Weber P, Mohajeri MH. Effects of vitamin E on cognitive performance during ageing and in Alzheimer's disease. Nutrients 2014;6(12):5453–72.
73. Löscher W. Animal models of intractable epilepsy. Prog Neurobiol 1997;53:239–58.
74. Volk HA, Matiasek LA, Feliu-Pascual LA, et al. The efficacy and tolerability of levetiracetam in pharmacoresistant epileptic dogs. Vet J 2008;176:310–9.
75. McDonald TJW, Cervenka MC. Ketogenic diets for adults with highly refractory epilepsy. Epilepsy Curr 2017;17:346–50.
76. Larsen JA, Owens TJ, Fascetti AJ. Nutritional management of idiopathic epilepsy in dogs. J Am Vet Med Assoc 2014;245:504–8.
77. Thavendiranathan P, Mendonca A, Dell C, et al. The MCT ketogenic diet: effects on animal seizure models. Exp Neurol 2000;161:696–703.
78. Chang P, Zuckermann AM, Williams S, et al. Seizure control by derivatives of medium chain fatty acids associated with the ketogenic diet show novel branching-point structure for enhanced potency. J Pharmacol Exp Ther 2015;352:43–52.
79. Chang P-S, Augustin K, Boddum K, et al. Seizure control by decanoic acid through direct AMPA receptor inhibition. Brain 2016;139:431–3.
80. Hughes SD, Kanabus M, Anderson G, et al. The ketogenic diet component decanoic acid increases mitochondrial citrate synthase and complex I activity in neuronal cells. J Neurochem 2014;129:426–33.
81. Law TH, Davis SS, Pan Y, et al. A randomised trial of a medium-chain TAG diet as treatment for dogs with idiopathic epilepsy. Br J Nutr 2015;114:1438–47.
82. Berk BA, Law TH, Packer RMA, et al. A multi-center randomized controlled trial of medium-chain triglyceride dietary supplementation on epilepsy in dogs. J Vet Intern Med 2020;34:1248–59.
83. Bauer JE. Evaluation and dietary consideration in idiopathic hyperlipidemia in dogs. J Am Vet Med Assoc 1995;206:1684–8.

Nutritional Concerns for Cancer, Cachexia, Frailty, and Sarcopenia in Canine and Feline Pets

Korinn E. Saker, MS, DVM, PhD

KEYWORDS

• Nutrition • Cancer • Cachexia • Frailty • Sarcopenia • Malnutrition • Aging

KEY POINTS

- Cancer, cachexia, frailty, and sarcopenia are interrelated, occur predominately in the aging pet, are associated with loss of muscle mass and functionality, and are initiated or perpetuated by inflammation and malnutrition.
- Early detection of these conditions can be challenging, but, when possible, targeted nutritional intervention can help slow progression and maintain a higher quality of life.
- Adjustment of selected dietary nutrients, especially protein, is necessary to help mitigate lean muscle loss, temper the inflammatory process, and help enhance nutrient utilization by patients with these conditions.

INTRODUCTION

Cachexia, including cancer cachexia, frailty, and sarcopenia, continues to be investigated and redefined in people to further the identification of potential therapeutic strategies to aid in patient care. As clarity regarding the pathophysiology of the conditions evolves, specific nutrient-focused interventions are being tested, particularly in aging men and women, with promising results. These syndromes recently have become a topic of interest in veterinary medicine.[1] Although a single commercial diet has not yet been formulated to address these clinical conditions/syndromes specifically in the canine and feline populations, individual nutrients and diet characteristics can be emphasized as to their benefit. Much of the nutritional research focused on these conditions has been published from a human study perspective. The pathophysiology of these conditions in companion pets shares similarities to that in people, allowing veterinarians to glean useful insight for nutritional management from what is recommended for humans. A universally acknowledged definition of these conditions is a reasonable starting point to understanding their interrelationship (**Box 1**). This article

Department of Molecular and Biomedical Sciences, NC State University College of Veterinary Medicine, 1060 William Moore Drive, Raleigh, NC 27606, USA
E-mail address: Korinn_saker@ncsu.edu

Vet Clin Small Anim 51 (2021) 729–744
https://doi.org/10.1016/j.cvsm.2021.01.012

Box 1
Definitions

- *Cancer* is commonly defined as a disease caused by the abnormal division of cells in the body, resulting in formation of a tissue mass referred to as a tumor.
- *Cachexia* is defined as a complex metabolic syndrome associated with underlying illness and characterized by loss of muscle mass with or without loss of fat mass. The prominent clinical feature of cachexia is weight loss in adults.[2] It is associated with a decreased QOL and poor prognosis.
- *Frailty* is a multidimensional syndrome characterized by decreased reserves and diminished resistance to stressors (homeostatic reserves) resulting from cumulative declines across multiple physiologic systems that collectively predispose an individual to adverse outcomes.[3,4] The literature consistently describes sarcopenia as the counterpart of physical frailty.
- *Sarcopenia* commonly has been defined as the progressive and generalized loss of skeletal LMM and function with aging in the absence of disease. A focus now includes the functionality of muscle as well as the mass; thus, a clinical definition would include decreased gait speed or grip strength in a person with low muscle mass.[5]

examines cancer, cachexia, and frailty as independent entities and as constituents of malnutrition and the aging process, with additional focus on lean muscle loss, referred to as *sarcopenia*.

Although cachexia, frailty, and sarcopenia, are referred to as *tissue loss syndrome,* this is not to imply a communal interrelationship. That noted, the tissue loss syndrome of cachexia or sarcopenia and frailty is more prevalent in the aging, senior-geriatric human population; although poorly defined in companion pets, these syndromes likewise are observed in aging pets.[1,6] Furthermore, a physical association undeniably exists between the cachexic patient and the onset of frailty, whereas frailty is appreciated as a consequence of ongoing sarcopenia. Both cachexic and sarcopenic patients exhibit muscle loss, but the presence of one does not preclude the onset of the other. From a medical perspective, delineation between muscle loss due to cachexia or sarcopenia helps to address patient prognosis and identification of beneficial and realistic patient management strategies. The similarity of nutrients involved in the onset as well as the progression and/or reversal of these 3 conditions more likely characterizes and links them as a syndrome. This article reveals the nutritional interconnectedness of cancer[4] and these conditions, highlighting malnutrition as an overarching theme.

CANCER: Malnutrition of Cancer and Current Nutritional Concerns

As with humans, cancer and its common accompanying clinical manifestations of cachexia and frailty are an unwelcome disease state in the canine and feline population. Palliative care, including nutrition support, can help slow progression of the inevitable changes in appetite, body weight and muscling, activity, attitude, and cognitive function that are observed. These progressive alterations inherent with most diagnoses of cancer can be exhausting on many levels for pets and their caregivers.

A multitude of tumor types have been identified in cats and dogs, many categorized as malignant, although some as benign. Chemotherapy, radiation, and surgery are common modalities employed to abrogate tumors or minimize their metastases. Remission is realized by some patients, yet many patients are not as fortunate and eventually succumb to the quietus of end-stage cancer. Early diagnosis and initiation of a patient management protocol that includes nutrition have been reported to slow disease progression, mitigate adverse physical and metabolic responses to tumor growth, and sustain a higher quality of life (QOL).[7] To date, nutritional intervention, as preventative, treatment modality, or component of palliative care, has greater evidence-based guidelines for humans compared with companion animals. This void directs reviewing the human literature to identify and extrapolate beneficial nutrition support strategies for canine and feline cancer patients. As is the case in people, under-nutrition or malnutrition effects mainly patients with gastrointestinal (GI) maladies. Those with oral, esophageal, gastric, small intestinal, or pancreatic cancer are at higher risk for inadequate nutrition, followed closely behind by patients with cholangiocellular, hepatocellular, and colon cancers.[7] Therefore understanding factors and clinical manifestations associated with these solid cancers is an ideal place to focus nutritional intervention strategies.

One aspect of cancer malnutrition can be attributed to a reduction in nutritional intake. Anorexia, often described by taste alterations, loss of appetite, and general malaise, is associated with poor nutrient intake; and that condition can be worsened by the side effects of cancer treatments. Dysphagia perpetuates the anorexia, especially when upper GI tract cancers are involved, whereas tumor masses causing a disturbance in GI motility result in nausea, vomiting, regurgitation, and reduced nutrient intake. Gastric, GI, and pancreatic surgery can result in hormonal and anatomic alterations, leading to nutrient maldigestion and malabsorption with ultimate malnutrition.[7]

The second aspect of cancer malnutrition can be characterized by the release of inflammatory mediators, including tumor necrosis factor α, interleukin (IL)-1, and IL-6, that can regulate both appetite and nutrient utilization in the body. It is this aspect of cancer that commonly leads to cachexia or cancer cachexia. Energy intake, controlled by the hypothalamus and its mix of orexigenic and anorexigenic hormones, influences food intake. Tumor-produced cytokines promote lean muscle mass (LMM) breakdown by interfering with normal protein degradation-synthesis pathways to increase proteolysis and hasten the cachexic state.[7,8] Eicosapentaenoic acid (EPA), an omega-3 fatty acid (n-3 FA), has been shown to preserve lean muscle by interfering with the ubiquitin-dependent protein degradation pathway.[9]

The impacts on cell signaling pathways in companion pets by n-3 FAs, specifically EPA and docosahexaenoic acid (DHA), along with antioxidants and bioflavonoids from functional foods, have been reported to mitigate the up-regulation of inflammatory mediators, which have been shown to stimulate metastases and promote the tissue wasting state of cachexia.[10,11] Other key nutrients identified in human and canine or feline cancer research, such as vitamin D[12] and select amino acids,[13,14] as well as more common supplements, turmeric and garlic, have been included in anticancer diets. Functional foods, such as green tea, red wine, fruits, and green and orange vegetables, likewise are recommended for human consumption to mitigate tumor growth, support systemic and GI health after chemotherapy and radiation therapy, and hasten recovery and minimize complications postsurgery.[15]

The question of nutrition-focused strategies to mitigate tumor growth still is controversial, particularly regarding carbohydrates. More than 60 years ago, it was recognized that the tumor cell has a distinctive ability to exhibit increased glycolysis and pentose phosphate cycle activity, while demonstrating reduced rates of respiration, which normally result in death of healthy cells.[9] These tumor cell survival mechanisms are reported to involve unhampered glucose uptake by cells; reduction in cellular mitochondria, forcing anerobic metabolism for energy to yield lactate versus pyruvate; and detoxification of intracellular oxidants. Thus, this glucose-dependent state of tumor cells suggests a potential target for inhibiting tumor cell growth. The earliest canine studies suggested that increasing the rate of glycolysis in tumor cells promotes tumor cell growth and hyperlactatemia in lymphoma dogs compared with control dogs,[13] leading to dietary recommendations of reducing digestible carbohydrate calorie intake for dogs with cancer. A more recent publication summarizing the role of dietary carbohydrates in the nutritional management of dogs and cats with cancer challenges these early recommendations, stating the evidence is not conclusive.[16] Moderation of highly digestible dietary carbohydrate intake in patients with insulin resistance from endocrine disease or critical illness/acute trauma should be considered to help counter the inflammation and protein catabolism aspects of these conditions.[8] Despite the lack of consensus regarding carbohydrate metabolism, the benefit of increased calories from protein, fat, or both, when carbohydrates are minimized in a diet, can have numerous anticancer cachexia benefits for pets based on their associated comorbidities. A particular benefit is the preservation of muscle, or slowing muscle protein degradation, to improve QOL. The question then, of whether a diet can be formulated to starve the tumor yet simultaneously feed the nontransformed cells, remains unanswered, especially so for veterinary patients. Veterinarians should stay mindful, however, that nutrition has shown to be a strong instrument in cancer management protocols for humans and, therefore, should be included in every cancer patient's care.

CACHEXIA: Pathophysiology, Detection, and Nutritional Concerns

A physical description of the cachectic state originally was introduced by Hippocrates in people suffering from congestive heart failure (CHF). There now is a better understanding and it is acknowledged as a complex metabolic syndrome observed in chronic diseases associated with systemic inflammation (**Box 2**). Cachexia is characterized by loss of muscle mass with or without loss of fat mass, with a prominent feature of cachexia being weight loss, specifically greater than or equal to 5% of body weight during the previous 12 months or less.[17] Systemic inflammation from these conditions often results in changes to metabolism and body composition; subsequently, cachexia is associated with increased mortality and poor QOL. Cachexia remains a contributing factor to the progressive decline in people because it is estimated that more than 5 million people in the United States have cachexia occurring with CHF and a variety of disease states, including cancer. Cachexia is diagnosed more easily in the advanced stages of disease when lean muscle loss is grossly apparent. Approximately 50% to 80% of cancer patients experience cachexia, termed

Box 2
Chronic disease states associated with systemic inflammation and progression to a cachexic state

Multiorgan
- Neoplasia

Organ-specific
- CKD
- CHF
- Hepatobiliary diseases
- Inflammatory bowel disease
- Systemic inflammatory response syndrome

cancer-cachexia, as the disease state worsens. Other common forms of cachexia include cardiac, renal, hepatic, and respiratory cachexia, which, together with cancer cachexia, have been observed in companion pets. Cachexia, when associated with cancer and other clinical states, is difficult to assess due to the lack of a clear definition for clinical application. Physical criterion of loss of lean (and often fat) tissue mass is the most common gross identifier in humans and pets. It has been reported that a 15% reduction in LMM interferes with organic and physiologic functions, and a 30% or greater reduction usually is fatal.[18] Biochemical measures regarded as important parameters of cachexia include serum protein status, electrolytes, history of anorexia, and increased C-reactive protein values,[19] but these currently are limited to human patients. C-reactive protein is a universal biomarker of inflammation, implying that inflammation plays a role in lean muscle homeostasis, particularly during disease states. To date, specific biomarkers for detection of cachexia in companion pets are not well documented. A clinical definition and quantitative measures of cachexia for companion animal patients would allow for earlier diagnosis, followed by medical and nutritional interventions to slow its progression and enhance the patient's QOL.

The pathophysiology of cachexia has been described to include 4 aspects: increased energy requirements, decreased nutrient absorption, decreased energy intake, and alterations in metabolism.[1] The underlying disease pathophysiology, form of cachexia, and subsequent clinical manifestations in the patient, to some degree, dictate total daily energy needs based on assumptions and clinician experience. Calculation of daily energy expenditure via bedside calorimetry provides the quantitative aspect, although this modality is not readily available in veterinary general practices. Increased respiratory effort, chronic inflammation, organ malfunction, current or desired body condition and muscling, activity level, and GI mucosal integrity can have an impact on daily energy expenditure, nutrient digestion, and absorption. Nausea or regurgitation, acquired food aversions, anorexia, loss of taste and smell senses, and compromises in food apprehension, chewing, and swallowing can have an impact on actual daily energy intake. Although a chronic, ongoing state of inflammation associated with cachexia and the underlying disease process likely is most influential in the loss of LMM, loss of fat mass is prompted by decreased energy intake and/or altered nutrient absorption.[2] Omega-3 fatty acids have been a primary focus to mitigate the cytokine storm, with reported benefit in the management of cardiac, renal, cancer, and other cachexia-related disease states for both people and pets.

SARCOPENIA: Pathophysiology, Detection, and Nutritional Concerns

Aging is associated with a progressive decline of muscle mass, quality, and strength, a condition referred to as sarcopenia. It develops during aging in the absence of disease. Sarcopenia begins early in adult life and progresses—a 30% reduction in LMM is reported from ages 20 years to 80 years,[1,20] although sarcopenic LMM begins during middle age in companion pets. Often the muscle loss is countered by added fat mass (sarcopenic obesity), evident in both humans and companion pets, and increases the challenge of appropriate nutritional management because there is no change in total body weight. A 256-cat survey of cats showed a linear loss of LMM beginning at 10 years of age, whereas a smaller 90-cat study indicated linear decreases in LMM starting at 7 years of age.[21] A similar trend was noted in aging dogs.[18] Advanced sarcopenia, as with cachexia, is associated with physical disability, poor QOL, and increased death risk for pets.[5,21,22]

The pathophysiology of sarcopenia has been reviewed in several excellent publications.[2,3,20] Briefly, in sarcopenic muscle, the rate of muscle injury exceeds that of repair and regeneration. There are several key factors that play a role in the muscle loss of aging; these factors lead to reduced muscle functionality with consequences of increased physical demise.

Detection of sarcopenia is more objective for people than for companion animals. Conversely, veterinary patients still are assessed subjectively using a published 4-point muscle mass score (MMS) to assess marked, moderate, mild, and no muscle wasting.[23] Although the subjective nature is a limitation, this MMS commonly is used while awaiting a more quantitative, cage-side measurement tools. Recently, 2 studies have utilized ultrasound to quantitate LMM thickness as a means to monitor changes in muscle mass in dogs,[24,25] a welcome step toward more accurate assessment for veterinary patients.

Nutritional concerns for sarcopenia overlap those for both cachexia and frailty. Along with adequate supply of dietary protein levels, evidence suggests (in people) that leucine and its bioactive metabolite, β-hydroxy-β-methylbutyrate, stimulate muscle protein synthesis more than nonessential amino acids and may be useful to maintain lean body mass and improve muscle function.[26] This can be important especially for hyperthyroid cats, because hyperthyroidism contributes to both protein catabolism and muscle wasting.

Vitamin D likewise is of interest in the aging sarcopenic patient because low serum vitamin D and subsequent increased parathyroid hormone concentrations have been reported. Increased parathyroid hormone, as a consequence of low vitamin D concentrations, disrupts muscle function/structure via elevated intracellular calcium levels and can lower muscle mass through the stimulated release of inflammatory mediators, such as IL-6.[27]

Acid-base balance is another reported factor that influences protein balance and muscle wasting. In short, acidosis perpetuates insulin resistance, which subsequently influences signaling pathways that trigger reduction of phosphoinositide 3-kinase (PI3K) activity. Reduced PI3K up-regulates the ubiquitin proteasome pathway, a prominent avenue for protein degradation.[28] The importance of acid-base balance can be appreciated from a pet food perspective, because common animal proteins in pet foods are metabolized to acidic residues. Dietary mineral content influences acid-base balance, where potassium, magnesium, and calcium are base-forming and sulfur, phosphorus, and iron are considered acidic minerals. Several lines of evidence suggest that a correction of dietary acid load could improve acid-base balance and thereby reduce chronic disease, such as osteoporosis, kidney stones, or sarcopenia.[29] Human studies have appreciated a greater lean body mass associated with individuals with a higher intake of alkaline foods and or supplementation with potassium bicarbonate.[30] To date, data are not available on pets that reflect the impact of an alkaline diet versus acidic diet on LMM but could be beneficial to address muscle wasting, especially in chronic kidney disease (CKD) pets.

N-3FAs are yet another dietary factor potentially influencing muscle mass that warrant comment. The benefit that EPA and DHA, the biologically active metabolites of n-3 FAs, have on mitigating inflammation has been well established. Furthermore, the influence that inflammation has on the mammalian target of rapamycin (mTOR) signaling pathway and its resultant impact on sarcopenia have been reviewed. Although publications regarding the impact of EPA/DHA on muscle mass or function in companion pets are nominal at best, human studies have reported enhanced mTOR activation and protein synthesis in a healthy, older population when given fish oil (high n-3 FAs) versus corn oil (high n-6 FAs).[26]

FRAILTY: Pathophysiology, Detection, and Nutritional Concerns

It would be short-sighted to discuss frailty without including its interrelationship to sarcopenia and cachexia, because all are linked to decreased muscle mass and function (**Fig. 1**). Frailty is regarded as a common clinical syndrome, seen most often in the geriatric population.[3] It appears to be a multidimensional entity comprised of physical, psychological, and sociologic components. Generally, because there is less inclination to evaluate the latter 2 components when assessing older companion animals, frailty is not commonly considered for its impact on QOL and medium-term to long-term outcomes. Clinical manifestations of frailty are related in a mutually exacerbating cycle of negative energy balance, sarcopenia, and diminished strength and tolerance for exertion.

Although the pathophysiology of frailty is not well defined, there are several identified components. Studies that concentrated on the relationship between frailty and nutrition have shown association with inadequate daily energy and protein intake as well as low or deficient levels of vitamins D, E, and B_{12} in the frail and prefrail older female population.[3] Inflammatory mechanisms have been associated with frailty. Increased fat mass, particularly evidenced as central obesity, along with high insulin resistance and likelihood for metabolic syndrome, are identified as important in the pathogenesis of frailty. Lastly, various age-related hormone changes, including decreases in testosterone, growth hormone, and insulinlike growth factor 1, which influence muscling, have been linked to frailty.[3]

Detecting frailty through quantitative measures is helpful when applying a clinical value. Two approaches commonly are discussed for people. First is a phenotypic definition developed by Fried and coworkers in the early twentieth century.[31] It proposes that frailty is diagnosed when 3 of 5 items, including weight loss, exhaustion, weakness, slow walking speed, and low levels of physical activity, are present. Alternatively, Rockwood and coworkers (2005)[32] introduced the frailty index (FI), whereby they identified 70 deficits by which to evaluate individuals for frailty. The deficits covered the categories of active diseases, abilities in the activities of daily living, and physical signs from clinical and neurologic examinations.[3] In clinical practice, identification of frailty

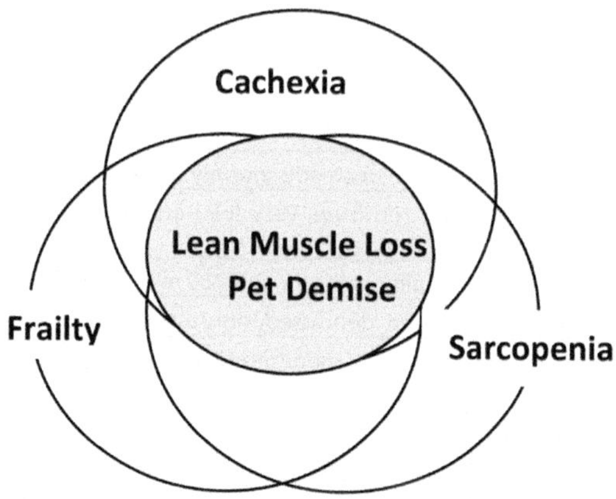

Fig. 1. Interrelationship between cachexia, frailty and sarcopenia. All three conditions lead to lean muscle mass loss or wasting via independent and overlapping mechanisms. Prolonged, irreversible lean muscle loss with ongoing comorbidities including malnutrition of cancer, CHF, CKD, hepatic and respiratory compromise will lead to the patients' demise.

using the Clinical Frailty Scale (CFS), a visual tool based on a comprehensive clinical assessment of a patient, enables assignment of a frailty category.[3] The CFS identifies where on a continuum the patient falls, from being physiologically robust and independent to being at high risk of hospitalization, institutionalization, and death. The more physiologically robust (low CFS), the higher the likelihood for full recovery following an insult compared with those with a high CFS.

There is an FI for laboratory animals and recently the first FI model for dogs has been developed.[33] The dog model is reported to exhibit a moderate correlation between age and the FI, with increased FI as age increases, but is not yet ready for practical clinical application. Development of a user-friendly questionnaire to obtain relevant frailty-related and disability-related information regarding a pet in its normal environment could be quite useful in clinical CFS assessment of pets, especially to institute appropriate nutrition support guidelines. Simple, basic screening criteria to assess for onset of frailty in companion pets are outlined in **Table 1**.

As discussed previously, the human frailty phenotype involves unintentional weight loss, exhaustion, weakness (low grip strength), slow walking speed, and low physical activity, many if not all of which are dependent on adequate muscle mass and function. Lean muscle health has an increasing importance in the management of cachexia and sarcopenia as well. A recent review of 5 studies on the nutritional determinants of frailty reported that frailty is associated with low intakes of specific micronutrients; and that higher protein intake, better diet quality, and high antioxidant capacity of diet were associated with a lower risk of frailty.[34] Additional nutritional factors related to frailty in people include poor oral health, dysphagia, anorexia, and polypharmacy via side effects of drugs that have an impact on nutrition.[35] Skeletal stability influences ability to perform activities, not to mention influence risk of falls. In that vein, adequate

Table 1
Suggested criteria screening to assess frailty in veterinary patients

Frailty Criteria	Maximum Value
Changes in body weight: 1 unit for each 2.5% change with maximum at >10%	4
Changes in fat mass (body condition score [BCS]) as more than 1 body condition score (±) from ideal[a] (assume 5 = ideal)	4
Circumference and shape changes[b] in epaxial, rear limb, forelimb, temporal muscles	4
Ambulation status[c]: stable on all limbs, unsteady, wobbly or, nonambulatory	4
Strength[d] (climbing up/down stairs, furniture, vehicle): normal, delayed, interrupted, unable	4
Exhaustion[e]: run >15 min, run <15 min, walk >15 and <30 min, walk <15 min	4
Demeanor[f]: bright and alert, lethargic, depressed, nonresponsive	4
Total score: not frail (0), mildly frail (1–14), moderately frail (15–21), severely frail (>21)	

[a] 1 point for each 1-unit decrease from 5.
[b] 1 point for each muscle area with observed change.
[c] 1 point for each progressive loss of ambulation.
[d] 1 point for each progressive loss of strength.
[e] 1 point for each decrease in time to exhaustion.
[f] 1 point for each worsening in demeanor.

mineral constituents (calcium, phosphorus, and magnesium) to maintain bone integrity are necessary. Although not reported in the scientific literature, these nutrients and diet characteristics logically would be relevant to frailty concerns in companion pets.

The role of gut microbiota in frailty is of growing interest, and recent literature suggests that a gut–muscle axis exists and that gut microbiota may act as a mediator for the effects of nutrition on muscle cells.[35] To date, only 1 published study exists for review. It describes changes in microbiota in frail nursing home residents. The benefit of supplemental probiotics partnered with dietary sources of prebiotics may help optimize gut microbiota in favor of lean muscle health and functionality. This is a fascinating area that deserves more research to provide useful clinical application.

Nutrition-focused and exercise-focused interventions play a significant role in management of frailty and sarcopenia because they reportedly have an impact on muscle mass and function. A combination of these 2 interventions is associated with better function, strength, and less inflammation in older sarcopenic, frail people.[35] This double-barreled approach likely would have benefit to companion pets in a similar scenario. Insight into aspects of physical activity to address in the aging pet is not covered in this article; rather, the focus is on nutritional considerations.

NUTRIENT TARGETS FOR CACHEXIA, SARCOPENIA, AND FRAILTY

The first step to reversing frailty and sarcopenia, as well as to slow cachexia, is early identification of these syndromes in clinical practice. Studies on reversing frailty with nutrition alone in the past 2 years are sparse and mainly involve protein, protein-energy mismatch, and micronutrient supplementation.[35,36] The role of protein, leucine, omega-3 fatty acids, and vitamin D in the prevention and treatment of sarcopenia and functional decline has been reviewed; and identifies specific targets for key nutrients in people that may represent an intervention strategy. These targets include protein intake of 1.0 g/kg/d to 1.2 g/kg/d evenly distributed during the day, vitamin D supplementation of 800 IU to 1000 IU, and approximately 3 g/d of omega-3 polyunsaturated

Box 3
General nutritional support considerations to manage the cachexic, frail, sarcopenic pet

- Increase protein intake by 1.5-times to 2-times maintenance intake level.
- Identify protein sources enriched in muscle-building amino acids (ie, whey, egg, and soy products). Enhance EPA and DHA intake from fish-based sources.
- Enhance oral vitamins E and C supplementation (except during chemotherapy or radiation cancer therapy).
- Monitor serum vitamin D levels; consider oral supplementation if low.
- Feed smaller meals more frequently across the day.
- Adjust diet texture according to the pet's dental health.
- Warm foods to enhance aroma and palatability.
- Utilize appetite stimulants when anorexia is noted for more than 3 days.
- Always consider assisted feeding when pet is not voluntarily consuming a minimum of 66% of its daily calories needs consistently.
- Incorporate interactive feeding practices to increase interest in diet, prompt activity, and stimulate cognitive functions in older pets.

Table 2
Practical feeding guidelines based on nutritional and frailty assessment

	Nutritional Assessment		
Clinical Criteria	**Well Nourished**	**Borderline Malnourished**	**Severe Malnourished**
Daily calorie intake	Consistent DER[b]	RER[c] ↔ DER[f,g]	≤66% RER
BW changes	Stable	<10% loss	≥10% loss
BCS	Optimal 3/5 or 5/9	Variable	Poor, ≤2.5/5 or 3/9
MMS	2–3	1–2	0–2
Albumin	Normal	Normal–mild ↓	Moderate–severe ↓
Nutrient losses[a]	None	Moderate, controlled	Ongoing, uncontrolled
Frailty screening	Refer to Table _ for details 0–7	8–21	>21
Practical recommendations	No diet or calorie intake change Overweight to obese: target calorie intake for BCS 3/5 or 5–6/9. Avoid harmful foods. Fresh water always Monitor daily intake.	Calculate and feed DER.[f,g] ID and meet specific nutrient concerns. Hand or tube feed[d]; keep head and upper body elevated for 15–30 min postmeal to minimize aspiration. Monitor daily intake.	Target RER to DER[j,k] intake. Meet specific nutrient concerns. Hand or tube feed. Institute PN[e] if NPO or combination feeding. Monitor daily intake.

Specific feeding guidelines	Calculate DER at current or ideal BW. Overweight to obese: calculate RER optimal BW. Choose appropriate commercial or CHP diet. Avoid supplemental AOX with anticancer therapy. Consider oral probiotics. Feed 2–3 times daily. Monitor daily intake.	Calculate DER.[f,g] Choose appropriate commercial or CHP diet. Human liquid diets can be considered.[h] Increase daily protein intake by 50% for nonrenal cachexia, frailty, sarcopenia. Consider oral probiotics Feed 2–4 times daily; combine VI and AF[i] as enteric tube feeding when needed to ensure DER intake. AF as bolus feeding Monitor daily intake.	Calculate DER.[j] Choose appropriate commercial or CHP diet. Double daily protein intake for nonrenal cachexia, frailty, sarcopenia. Consider oral probiotics. Feed 3–6 times daily. AF as bolus or CRI feeding; utilize PN ± enteric tube feeding. Monitor daily calorie delivery.
Feeding approach	VI	VI ± AF	AF

Abbreviations: AF, assisted feeding; AOX, antioxidants; BCS, body condition score; BW, body weight; CHP, cooked home-prepared; CRI, constant rate infusion; DER, daily energy (calorie) requirement; ID, identify; ME, metabolizable energy; MMS, MMS where 1/3 = severely muscle wasted and 3/3 = normal muscling; PN, parenteral nutrition; RER, resting energy (calorie) requirement; VI, voluntary intake ↓, decreased ↔, ranging between.

[a] Nutrient losses from vomiting, regurgitation, diarrhea.

[b] DER for well-nourished pet, derived from a mathematical calculation: DER (kcal ME/d) = dogs: $DER_{optimal\ BW} = RER \times 1.6$; cats: $DER_{optimal}$ $BW = RER \times 1.2$. Dogs: $DER_{overweight\ to\ obese} = RER \times (1.2 \rightarrow 1.0)$; cats: $DER_{overweight\ to\ obese}$ $BW = RER \times (1.0 \rightarrow 0.8)$. Note: DER calculations are considered a starting point and may need adjustment based on individual metabolism.

[c] RER derived as RER (kcal ME/d) = $(BW_{kg})^{0.75} \times 70$.

[d] Enteric tube feeding options include nasoenteric, esophagostomy, gastrostomy, and jejunostomy feeding tubes; esophagostomy and gastrostomy tube feeding can be included in home care.

[e] Parenteral feeding performed most commonly via a central or peripheral venous catheter and requires hospitalization and specific monitoring for metabolic and mechanical concerns.

[f] DER for borderline malnourished dogs: DER = RER × (1.6–2.5).

[g] DER for borderline malnourished cats: DER = RER x (1.2–2).

[h] Human liquid diets not ideal for cats. Require supplementation with arginine, taurine, and arachidonic acid if feeding longer than 24 h.

[i] AF includes hand feeding, enteric feeding tube, or parenteral (intravenous IV) feeding.

[j] DER for severely malnourished dogs: DER = RER x (1.6–3.0).

[k] DER for severely malnourished dogs: DER = RER x (1.6–3.0).

fatty acid supplements. This was confirmed by a study in Japan that showed increased consumption of meat and dairy products provide sufficient protein and energy intake to reduce the odds of incident frailty by approximately 30%. Observational studies continue to support the role of nutrition in preventing frailty. In a cross-sectional study of 5638 community-living Japanese men and women, higher protein intake was associated with lower prevalence of prefrailty in women and of frailty in both men and women. In a study of 722 community living older people ages 85 years and over in the United Kingdom, protein intake of less than 1 g/kg of body weight negatively affected muscle strength and physical performance, independent of other covariates. A National Health and Nutrition Examination Study (NHANES) conducted in the United States involving 707 sarcopenic individuals found vitamin C and vitamin E supplementation influenced physical functioning differently between older men and women. The greatest improvements from nutritional intervention in the frail older adult population was seen in those with preexisting malnutrition,[35] which corroborates previous implications of the cachexia-sarcopenia-frailty relationship with malnutrition reviewed herein.

β-Alanine has become a popular dietary supplement among athletes based on evidence that it increases intramuscular L-carnosine concentrations. Enhanced levels of L-carnosine, a cytoplasmic dipeptide, is associated with improved performance in high-intensity exercises via its ability to improve calcium delivery to and protein removal out of the muscle sarcomere site.[37] Further research could reveal that muscle function in older frail, cachexic, or sarcopenic pets may glean benefit from β-alanine supplementations.

Because protein is used as a primary energy substrate when calorie deficits exist, intake of adequate nonprotein calories is paramount to addressing sarcopenia as well as cachexia, frailty, and malnutrition. Increased intake of non-protein calories can present challenges though when patients are obese, anorexic, or unable to voluntarily eat or have existing comorbidities that necessitate specific dietary nutrient profile alterations. Other nutrients and diet characteristics with potential to influence muscle mass include antioxidants, diet digestibility, select microminerals, B vitamins, and diet caloric density.

CLINICAL RELEVANCE AND APPLICATION

Published recommendations for the nutritional management of companion pets are not specific for cachexia, frailty, and sarcopenia, and the cancer nutrition literature still is rather nebulous. The commonality of LMM loss and inflammation can help direct nutrition intervention strategies. Considerations, supposed from the human literature, are summarized later (**Box 3**).

Table 3
Suggested nutrient levels[a] for the frail, sarcopenic, disease-free older canine and feline

Nutrient	Canine	Feline
Protein (g)	≥9	12–16
Fat (g)	>5	4.5–6.5
Taurine (mg)	—	25, canned diet, and 80, extruded diet

—, implies that specific guidelines have not yet been reported in the literature for that nutrient–condition.

[a] Nutrient values listed as grams, milligrams, or international units per 100-kcal basis.

Table 4
Suggested nutrient level[a] guidelines for cachexic, frail, and/or sarcopenic aging canine and feline pets with chronic disease states

Nutrient (Units/100 kcal)	Species	Congestive Heart Failure	Renal (Stages 11–IV)	Hepatic/ Cholangitis	Respiratory Compromise
Protein (g)	C	6–10	3–6	5–10 3.5–5, HE	≥10
	F	6–8	6–7, advanced 7.5–9.5, early	8–12 6–7, HE	14–16
Fat (g)	C	3.5–6	3.5–6.2	3.5–6, hepatic ≤3, cholangitis	>5
	F	4–6	3.5–6.5	4–6.5, hepatic 4–5, cholangitis	>6
Omega-3 fatty acids (mg)	C	150–350 (90–150]	150–350 [90–150)	150–350 (90–150)	150–350 (90–150)
(EPA + DHA) (mg)	F	80–200 (40–150)	80–200 (40–150)	80–200 (40–150)	80–200 (40–150)
Phosphorus (mg)	C	—	<120	—	—
	F	—	80–125	—	—
Sodium (mg)	C	40–110	40–110	40–150	—
	F	50–100	50–100	110–150	—
Carnitine (mg)	C	7–9	7–9	7–9	7–9
	F	5, HL, cholangitis	5, HL, cholangitis	5, HL, cholangitis	5, HL, cholangitis
Taurine (mg)	C	≥25, hepatic	—	—	—
	F	≥68, hepatic	—	—	—
MCT (g)	C	—	—	0.4–0.9	0.4–0.9
Soluble fiber (g)	C	—	0.3–1.4	0.3–1.4	—
	F	—	0.3–1.6	0.3–1.6	—
Antioxidants	C/F	15–20, vitamin E (IU) 3–6, vitamin C (mg)			
Energy density (kcal/g)	C	1.2–1.5, moist, and 3.5–4.2, dry			
	F	1.0–1.1, moist, and 3.8–4.2, dry			

—, implies that specific guidelines have not yet been reported in the literature for that nutrient–condition.
Abbreviations: C, canine; F, feline; HE, hepatic encephalopathy; HL, hepatic lipidosis; MCT, medium-chain triglycerides.
[a] Nutrient values listed as grams, milligrams, or international units per 100-kcal basis.

Tables 2–4 provide suggested nutrient levels and diet characteristics for canine and feline patients identified with cachexia, frailty, and sarcopenia. The values are derived from reviewing the human and veterinary literature as well as from years of clinical experience. There is no established consensus in veterinary nutrition as to exactly what the guidelines should be; therefore, they should be considered a starting point by which to help identify diets that can impart some benefit and yet do no harm. Although early detection protocols of tissue loss syndromes for veterinary patients are lacking, the guidelines provided in **Table 2** may be useful as a starting point. Specific dietary targets for protein and other nutrients, identified in the literature as beneficial to cachectic, sarcopenic, and/or frail humans, currently are not summarized for companion animals with these syndromes. Therefore, **Tables 3** and **4** provide suggested dietary nutrient levels for cachexic, frail, and/or sarcopenic aging canine and feline pets, when disease-free or disease-afflicted.

SUMMARY

The interrelationship of cachexia (cancer-cachexia), sarcopenia, and frailty in the aging senior population can be appreciated clinically as loss of body mass, mainly lean muscle body tissue. The overlapping mechanisms driving this LMM loss appears to be primarily inflammatory cytokines altering protein turnover. The loss is reported to be both a decline in synthesis and an increase in degradation. Key nutrients have been identified for aging humans help to slow, reverse, and possibly prevent this tissue wasting. Adapting these findings to veterinary companion pets currently is being investigated.

CLINICS CARE POINT

- Due to the emerging nature of this topic, little clinical evidence is available specifically focused on companion pets. Therefore, it is suggested to review the information included in **Tables 2–4** that provide clinical care points relevant to the nutritional concerns of cancer cachexia, frailty, and sarcopenia in dogs and cats.

DISCLOSURE

The author is an advisory council member for Purina Pet Care. This organization has not funded any studies done in my lab associated with the topics of cachexia, frailty or sarcopenia.

REFERENCES

1. Freeman LM. Cachexia ad sarcopenia: Emerging syndromes of importance in dogs and cats. J Vet Intern Med 2012;26:3–17.
2. Rolland Y, Van Kan GA, Gillette-Guyonnet S, et al. Cachexia versus sarcopenia. Curr Opin Clin Nutr Metab Care 2011;14:15–21.
3. Bauer JM, Sieber CC. Sarcopenia and frailty: A clinician's controversial; point of view. Exp Gerontol 2008;4:674–8.
4. Aapro M, Arends J, Bozzetti F, et al. ESMO (European School of Medical Oncology) Early recognition of malnutrition and cachexia in the cancer patient: A position paper of the European School of Oncology Task Force. Ann Oncol 2014;25:1492–9.
5. Cederholm T, Morley JE. Sarcopenia: the new definition. Curr Opin Clin Nutr Metab Care 2015;18:18–24.

6. Gingrich A, Volkert D, Kiesswetter E, et al. Prevalence and overlap of sarcopenia, frailty, cachexia and malnutrition in older medical inpatients. BMC Geriatr 2019; 19:120.
7. Ockenga J, Valentini L. Review article: anorexia and cachexia in gastrointestinal cancer. Aliment Pharmacol Ther 2005;22:583–94.
8. Cederholm T, Morley JE. Nutrient interface with biology and aging. Curr Opin Clin Nutr Metab Care 2016;19:1–4.
9. Saker KE. Principles of nutrition of the cancer patient. In: Dobson JM, Lascelles DBX, editors. BSAVA manual of canine and feline oncology. Glouchester (England: BSAVA Woodrow House; 2010. p. 102–10.
10. Cowing BE, Saker KE. Polyunsaturated fatty acids and EGFR - MAPK signaling in mammary cancer. J Nutr 2001;131:1125–8.
11. Tanner AE, Saker KE, Ju Y, et al. Cell proliferation of feline and human breast cancer cell types is inhibited by pomegranate juice. J Anim Physiol Anim Nutr 2008; 92(2):221–3.
12. Weidner N, Woods JP, Conlon P, et al. Influence of various factors on circulating 25(OH) Vitamin D concentrations in dogs with cancer and healthy dogs. J Vet Med 2017;31(6):1796–803.
13. Ogilvie GK, Fettman MJ, Mallincrod CH, et al. Effect of fish oil, arginine, and doxorubicin chemotherapy on remission and survival time of dogs with lymphoma: a double-blind, randomized placebo-controlled study. Cancer 2000;88: 1916–28.
14. Phang JM, Liu E, Hancock CN, et al. Proline metabolism and cancer: emerging links to glutamine and collagen. Curr Opin Clin Nutr Metab Care 2015;18:71–7.
15. Islam SMR, Siddiqua TJ. Functional foods in cancer prevention and therapy: Recent epidemiological findings. In: Kabir Y, editor. Functional foods in cancer prevention and therapy Academy Press. Elseiver Inc; 2020. p. 405–33. https://doi.org/10.1016/C2017-0-04743-2.
16. Mauldin GE. The role of dietary carbohydrate in the nutritional management of dogs and cats with cancer. In: Gerontology: an inside out perspective. St Louis (MO: Purina Institute; 2018. p. 101–4.
17. Evans WJ, Morley JE, Argiles J, et al. Cachexia: a new definition. Clin Nutr 2008; 27:793–9.
18. Laflamme D. Effects of diet on loss and preservation of lean body mass in aging dogs and cats. In: Gerontology: an inside out perspective. St Louis (MO: Purina Institute; 2018. p. 51–6.
19. Mallard J, Gagez A-L, Baudinet C, et al. C-Reactive Protein Level: A Key Predictive Marker of Cachexia in Lymphoma and Myeloma Patients. J *Hematol* 2019; 8(2):55–9.
20. Sakuma K, Yamaguchi A. Sarcopenia and cachexia: the adaptations of negative regulators of skeletal muscle mass. J Cachexia Sarcopenia Muscle 2012;3: 77–94.
21. Peterson ME, Little SL. Cachexia, sarcopenia and other forms of muscle wasting: common problems of senior and geriatric cats with endocrine disease. In: Gerontology: an inside out perspective. St Louis (MO: Purina Institute; 2018. p. 67–75.
22. Peterson ME, Eirmann L. Dietary management of feline endocrine disease. Vet Clin North Am Small Anim Pract 2014;44:775–88.
23. Freeman L, Becraova I, Cave N, et al. WASAVA Nutritional Assessment Guidelines. J Small Anim Pract 2011;52.

24. Bullen L, Evola M, Griffith E, et al. Validation of ultrasonographic muscle thickness measurements as compared to the gold standard of computed tomography in dogs. PeerJ 2017;5:e2926.
25. Freeman L, Sutherland-Smith J, Prantil LR, et al. Quantitative assessment of muscle in dogs using a vertebral epaxial muscle score. Can J Vet Res 2017;81:255–60.
26. Robinson SM, Reginster JY, Rizzoli R, et al. Does nutrition play a role in the prevention amd management of sarcopenia? Clin Nutr 2018;37(4):112101132.
27. Visser M, Deeg DJH, Lips P. Low vitamin D and high parathyroid hormone levels as determinants of loss of muscle strength and muscle mass (sarcopenia): The Longitudinal Aging Study Amsterdam. J Clin Endocrinol Metab 2003;88:5677–772.
28. Garibotto G, Sofia A, Russo R, et al. Insulin sensitivity of muscle protein metabolism is altered in patients with chronic kidney disease. Kidney Int 2015;88:1419–26.
29. Konig D, Muser K, Dickhuth H-H, et al. Effect of a supplement rich in alkaline minerals on acid-base balance in humans. Nutr J 2009;8:23.
30. Dawson-Hughes B, Harris SB, Caglia L. Alkaline diets favor lean tissue mass in older adults. Am J Clin Nutr 2008;87:662–5.
31. Fried L, Tangen CM, Walston J, et al. Frailty in older adults: evidence for a phenotype. J Gerontol A Biol Sci Med 2001;56:M146–56.
32. Rockwood K, Song X, MacKnight C, et al. A global clinical measure of fitness and frailty in elderly people. CMAJ 2005;173(5):489–95.
33. Banzato T, Franzo G, DiMaggio R, et al. A Frailty Index based on clinical data to quantify mortality risk in dogs. Sci Rep 2019;9:16749.
34. Lorenzo-Lopez L, Maseda A, de Labra C, et al. Nutritional determinants of frailty in older adults: a systematic review. BCM Geriatr 2017;17:108–21.
35. Cruz-Jentoft AJ, Woo J. Nutritional interventions to prevent and treat frailty. Curr Opin Clin Nutr Metab Care 2019;22:191–5.
36. McKendry J, Thomas ACG, Phillips SM. Muscle mass loss in older critically ill population: Potential therapeutic strategies. Nutr Clin Pract 2020;35(4):607–16.
37. Blancquaert L, Everaert I, Derave W. Beta-alanine supplementation, muscle carnosine and exercise performance. Curr Opin Clin Nutr Metab Care 2015;18:63–70.

Printed and bound by CPI Group (UK) Ltd, Croydon, CR0 4YY
14/09/2026
02216284-0001